AOSpine Masters Series

Back Pain

Thieme

AOSpine Masters Series

Back Pain

Series Editor:
Luiz Roberto Vialle, MD, PhD
Professor of Orthopedics, School of Medicine
Catholic University of Parana State
Spine Unit
Curitiba, Brazil

Guest Editors:
Jeffrey C. Wang, MD
Chief, Orthopaedic Spine Service
Co-Director USC Spine Center
Professor of Orthopaedic Surgery and Neurosurgery
USC Spine Center
Los Angeles, California

Claudio Lamartina, MD
Chief, GSpine4 Department
Director, Spinal Research Program
I.R.C.C.S. Istituto Ortopedico Galeazzi
Milan, Italy
Professor, Specialization School in Orthopaedics and Traumatology
Milan and Turin Universities

With 133 figures

Thieme
New York • Stuttgart • Delhi • Rio de Janeiro

Thieme Medical Publishers, Inc.
333 Seventh Ave.
New York, NY 10001

Executive Editor: William Lamsback
Managing Editor: Sarah Landis
Director, Editorial Services: Mary Jo Casey
Editorial Assistant: Haley Paskalides
Production Editor: Barbara A. Chernow
International Production Director: Andreas Schabert
Vice President, Editorial and E-Product Development: Vera Spillner
International Marketing Director: Fiona Henderson
International Sales Director: Louisa Turrell
Director of Sales, North America: Mike Roseman
Senor Vice President and Chief Operating Officer: Sarah Vanderbilt
President: Brian D. Scanlan
Compositor: Carol Pierson, Chernow Editorial Services, Inc.

Library of Congress Cataloging-in-Publication Data
Names: Wang, Jeffrey C., editor. | Lamartina, Claudio, editor. | AOSpine International (Firm), issuing body.
Title: AOSpine masters series. Volume 8, Back pain / guest editors, Jeffrey C. Wang, Claudio Lamartina.
Other titles: Back pain
Description: New York : Thieme, [2017] | Includes bibliographical references and index.
Identifiers: LCCN 2016029831| ISBN 9781626232297 (alk. paper) | ISBN 9781626232303 (eISBN)
Subjects: | MESH: Back Pain
Classification: LCC RD771.B217 | NLM WE 720 | DDC 617.5/64—dc23
LC record available at https://lccn.loc.gov/2016029831

Important note: Medicine is an ever-changing science undergoing continual development. Research and clinical experience are continually expanding our knowledge, in particular our knowledge of proper treatment and drug therapy. Insofar as this book mentions any dosage or application, readers may rest assured that the authors, editors, and publishers have made every effort to ensure that such references are in accordance with **the state of knowledge at the time of production of the book.**

Nevertheless, this does not involve, imply, or express any guarantee or responsibility on the part of the publishers in respect to any dosage instructions and forms of applications stated in the book. **Every user is requested to examine carefully** the manufacturers' leaflets accompanying each drug and to check, if necessary in consultation with a physician or specialist, whether the dosage schedules mentioned therein or the contraindications stated by the manufacturers differ from the statements made in the present book. Such examination is particularly important with drugs that are either rarely used or have been newly released on the market. Every dosage schedule or every form of application used is entirely at the user's own risk and responsibility. The authors and publishers request every user to report to the publishers any discrepancies or inaccuracies noticed. If errors in this work are found after publication, errata will be posted at www.thieme.com on the product description page.

Some of the product names, patents, and registered designs referred to in this book are in fact registered trademarks or proprietary names even though specific reference to this fact is not always made in the text. Therefore, the appearance of a name without designation as proprietary is not to be construed as a representation by the publisher that it is in the public domain.

Printed in China by Everbest Printing Ltd.
5 4 3 2 1
ISBN 978-1-62623-229-7

Also available as an e-book
eISBN 978-1-62623-230-3

MIX
Paper from responsible sources
FSC www.fsc.org FSC® C124385

AOSPINE INTERNATIONAL

AOSpine Masters Series

Luiz Roberto Vialle, MD, PhD
Series Editor

Volume 1 Metastatic Spinal Tumors

Volume 2 Primary Spinal Tumors

Volume 3 Cervical Degenerative Conditions

Volume 4 Adult Spinal Deformities

Volume 5 Cervical Spine Trauma

Volume 6 Thoracolumbar Spine Trauma

Volume 7 Spinal Cord Injury and Regeneration

Volume 8 Back Pain

Volume 9 Pediatric Spinal Deformities

Volume 10 Spinal Infection

Contents

Series Preface

Spine care is advancing at a rapid pace. The challenge for today's spine care professional is to quickly synthesize the best available evidence and expert opinion in the management of spine pathologies. The AOSpine Masters Series provides just that—each volume in the series delivers pathology-focused expert opinion on procedures, diagnosis, clinical wisdom, and pitfalls, and highlights today's top research papers.

To bring the value of its masters level educational courses and academic congresses to a wider audience, AOSpine has assembled internationally recognized spine pathology leaders to develop volumes in this Masters Series as a vehicle for sharing their experiences and expertise and providing links to the literature. Each volume focuses on a current compelling and sometimes controversial topic in spine care.

The unique and efficient format of the Masters Series volumes quickly focuses the attention of the reader on the core information critical to understanding the topic, while encouraging the reader to look further into the recommended literature.

Through this approach, AOSpine is advancing spine care worldwide.

Luiz Roberto Vialle, MD, PhD

Guest Editors' Preface

The complex nature of the topic of this AOSpine Masters Series volume, entitled *Back Pain*, is reflected in the lack of established, shared opinions. For example, the reported prevalence of back pain ranges from 70% to 85%, according to different analyses. This variability reflects the lack of consensus even in the basic descriptive statistics. This is why we asked ourselves if an AOSpine Master Series book could help, both on the cultural and practical side. This volume, and the work behind it, is our attempt to answer that question. Given the serious and often confounding nature of the subject matter, we wanted to distinguish the topic with clever chapter titles that would pique the interest of the readers. Therefore, the editors have given a "playful" name to each chapter that is consistent with the specific subject being discussed. These "extra" titles are separate from the authors' titles and appear in the upper lefthand corner of every chapter opening page. We hope you will be able to interpret their meaning and that they will make your reading more pleasurable.

Back pain is an increasing medical problem and a large economic issue, and this book tries to convey the most current knowledge in the field. This is a highly controversial area among scientific and clinical experts, as evidenced in Chapter 1, "Back Pain No Gain." Advances in the basic sciences and understanding of the pathogenesis of disk degeneration are rapidly progressing, and novel concepts are described in Chapter 6, "DiscOver." Chapter 4 on imaging techniques, "The Eye of the Tiger," provides more information, but we are strongly convinced that a good physical exam, as discussed in Chapter 3, "Touching with Hands," is mandatory for this patient population. In this complex arena, an integrated clinical evaluation is the only possible way to decipher the optimal treatment options for patients with complex back pain.

The possible scenarios range from the pediatric and young adult with back pain, described in Chapter 8, "Young and Painful," to older patients with degenerative conditions, discussed in Chapter 9, "The Golden Ageing." Chapter 7, "NeuroBureau," examines where neurological and neuromuscular settings of back pain. A dedicated space is given to sacroiliac pathology in Chapter 5, "Under the Bridge." Inflammatory disease and infections are covered in Chapter 10, "Germination."

Special attention is then given to some emerging or recently acquired causes for back pain. Chapter 14, "Bended and Blended," focuses on back pain and sagittal malalignment, an underestimated and surgically manageable condition. Chapter 15, "Scar Wars," discusses the endless struggle with multioperated patients who do not improve with further revision surgeries. In these patients, a thorough, logical, and systematic analysis of the primary reasons for failure is mandatory. The chapter is built on the analysis of several clinical cases and presents many practical operative tips. Unfortunately, there is a group of patients who will never improve, as described in Chapter 16, "The End of the Road." However, even for this group, some practical clinical management tips are given that may prove helpful.

Finally, the crucial issue of outcome evaluation is covered in Chapter 12, "Happily Ever After." It represents a valuable tool for spine specialists in the global community to compare results and subsequently build evidence for efficacy.

As you can guess from this brief overview of the chapters, we avoided standard formats and tried to be practical and to provide valuable answers from current expert opinions. This is a contempory and up-to-date set of opinions, representing the most recent achievements and evidence in every topic. We have tried to give the reader the opinions of international spine clinical experts and basic science researchers, clustered in a multidisciplinary spine expert group. The hope is to pique your interest and to provide information for the best current treatment options for patients with low back pain.

Jeffrey C. Wang, MD
Claudio Lamartina MD

Contributors

Max Aebi, MD, DHC, FRSC, FMHOrth
Professor and Chair Emeritus
Orthopaedic Surgery
Das Rückenzentrum
Hirslanden-Salem Hospital
Bern, Switzerland

Mauro Alini, PhD
Professor
AO Research Institute Davos
Davos Platz, Switzerland

Roberto Bassani, MD
Head
2nd Spinal Surgery
I.R.C.C.S. Istituto Ortopedico Galeazzi
Milan, Italy

Pedro Berjano, MD, PhD
Director
GSpine4 Spine Surgery Division
I.R.C.C.S. Instituto Ortopedico Galeazzi
Milan, Italy

Marco Brayda-Bruno, MD
Director
Spine Care Group
Spine Surgery III–Scoliosis Department
I.R.C.C.S. Istituto Ortopedico Galeazzi
Milan, Italy

Roberto Chapa Sosa, MD
Assistant Professor
Ortopedia–Cirugía de Columna
Monterrey, México

Alessandra Colombini, MSc
Specialist
Clinical Biochemistry
Researcher
Orthopaedic Biotechnology Lab
I.R.C.C.S. Istituto Ortopedico Galeazzi
Milan, Italy

John P. Dormans, MD
Chief, Division of Pediatric Orthopaedic Surgery
Department of Surgery
Texas Children's Hospital
Tenured Professor, Orthopaedic Surgery
Baylor College of Medicine
Houston, Texas

Asdrubal Falavigna, MD, PhD
Coordinator
Medical School and Postgraduate Program in Health Science
Department of Neurosurgery
Caxias do Sul University
Caxias do Sul, Rio Grande do Sul, Brazil

Fabio Galbusera, MD
Director of the Laboratory of Biological Structures Mechanics
I.R.C.C.S. Istituto Ortopedico Galeazzi
Milan, Italy

Erica E. Gonzalez, BA
Research Assistant, Division of Pediatric Orthopaedic Surgery
Department of Surgery
Texas Children's Hospital
Houston, Texas

Sibylle Grad, MD
Principal Scientist
AO Research Institute Davos
Davos, Switzerland

Andre M. Jakoi, MD
Spine Fellow
Department of Orthopedic Surgery
Keck School of Medicine
University of Southern California
Los Angeles, California

Kristen E. Jones, MD
Adjunct Assistant Professor
Department of Neurosurgery
University of Minnesota
Minneapolis, Minnesota

Rishi Mugesh Kanna, MS, MRCS, FNB Spine
Associate Consultant Spine Surgeon
Department of Spine Surgery
Ganga Medical Centre and Hospital
Coimbatore, Tamilnadu, India

Claudio Lamartina, MD
Chief, GSpine4 Department
Director, Spinal Research Program
I.R.C.C.S. Istituto Ortopedico Galeazzi
Professor, Specialization School in Orthopaedics and Traumatology
Milan and Turin Universities
Milan, Italy

Lawrence G. Lenke, MD
Professor and Chief of Spinal Surgery
Department of Orthopedic Surgery
Columbia University College of Physicians and Surgeons
Surgeon-in-Chief
Spine Hospital
New York Presbyterian/Allen Hospital
New York, New York

Carlo Domênico Marrone, MD
Neurologist and Clinical Neurophysiologist
Neuromuscular Disorders Specialist
Clìnica Marrone
Porto Alegre, Brazil

Carlotta Martini, MD
I.R.C.C.S. Istituto Ortopedico Galeazzi
Milan, Italy

Christopher C. Ornelas, MD
Assistant Professor
Clinical Orthopaedic Surgery
Department of Orthopaedic Surgery
Keck School of Medicine
Los Angeles, California

Neil N. Patel, MD
Orthopaedic Spine Surgery Fellow
Department of Orthopaedic Surgery
University of Southern California
Los Angeles, California

Martin H. Pham, MD
Fellow
Department of Neurosurgery
University of Southern California
Los Angeles, California

David W. Polly, Jr., MD
Professor and Chief of Spine
Department of Orthopaedic Surgery
University of Minnesota
Minneapolis, Minnesota

Shanmuganathan Rajasekaran, MS, DNB, FRCS(Ed), MCh(Liv), FACS, FRCS(Eng), PhD
Chairman
Department of Orthopaedic and Spine Surgery
Ganga Hospital
Coimbatore, Tamilnadu, India

Katherine M. Schroeder, MD
Pediatric Orthopaedic Surgery Fellow
Department of Orthopaedic Surgery
Baylor College of Medicine
Houston, Texas

Elena Serchi, MD
Consultant
Department of Neurosurgery
I.R.C.C.S. of Neurological Sciences
Bologna, Italy

Ajoy Prasad Shetty, MS (Ortho), DNB (Ortho)
Consultant Spine Surgeon
Department of Orthopaedics, Traumatology and Spine Surgery
Ganga Medical Centre & Hospitals Pvt. Limited
Coimbatore, Tamil Nadu, India

Emiliano Vialle, MD
Head of Spine Surgery
Department of Orthopedics and Traumatology
Cajuru Hospital, Catholic University of Paraná
Curitiba, PR, Brazil

Jeffrey C. Wang, MD
Chief, Orthopaedic Spine Service
Co-Director USC Spine Center
Professor of Orthopaedic Surgery and Neurosurgery
USC Spine Center
Los Angeles, California

Hans-Joachim Wilke, PhD
Co-Director
Head of Spine Research
Institute of Orthopaedic Research and Biomechanics
Director and Chair, Prof. Dr. Anita Ignatius
Center of Musculoskeletal Research Ulm
University Hospital Ulm
Ulm, Germany

Mona Zall, DO
Fellow
Department of Orthopaedics
University of California
Los Angeles, California

Gustavo Zanoli, MD, PhD
Orthopaedic Surgeon
Ferrara, Italy

Alberto Zerbi, MD
EFM Professor of Radiology
University of Milan
University of Monza Bicocca
Chief, Department of Radiology
I.R.C.C.S. Istituto Ortopedico Galeazzi
Milan, Italy

1 Economic Issues, Risk Factors, and Litigation

Marco Brayda-Bruno

Introduction

The epidemiological burden of low back pain (LBP) and its socioeconomic impact in developed countries have been well analyzed and widely discussed in the past 40 years. Hundreds of basic research studies, clinical studies, multidisciplinary treatment proposals, analytic epidemiology papers, book chapters, and review articles have addressed this crucial problem. Low back pain (LBP), particularly in its chronic phenotype (CLBP), diminishes the patients' quality of life (QoL), with major consequences for their careers and social activities. In my 30 years of experience as a spine specialist, not much has changed in our understanding of the epidemiology of, risk factors for, and treatment of back pain.

Recent epidemiological research suggests that LBP is a leading cause of disability.[1] It presents a substantial societal burden in terms of health care costs and reduced work productivity to the tune of billions of dollars annually in many western countries. Lifetime prevalence rates of LBP are high, and a significant proportion of patients develop chronic symptoms lasting 3 months or longer. Chronic LBP results in extensive personal suffering and substantial economic costs for patients and society.

Background

Forty Years Ago

In a milestone paper published in the first issue of *Spine* in March 1976, Alf Nachemson[2] presented the issues and controversies in the treatment of LBP that have continued to be discussed by practitioners and researchers in the following decades:

> Low back pain is, in patients aged 30 to 60 years, the most expensive ailment from a socio-economic viewpoint.... At present the etiology is unknown ... and only symptomatic treatment is available.... So far no convincing evidence exists that any type of conservative treatment for the patient with low back pain is superior to nature's own course.... There are no more than 50 scientists in the world today at work on elucidating the cause of our most expensive disease. This is truly the orthopaedic superchallenge.[2]

Has the situation changed much since that paper was published? Certainly the number of researchers, clinicians, and surgeons engaged in LBP issues has increased tremendously, but it is not clear that this work has resulted in a definitive improvement in LBP patients' perceived QoL or in a reduction in the costs to society.

Thirty Years Ago

Based on epidemiological studies performed during the 1980s, it was already evident that the only illness occurring more frequently than LBP is the common cold! It is estimated that 75 to 85% of the world's population has experienced or will experience LBP at some point during their lifetime, generally as a short-term condition that, for 90% of patients, resolves within 2 months.

An editorial in *Acta Orthopaedica Scandinavica* entitled "The Back Pain Epidemic"[3] addressed the medico-social paradox of back pain: "Disability due to backache has reached epidemic proportion while heavy physical labor has decreased dramatically" in modern western countries. The editorial went on to state that the basic cause of CLBP

> is not due to physical work-related factors or to a universal weakening of the locomotor system. Rather, the culprits are (a) the idea that back problems generally improve with rest, and (b) the social-security reaction to this idea with prolonged sick leave and early retirement.[3]

Twenty Years Ago

In view of its high prevalence in developed countries, its heavy psychosocial and financial burden, and the burden imposed on health services, CLBP has become a severe public health problem. Consequently, the World Health Organization (WHO) established in the 1990s a working group to address the main diagnostic issues related to LBP and to review the epidemiology. Analyzing data obtained from the International Classification of Diseases (ICD-10) in 1993, the WHO report concluded that "low back pain is a general symptom" in at least 18 diagnostic categories![4]

The Present

Despite recent advances in technology that have aided diagnosis and treatment, as well as the abundance of epidemiological studies in the literature, no definitive solution for LBP has been proposed, and it continues to have a severe impact on the individual, the family, and society.

Epidemiology, Prevalence, Incidence, and Persistence and Recurrence of Low Back Pain

Box 1.1 provides definitions of epidemiology, prevalence, incidence, and persistence and recurrence. The following text subsections address these concepts with regard to LBP.

Incidence

The 1-year incidence of a first-ever episode of LBP ranges between 6.3% and 15.4%, whereas estimates of the 1-year incidence of any episode of LBP range between 1.5% and 36%. Meta-analytical incidence rates for first-time LBP and transition to pain from a pain-free state were similar (~ 25%), regardless of the community or occupational population.[5] Estimates of recurrence at 1 year range from 24% to 80%.

Prevalence

About 75 to 85% of all individuals will experience LBP at some point in their lifetime (lifetime prevalence). The yearly prevalence of back pain is estimated to range from 15 to 20% in the United States and from 25 to 45% in Europe. The prevalence of LBP was higher among women than among men. LBP was observed more frequently among older people and among those who were overweight.

Box 1.1 Definitions

Epidemiology

- Epidemiology refers to the frequency and causes of diseases or syndromes in different populations, and estimates the association between risk factors and diseases in statistical terms. A significant goal of epidemiology is to contribute to the planning and evaluation of primary prevention. The number of individuals who suffer from a disease or a syndrome is expressed in terms of prevalence rates, and the number of new cases is expressed in incidence rates.

Prevalence

- Prevalence refers to the percentage of a population that is affected with a particular disease for a given time period. This could be an entire lifetime (lifetime prevalence) or a specified number of months before the assessment (current prevalence rates).

Incidence

- Incidence refers to the number or rate of new cases of the disorder per number of persons at risk (usually 100 or 1,000) during a specified period of time (usually 1 year).

Persistence and Recurrence

- Because of its high prevalence and incidence rates, the burden of back pain in adult populations is better estimated with measures of the persistence (duration of pain episodes) and recurrence (number of episodes). Disability is of longer duration in recurrent LBP than in a single episode of LBP.

Source: Boos N, Aebi M, eds. Spinal Disorders: Fundamentals of Diagnosis and Treatment. New York: Springer; 2008.

Types of Pain

Most epidemiological studies do not differentiate between types of pain. It is well known that the natural history of LBP is usually favorable, and most individuals recover within 2 to 6 weeks, and more than 90% resolve within 3 months.

In the 1980s, Gordon Waddell[6] distinguished acute/subacute LBP from chronic LBP:

> CLBP is a completely different clinical syndrome from acute back pain, not only in time scale as per definition, but in kind. While acute pain could be relieved with efficacy if the underlying physical disorder is treated, chronic LBP becomes progressively dissociated from its original physical basis. The subsequent chronic disability and illness behaviour are increasingly coped with emotional distress, depression, and adoption of a sick role. CLBP becomes a self-sustaining condition that could be resistant to any medical management.

A very important contribution to our understanding of LBP and to the classification of the epidemiological characteristics of LBP was a 1988 article in the *New England Journal of Medicine* by John Frymoyer[7] that proposed the following definitions of acute, subacute, and chronic LBP, which subsequently were widely adopted: Acute LBP lasts up to 6 weeks and is generally unspecific, with only 10 to 20% of cases having a precise pathoanatomic cause. Subacute LBP lasts more than 6 weeks and up to 3 months; its cause is often elusive. Acute and subacute backache are transitory symptoms, having resolution within 2 months in 90% of patients. Chronic LBP lasts longer than 3 months. It occurs in 5% of patients, and accounts for 85% of the social costs in terms of reduced work productivity and lost compensation.

These findings have been frequently questioned, as the condition tends to relapse, and most patients experience multiple episodes years after the initial attack.

With respect to the cause of back pain, the so-called diagnostic triage classification has become standard. It categorizes LBP as (1) a specific spinal pathology, (2) nerve root pain/radicular pain, or (3) nonspecific.[8]

Pain, Impairment, and Disability

Chronic pain is very common. Epidemiological studies show a prevalence of chronic pain of 24 to 46% in the general population. The incidence of musculoskeletal pain in industrialized countries is reported to vary from 21% for shoulder pain to 85% for LBP; axial pain is very frequent, and studies have shown that it often becomes chronic.

Impairment is an abnormality in a body structure or in functioning that may include pain. Disability entails a reduction in the performance of activities. Disability at work and in one's personal life entails restrictions in the individual's major roles and limitations in social and recreational activities. Disability causes loss of productivity at home and at work, and the economic burden of chronic disability has become enormous in both developing and industrialized countries.

The Glasgow Illness Model (**Fig. 1.1**) is an operational clinical model of low back disability that includes physical, psychological, and social elements. It assumes that most back and neck pain starts with a physical problem, which causes nociception, at least initially. Psychological distress may significantly amplify the subjective pain experience and lead to abnormal illness behavior. This distress could alter social functions, and the individual may adopt the role of being a sick person; a small minority of patients with this "sick role" experience high levels of pain, even though the initial cause of nociception should have ceased and healing should have occurred.[8]

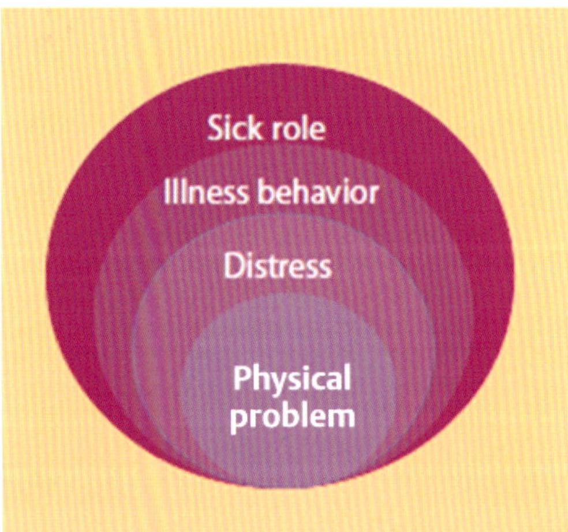

Fig. 1.1 The Glasgow Illness Model of Disability is an operational model of low back pain disability, as it develops from a physical problem to an illness behavior to a social sick role. (From Boos N, Aebi M, eds. Spinal Disorders: Fundamentals of Diagnosis and Treatment. Berlin: Springer; 2008. Reprinted by permission.)

Risk Factors

Models of back pain are multifactorial, and include genetic, biological, physical, psychological, sociological, and health policy factors. Occupational psychosocial variables are clearly linked to the transition from acute to chronic LBP, and from work disability, to recovery, to return to work. A relevant distinction regarding LBP is related to the perception of risk factors; although it was previously thought that work-related factors should be most strongly related to disk degeneration, there is increasing evidence that genetic factors influence disk degeneration more than any other factor. Other commonly reported risk factors include low educational status, stress, anxiety, depression, job dissatisfaction, low levels of social support in the workplace, and whole body vibration.

Risk factors can be categorized into several clusters: individual factors, morphological factors, general psychosocial factors, occupational physical factors, occupational factors, and psychological factors. They are described in the following subsections.

Individual Factors

There are multiple physical and psychosocial risk factors for a first-time LBP, but a history of a previous episode of back pain is by far the most strongly predictive and consistent risk factor for transition from a pain-free state to CLBP.[9]

Genetics

The genetic predisposition is clearly evident in disk degeneration, whereas the genetic predisposition in back pain is less clear and seems to depend on age. The influence of genetic predisposition has been established in several studies and in such multicenter European studies as Eurodisc and Genodics. It is likely that many genes are involved, and we are only beginning to unravel the molecular background of pain. Genetic factors could also affect pain perception. With the advance of molecular biological techniques, research has focused on exploring the genetic predisposition of interindividual differences. The influence on back pain, therefore, might be indirect, via spine morphological factors, or via a genetically determined tendency for psychological distress.[8]

Other individual characteristics indicating a susceptibility to spinal disorders include advanced age (> 50 years) and gender: females are more susceptible than males, but males are more likely to have a higher number of absences from work

Age and Gender

Hoy et al,[10] in a recent systematic review of the global prevalence of LBP, analyzed 165 general population studies from 54 countries, published between 1980 and 2009. LBP was shown to be a major problem throughout the world, with the highest prevalence among females and those of ages 40 to 80 years. Other studies have found that the incidence of LBP is highest in the third decade of life, whereas overall prevalence increases with age until the 60- to 65-year age group, and then gradually declines. Thus, as the population ages, the number of individuals with LBP worldwide is likely to increase substantially over the coming decades, as confirmed also by the study of Ghanei et al[11] that has shown a 1-year prevalence of LBP of close to 50% in community-living men of ages 69 to 81 years.

Many other environmental and personal risk factors may influence the onset and course of LBP. Being overweight, having a lower general health status and more comorbidities, smoking, and leading a sedentary lifestyle could be risk factors for LBP.

Morphological Factors

In the past, anatomic anomalies and structural spine modifications, together with their consequent mechanical or inflammatory processes, were thought to be crucial factors in causing back pain.[2] But now we know that such morphological factors are poorly correlated with LBP. Disk herniation or degeneration is often present in asymptomatic individuals; spina bifida, transitional vertebrae, spondylosis, and Scheuermann's disease do not appear to be associated with specific LBP. Similarly, patients with spondylolysis and spondylolisthesis are often considered to have nonspecific LBP.[8]

From an anatomic point of view, LBP commonly appears as pain, muscle tension, or stiffness localized below the costal margin and above the inferior gluteal folds, with or without leg pain (sciatica). Pain location is fairly consistent, with the immediate paraspinal region being the most common.

Psychosocial Factors

Since the very first studies on LBP,[2] psychosocial factors were known to influence low back disability, and, in accordance with the Glasgow Illness Model, recent epidemiological research confirms that these factors are an integral part of the pain disability process and have more impact on LBP disability than do biomechanical factors. Depression and anxiety are the most studied risk factors, and there is strong evidence that psychosocial variables are associated with the transition from acute to chronic pain and disability; inappropriate attitudes and beliefs about LBP, inappropriate pain behavior, low work satisfaction, and emotional problems are strongly linked to the development of chronic pain.[8]

Occupational Physical Factors

Heavy physical work is associated with LBP; in the past, it was considered as a major factor in inducing back pain,[2] but there is evidence of only a moderate association between the incidence (onset) of back pain and heavy physical work. Interestingly, although the proportion of people involved in heavy work has decreased in industrialized countries, there has been an increase in the number of people with work disability. Heavy physical labor may be a contributory factor in the onset of nonspecific back pain, but it is not a cause in many cases of work disability.

Physical risk factors for occupational back pain include heavy physical labor that entails positions of overextension, repetitive motion, twisting and bending, frequent lifting, awkward postures, and whole body vibration.[8]

Several recent studies on the specific occupational incidence of LBP provide an interesting overview based on work categories. Military personnel have an increased risk during training and combat deployment; approximately three quarters of duty-related burdens incurred during combat involve low back problems.[12] Low back symptoms are common and persistent among firefighters.[13] Nurses have reported the highest prevalence of LBP involving musculoskeletal pain problems,[14] as have farmers, who show a greater prevalence of musculoskeletal disorders than do nonfarmer populations, with LBP being the most common.[15]

Occupational and Psychological Factors

There is increasing evidence that the work factors leading to chronic disability are more psychosocial than biomechanical, and that they are strongly associated with disability itself and the consequent delay of return to work. The work-related psychosocial factors associated with spinal disorders are a rapid work rate, monotonous work, low job satisfaction, low social support, low decision attitude, and job stress.[8]

Other Issues

Epidemiological studies identify other issues to address in the development of LBP for which there is currently a lack of research evidence, such as (1) the limited diagnostic and prognostic value of medical imaging in nonspecific back pain, (2) the nonpositive but negative effect of bed rest, (3) the nonnegative but positive effect of early return to work, and (4) LBP in children and adolescents. The latter occurs more commonly than previously thought; recent epidemiological studies have shown that the prevalence of nonspecific LBP in childhood is high, matching that of adults by the end of the growth period, and it is becoming a public health concern. A meta-analytic investigation found that the most recent studies showed higher prevalence rates than the oldest studies, and studies with a better methodology exhibited higher lifetime prevalence rates.[16]

Geographic Variation

The reporting of back pain exhibits some geographic variations, even though there is little epidemiological information about the prevalence of back pain in developing countries.

According to some recent studies, LBP demonstrates a bimodal distribution in the United States, with peaks between 25 and 49 years in men and 65 to 94 years in women; black and Caucasian patients were found to have significantly higher rates of back pain than Asians.[17] In a Canadian population, the prevalence of claims-based recurrent LBP progressively decreased between 2000 and 2007 for younger adults (< 65 years), whereas older adults (≥ 65 years) showed an increase.[18] In a large Latin American study, the estimated prevalence of LBP is 16.7% for the population exposed to few risk factors, up to 65% for the higher risk subgroup,[19] with the most significant risk factors being long periods of time in the sitting position, obesity, pregnancy, smoking, advanced age, lifting and carrying heavy loads, domestic work, sedentary lifestyles, and longer duration of current employment. In Japan, LBP prevalence was highest in people in their 30s to 50s, and it specifically correlated with losing a job, leaving school, or changing jobs; up to 30% reported unchanged or aggravated symptoms and dissatisfaction with treatment.[20] An Australian study based on twin analysis (the AUstralian Twin low BACK pain [AUTBACK] study) has found that heavy domestic physical activity (PA) is associated with an increased probability of LBP, and the combination of heavy domestic and recreational PA might increase the probability of LBP more than heavy domestic or recreational PA alone.[21]

Costs

The CLBP patient population engenders enormous costs for the health care system in terms of medical consultations, diagnostic and therapeutic procedures, hospitalizations, and pharmaceuticals such as analgesics.[8]

Papageorgiou and Rigby[22] characterized the back pain–related contact with medical services by applying a one-in-five rule of thumb: one in five of the population experience back pain at any given period of time; of these patients, one in five consult their general practitioner (GP); and one in five of those consulting their GP are referred to a specialist. One in five of those attending outpatient clinics are admitted to the hospital, and one in five of those admitted undergo surgery for any kind of back pain.

The total costs of LBP are thus enormous, and are predominantly caused by disability; only a minority of patients are chronically disabled, but such cases engender most of the costs, because patients with LBP consume close to twice as much health care as the general population.

The economic burden of spinal disorders includes direct, indirect, and intangible costs, as follows:

- Direct costs consist of medical expenditures, such as the costs of prevention, detection, treatment, rehabilitation, and long-term care.
- Indirect costs consist of lost work output attributable to a reduced capacity for activity, and result from lost productivity, lost earnings, lost earnings and opportunities for family members, and lost tax revenue. Over 50% of the costs of spinal disorders are related to indirect societal costs.
- Intangible costs consist of psychosocial burdens resulting in reduced quality of life, such as job stress, financial stress, family stress, and suffering. Intangible costs are the most difficult to estimate.

Treatment

A general treatment concept is to prevent pain from persisting and becoming chronic, by the use of an aggressive, multimodal, preemptive approach for the treatment of acute pain.[8] Bed rest for longer than 3 days is ill-advised for patients with chronic LBP. Instead, patients should be instructed to stay as active as possible: “Pain does not hurt so much if you have something to do.”

Another important concept is that the pure distinction between organic and psychogenic or functional CLBP can be difficult to make and it is too simplistic, especially when deciding on treatment. Thirty years ago, Menges[23] proposed a three-part classification for CLBP patients consisting of a somatic part, a depressive part, and a “role” part. When the somatic aspect is predominant, role and psychological profile do not present specific problems; generally, the patient demonstrates satisfactory compliance with treatment, which is primarily medical or surgical. When the depressive part is predominant, patients are masking their problems through pain, and the onset of symptoms often corresponds with particular life events; psychological counseling is of primary importance in these patients, and the medical/surgical approach is secondary pending the resolution of the psychological disturbance. When the “role” aspect is dominant, the other two parts are not absent; there is a long history of interpersonal conflicts, life complications, and clashes with others. Usually after an episode of illness, pain is incorporated into the complex pattern of problems, and the patient’s “sick role” justifies other behavioral components (e.g., sexual problems, a compensatory strategy, etc.). These patients generally have extensive medical records, but medicalization of their pain, especially invasive treatments, could reinforce the patients’ pain behavior and thus are contraindicated; the best management for these patients is behavioral psychotherapy, not surgery.

Research evidence confirms that biopsychosocial interventions are effective in chronic LBP pain. This research has resulted in the development of various new treatment approaches, such as behavioral and cognitive-behavioral treatments. There is conflicting evidence on the effectiveness of so-called back schools, exercise therapy, and spinal manipulation, and the surgical treatment of chronic nonspecific spinal LBP continues to be very controversial, because there is no evidence of success.

Litigation

Litigation refers both to seeking compensation and to medical forensic problems. This issue has not been widely addressed in the recent literature, but it is a factor in our daily practice.

The seeking of compensation is a significant psychosocial factor in back pain becoming chronic. Social protections and guarantees for employees in Western European welfare systems have promoted "sick behavior" in back pain patients who have low job satisfaction or social problems. Twenty years ago, Blake and Garrett[24] discussed the effects of litigation on outcome, comparing two small groups of patients with LBP who were treated with a psychological and physical approach to rehabilitation; significant improvements were achieved in terms of flexibility, muscle endurance, pain reduction, and exercise fitness in both litigants and nonlitigants alike. But, despite reduced impairment and disability, the litigants showed no change in handicap, allowing the authors to speculate that, in the presence of ongoing litigation, patients are less amenable to restoration of function in their daily lives. Therefore, the authors' findings suggest that litigants fail to translate the gains achieved in impairment and disability measures into improved function.[24]

Medical forensic issues have increasing impact on the clinical practice of spine specialists, mostly related to the unsatisfactory outcomes of medical and especially surgical procedures performed on CLBP patients. No significant literature is available on this topic, apart from a couple of case reports, but nonetheless there is a general perception that this growing litigation affects the practice of clinical medicine. No specific advice can be given to spine surgeons, except to critically analyze the demands and expectations of CLBP patients, as well as to review their psychosocial situation. It is crucial to assess whether a single-discipline approach is suitable to improve the patients' condition, or whether a more holistic multidisciplinary biopsychosocial rehabilitation (MBR) approach should be recommended. If so, it is important to explain to patients the reason for this approach and to discourage them from seeking surgery.

The Nature of Pain and the Search for an Appropriate Treatment Modality

Often the nature of pain is dependent on the patient's subjective experiences. Many factors influence the onset of pain and pain-affected behavior, such as cultural factors, the doctor–patient relationship, and the patient's educational level, socioeconomic status, history, current psychological problems, and employment situation.

By its natural history, acute or subacute LBP appears to be a universal, benign, self-limiting condition. The majority of the LBP population copes with it and does not seek medical treatment, because the symptoms are interpreted as minor nociceptive stimuli, and are managed either by ignoring them or by resting periodically. Whether the person seeks medical treatment seems to depend on the person's pain perception, care expectation, and cultural patterns of illness behavior.

In contrast, disability due to CLBP, as opposed to LBP, appears to be an epidemic that is not explained by any demonstrable physical disorder or degeneration. For 30 years, CLBP has been known to have enormous worldwide impact on individuals, families, communities, businesses, and society. CLBP is a multidimensional process associated with comorbidities such as anxiety and depression. Recent research using advanced in vivo brain imaging technologies has found increasing insights into the etiology and pathogenesis of chronic pain. Psychometric measures have found significantly higher scores on depression and anxiety scales in the patient population. *Voxel-based morphometry* (*VBM*) analysis has demonstrated significant decreases in gray matter density in areas associated with pain processing and modulation (e.g., the dorsolateral prefrontal cortex, the thalamus, and the middle cingulate cortex). Thus, compelling evidence exists that alterations of gray matter architecture in brain regions in CLBP patients should play a major role in pain modulation and control; these results could confirm the hypothesis of a "brain signature" in chronic pain conditions, although the exact mechanisms by which LBP becomes chronic remain unclear.[25]

The Global Burden of Disease Study 2010 addressed LBP in relation to impairment and activity limitation. Other studies aimed to quantify the burden arising from LBP due to occupational exposure to ergonomic risk factors, and estimated the work-related burden in disability-adjusted life years (DALYs). This analysis was made for each of 21 world regions and 187 countries, separately for 1990 and 2010, using consistent methods. The conclusions were that worldwide, LBP arising from ergonomic exposures at work was estimated to cause 21.7 million DALYs in 2010. The overall population-attributable fraction was 26%, varying considerably with age, sex, and region; 62% of LBP DALYs were in men (mostly of ages 35 to 55 years), and the highest relative risk was in the agricultural sector. There was a 22% increase in overall work-related LBP DALYs between 1990 and 2010 due to population growth.[26] There is a need for further information on exposure distributions and relative risks, particularly in developing countries, because LBP arising from ergonomic exposures at work is an important cause of chronic disability.

Treatment of CLBP remains a challenge, as its success is influenced more by the patient's functioning than by physical problems. No treatment modality or CLBP has demonstrated a clear superiority over other options.[6] Chronic back pain has multiple etiologies, including neurologic, physiological, psychological, sociocultural, motivational, cognitive, and behavioral factors—all of which should be addressed in a holistic approach.

One treatment approach conceptualizes LBP as a biopsychosocial problem. This approach is supported by the observation that LBP, particularly at the chronic stage, is caused by a combination of factors, and psychological and social factors may play a role in the development and maintenance of pain and disability. Interestingly, several research studies from 25 years ago were already suggesting that a multidisciplinary team approach should be used in managing pain, because there was considerable evidence that MBR could be the most effective method for treating chronic pain. Wider acceptance of the biopsychosocial model and the ineffectiveness of monotherapies have led to increased use of a multidisciplinary approach, which has resulted in promising reports from clinical practice. MBR can be offered in multidisciplinary pain clinics, rehabilitation centers, and outpatient settings. MBR includes elements aimed at improving back-related physical dysfunction as well as addressing psychological issues and targeting social and work-related behaviors. There is some evidence from systematic reviews to suggest that these interventions may have a positive effect on long-term work participation outcomes.[27] In the past 10 years, despite the large volume of clinical research focused on identifying the most effective treatments for CLBP, finding the optimal management approach has proved to be elusive.

The Cochrane Collaboration recently conducted a systematic review of LBP studies.[27] Previous Cochrane reviews had addressed behavioral treatment for CLBP, physical conditioning programs for improving work outcomes in workers with back pain, and individual patient education for LBP. But these earlier studies are now out of date. The recent review analyzed 41 studies reporting on a total of 6,858 participants. The authors conclude that an MBR intervention for CLBP patients has a more positive effect on pain and disability outcomes than does the standard care or a physical treatment program. It is also likely that MBR will have a beneficial effect on work outcomes compared with physical treatment. However, given the moderate size of these effects and the potentially high cost of an intensive intervention, there is little to gain by using MBR on patients whose condition does not entail a substantial physical and psychosocial impact. Clinical practice guidelines commonly recommend assessment and treatment of physical and psychosocial factors, and then referral to MBR programs only for those patients in whom these factors are present. MBR should not be recommended solely on the basis of chronicity of symptoms.

Past, Present, and Future Research Trends

Past

In 1988, in a visionary report, Frymoyer[7] suggested that researchers "study degenerative changes in spinal tissues, especially disc and support structures, . . . to distinguish degeneration from injury and disease." Research studies could include magnetic resonance imaging scans in vivo, genetic linkage with lumbar disk degeneration, disk biology, macromolecules, disk cell phenotypes, markers for disk degeneration, disk nutrition and vascular supply, bioengineering disk models, animal models of disk degeneration, biomechanical studies of kinematics after bony structure excision, instability and facet anatomy, animal models in instability, mathematical models of instability, and load sharing on facet joints.

Present

Traeger et al[28] propose a screening tool to predict the risk of chronic LBP in patients presenting with acute LBP. The early identification of at-risk patients will enable clinicians to make informed decisions based on a prognostic profile, and will enable researchers to address a specific clinical phenotype of individuals. Prevention of CLBP must be emphasized. In many patients, an optimal approach at an early stage might prevent pain from becoming chronic, because protracted symptoms promote the development of pain behavior and the so-called pain identity. Recently, Mehling et al[29] reported on a 2-year prospective cohort study of risk factors for the progression to chronic pain. The study enrolled 605 patients; 13% had chronic pain at 6 months and 19% at 2 years. A clinical decision rule (CDR) was developed that may help primary care clinicians to classify patients with strictly defined acute LBP into low-, moderate-, and high-risk groups for developing chronic pain. This CDR should have an important future application by general practitioners and by spine specialists.

Future

Future epidemiological research should address the classification of spinal disorders with standardized, reliable, and valid methods, to reach greater agreement on definitions and staging. In addition, using a population-based registries approach, a standard assessment of risk, treatment, and outcomes needs to be developed. Furthermore, a standardized costing methodology is urgently needed, to help estimate the long-term economic consequences of treatment.

Conclusions

- Low back pain, and especially its chronic evolution (CLBP), represents a major public health problem in developed countries.
- The medico-social aspect of LBP arises from sociocultural factors in modern societies and by the compensation role of welfare systems. These factors could increase the perception of pain and its threshold among patients with LBP, and could promote the adoption of the socially recognized status of "sick" person.

- The person at risk of developing a disability should be identified as early as possible in the course of an episode of LBP to prevent the morbidity and high costs associated with chronic disability. The most important factors in predicting disability relate less to physical findings and more to the duration of the current impairment, the history of previous disability, psychosocial factors, occupational requirements, and job satisfaction. It is not surprising, therefore, that these same factors are highly associated with perceived failures of both operative and nonoperative treatment of CLBP.
- There is moderate evidence that multidisciplinary treatments such as MBR result in larger improvements in pain and daily function than the standard care or treatments aimed only at physical factors. This may be important for people whose symptoms are not responding to other treatments, but the effects of MBR need to be balanced with their costs in terms of resources and time. Because MBR programs are often intensive and expensive, they are most appropriate for patients with severe or complex problems who have passed a preliminary triage.
- Conventional medical treatments and surgical approaches for CLBP have largely failed.
- Surgery is a single-discipline treatment, not a multidisciplinary treatment. In a visionary report in 1976, Alf Nachemson[2] stated, "For 98% of patients, the present knowledge of the psychologic, social and mechanical stress factors ... should be utilized for proper counselling, together with attempts at correction with any type of noninvasive modality, according to the preference of the individual physician." The situation has not changed much in the subsequent 40 years. No noninvasive or minimally invasive treatment has provided evidence of its effectiveness. The risk factors for CLBP disability remain the same.
- A single-discipline medical or surgical treatment for CLBP is inappropriate.

Chapter Summary

Low back pain, and especially if it is chronic, represents a major public health problem of epidemic proportions in developed countries. The medico-social paradox—more back pain patients even though there are fewer manual labor jobs—is partially explained by sociocultural aspects of modern welfare systems. The compensation role of these systems encourage LBP patients to increase their perception of pain, thus promoting the adoption of the socially recognized status of "sick" person.

Because the patient population suffering from CLBP has been found to be responsible for an enormous proportion of health care costs, the person at risk of chronicity should be identified early in the course of a first episode of LBP, to prevent morbidity and the costs associated with chronic disability.

The factors that predict the development of a disability relate less to physical findings than to the duration of the current back impairment, psychosocial issues, occupational requirements, and job satisfaction. These same factors are associated with the perceived failures of both operative and nonoperative treatment of CLBP.

Conventional medical and surgical treatments of CLBP have demonstrated little success. A holistic approach to CLBP patients is indicated, using preliminary psychosocial triage to identify the nonorganic factors that could influence the perception of back pain as a chronic lifelong problem. There is evidence that multidisciplinary biopsychosocial rehabilitation (MBR) can provide improved results in terms of pain and daily functioning when compared with treatments that address only physical factors. Nevertheless, despite recent advances in diagnosis and treatment, and the evidence provided by epidemiological studies, no definitive treatment has been proposed for LBP, which continues to have a severe impact on individuals, families, and society.

Pearls

- Chronic LBP represents a major public health problem that entails enormous direct and indirect costs.
- The compensation role of welfare systems promotes the adoption of a status of "sick" person in CLBP patients.
- A person at risk of disability should be identified early to prevent morbidity and the costs associated with CLBP disability.
- Some evidence exists that multidisciplinary treatments such as MBR can induce improvement in pain and daily function. Due to its high costs in resources and time, it should be adopted only in severe or complex CLBP cases.

Pitfalls

- In CLBP patients, conventional and innovative medical or surgical treatments have most often failed.
- A single-discipline approach (such as surgery) is not advisable in CLBP treatment.

References

Five Must-Read References

1. Vos T, Flaxman AD, Naghavi M, et al. Years lived with disability (YLDs) for 1160 sequelae of 289 diseases and injuries 1990-2010: a systematic analysis for the Global Burden of Disease Study 2010. Lancet 2012; 380:2163–2196
2. Nachemson AL. The lumbar spine: an orthopaedic challenge. Spine 1976;1:10–21
3. Editorial. The back pain epidemic. Acta Orthop Scand 1989;60:633–634
4. de Girolamo G. Epidemiology and social costs of low back pain and fibromyalgia. Clin J Pain 1991;7(1, Suppl 1):S1–S7
5. Hoy D, Brooks P, Blyth F, Buchbinder R. The Epidemiology of low back pain. Best Pract Res Clin Rheumatol 2010;24:769–781
6. Waddell G. 1987 Volvo award in clinical sciences. A new clinical model for the treatment of low-back pain. Spine 1987;12:632–644
7. Frymoyer JW. Back pain and sciatica. N Engl J Med 1988;318(5):291–300
8. Boos N, Aebi M, eds. Spinal Disorders: Fundamentals of Diagnosis and Treatment. Berlin: Springer; 2008
9. Taylor JB, Goode AP, George SZ, Cook CE. Incidence and risk factors for first-time incident low back pain: a systematic review and meta-analysis. Spine J 2014; 14:2299–2319
10. Hoy D, Bain C, Williams G, et al. A systematic review of the global prevalence of low back pain. Arthritis Rheum 2012;64:2028–2037
11. Ghanei I, Rosengren BE, Hasserius R, et al. The prevalence and severity of low back pain and associated symptoms in 3,009 old men. Eur Spine J 2014;23: 814–820
12. Cohen SP, Gallagher RM, Davis SA, Griffith SR, Carragee EJ. Spine-area pain in military personnel: a review of epidemiology, etiology, diagnosis, and treatment. Spine J 2012;12:833–842
13. Lusa S, Miranda H, Luukkonen R, Punakallio A. Sleep disturbances predict long-term changes in low back pain among Finnish firefighters: 13-year follow-up study. Int Arch Occup Environ Health 2015;88:369–379
14. Davis KG, Kotowski SE. Prevalence of musculoskeletal disorders for nurses in hospitals, long-term care facilities, and home health care: a comprehensive review. Hum Factors 2015;57:754–792
15. Osborne A, Blake C, Fullen BM, et al. Prevalence of musculoskeletal disorders among farmers: A systematic review. Am J Ind Med 2012;55:143–158
16. Calvo-Muñoz I, Gómez-Conesa A, Sánchez-Meca J. Prevalence of low back pain in children and adolescents: a meta-analysis. BMC Pediatr 2013; 13:14
17. Waterman BR, Belmont PJ Jr, Schoenfeld AJ. Low back pain in the United States: incidence and risk factors for presentation in the emergency setting. Spine J 2012;12:63–70
18. Beaudet N, Courteau J, Sarret P, Vanasse A. Prevalence of claims-based recurrent low back pain in a Canadian population: a secondary analysis of an administrative database. BMC Musculoskelet Disord 2013; 14:151
19. Garcia JB, Hernandez-Castro JJ, Nunez RG, et al. Prevalence of low back pain in Latin America: a systematic literature review. Pain Physician 2014;17: 379–391 Review
20. Nakamura M, Nishiwaki Y, Ushida T, Toyama Y. Prevalence and characteristics of chronic musculoskeletal pain in Japan. J Orthop Sci 2011;16:424–432
21. Hübscher M, Ferreira ML, Junqueira DR, et al. Heavy domestic, but not recreational, physical activity is associated with low back pain: Australian Twin low BACK pain (AUTBACK) study. Eur Spine J 2014;23: 2083–2089

22. Papageorgiou AC, Rigby AS. Review of UK data on the rheumatic diseases—7. Low back pain. Br J Rheumatol 1991;30:208–210
23. Menges LJ. Chronic low back pain: a medical-psychological report. Soc Sci Med 1983;17:747–753
24. Blake C, Garrett M. Impact of litigation on quality of life outcomes in patients with chronic low back pain. Ir J Med Sci 1997;166:124–126
25. Ivo R, Nicklas A, Dargel J, et al. Brain structural and psychometric alterations in chronic low back pain. Eur Spine J 2013;22:1958–1964
26. Driscoll T, Jacklyn G, Orchard J, et al. The global burden of occupationally related low back pain: estimates from the Global Burden of Disease 2010 study. Ann Rheum Dis 2014;73:975–981
27. Kamper SJ, Apeldoorn AT, Chiarotto A, et al. Multidisciplinary biopsychosocial rehabilitation for chronic low back pain. (review) Cochrane Database Syst Rev 2014;9:CD000963
28. Traeger A, Henschke N, Hübscher M, et al. Development and validation of a screening tool to predict the risk of chronic low back pain in patients presenting with acute low back pain: a study protocol. BMJ Open 2015;5:e007916
29. Mehling WE, Ebell MH, Avins AL, Hecht FM. Clinical decision rule for primary care patient with acute low back pain at risk of developing chronic pain. Spine J 2015;15:1577–1586

2

Decision Making and Flag Systems

Gustavo Zanoli

Introduction

Back pain has become a standard indication for a broad group of conditions in the biomedical literature, as if it were a diagnosis rather than a simple descriptive symptom. This has many advantages from a general medicine and epidemiological perspective, but sometimes it makes it difficult for the specialist to correctly identify and treat different types of back pain. Moreover, this difficulty is reflected in clinical research, where very often the effects of treatments cannot be clearly established due to a great number of confounding factors in a sometimes very inhomogeneous sample of patients.

For these reasons, it is very important for the clinician to undertake a thorough anamnestic interview and to follow defined clinical pathways from the early steps of the decision-making process. As an aid to "navigate" the complexity of these syndromes, several flag systems have been introduced, which aim to quickly identify risk factors for more serious conditions or prognostic factors that might interfere with the recovery from a back pain episode.

This chapter reviews the literature regarding the use of flag systems and history-taking algorithms, and offers some practical advice for the clinician.

A Brief History of the Use of Flags in the Assessment of Low Back Pain

In the early 17th century, a solid red flag was used by military forces to indicate that they intended to start a battle, as seen in poems and paintings that can be easily found on Wikipedia.[1]

According to Welch,[2] in medical practice, the term *red flag* was originally associated with back pain. The first catalogue of red flags for back pain appeared in the literature in the early 1980s, and since then numerous lists have been compiled. At the same time, Waddell introduced the study of nonorganic signs[3] and the biopsychosocial model[4] in low back pain (LBP), and the great research interest in psychosocial risk and prognostic factors started. The term *yellow flag* was introduced by Kendall et al[5] in 1997 to cover psychological, social, and environmental risk factors (in contrast to red flags indicating physical risk factors) for long-term disability and work loss and was then adopted in some guidelines. The original list of yellow flags contained many domains, including attitudes and beliefs about back pain and work. Subsequently, in 2002, the system was refined by Chris Main[6] so that workplace factors that were originally considered as yellow flags were reclassified in two separate categories: black flags for workplace organizational (objective) conditions, and blue flags for individual (subjective) perceptions about work issues. In 2005, Main et al[7] suggested that orange flags should also be added to the toolbox, to identify signs of a more serious mental disorder that requires referral to a psychiatric treatment center (**Table 2.1**).

Red Flags

Silvano Boccardi, one of the fathers of Italian rehabilitation medicine, is credited with creating a list of more than 800 different causes of back pain. (I learned this from Francesco Greco, head of the school of orthopedics that I attended, and the list can be found in several Italian Web sites and publications, even though I could not find the original reference; it was probably just a paradoxical speculation, calculated by multiplying the possible anatomic sites of pain in 33 vertebrae with the different underlying pathologies, such as traumatic, neurologic, inflammatory, degenerative, neoplastic, infective, and others.) Of course, the intent of Boccardi's estimate of 800 causes was to be provocative, to emphasize the difficulties of a merely physiological model of conditions such as LBP. In fact, specific back pain, that is, back pain that can be the presenting symptom of a serious underlying pathology, accounts for a minority of cases (less than 10 to 20% according to different reports in specialized settings,[8] and 1 to 5% in primary care[9]). However, given the possibly severe consequences of missing or delaying the diagnosis of an etiologic condition with unfavorable outcomes, it would be highly advisable to exclude those few patients from the start. Furthermore, the vast majority of studies in the literature focus on aspecific LBP, which can be defined only after ruling out other known relevant pathologies. Finally, it can never be assumed by any health care provider that others have already excluded the presence of these conditions, because even the most skilled practitioner can miss them, and clinical situations might change over time. For all these reasons it would be ideal to have a simple and reproducible tool to rapidly (and repeatedly, if necessary) detect the few cases requiring a separate diagnostic workout. This explains the success of the red flag system and its subsequent impact on clinical reasoning and on other sites of musculoskeletal pain.

The consensus on the importance of assessing red flags is not reflected in its practical implementation. In a retrospective review of clinic charts for 160 patients with LBP seen at six outpatient physical therapy clinics, Leerar et al[10] found that only seven of the 11 red flag items investigated were documented over 98% of the time. They also noted that experts had provided varied opinions as to what constitutes a red flag finding for patients with LBP, with differences varying from item formulation (e.g., duration of symptoms, specified as over 1, 1.5 or 3 months in the different sources) to including or not including a specific item such as history of trauma, or even to using a cluster of red flags to identify high-risk patients to refer for medical evaluation. Major conditions investigated by red flags can be summarized in five areas: fracture, tumor, infection, inflammatory disease, and cauda equina syndrome.

In a review performed by Zanoli et al[11] for the Italian Orthopedic Society in 2011, all six international LBP guidelines reviewed recommended using red flags in the initial assessment, but this recommendation seemed to be opinion based, and the red flag lists differed in the various guidelines. A previous systematic review with a slightly different methodology analyzed 10 different guidelines and found that the number of red flags specified in each guideline ranged from seven to 17, with a mean of 11.[12] Overall, 22 red flags were identified, only three of which were included in nine of 10 guidelines: age > 50 years, history of cancer, and steroid use. Eight red flags were potentially associated with spinal cancer, six with cauda equina syndrome, five with spinal fracture, and five with spinal infection, for a total is 24, but

Table 2.1 Possible Factors to Investigate During the Anamnestic Process, Categorized by Their Respective Flag Group

Biomedical/Organic Factors	Psychosocial Factors	Psychiatric Factors	Subjective Work Factors	Objective Work Factors
Presence of at least two of five indicates risk of possible fracture: • History of significant trauma (major in young patients, minor in elderly patients) • Prolonged corticosteroid use • Older age • Female gender • Osteoporosis *Two most relevant factors to consider when screening for malignancy:* • History of cancer • Older age	• Distress/depression, feeling useless and not needed because of pain • Reduced activity level, withdrawal from ADL, avoidance of personal and social activity, extended rest • Preexisting chronic pain, either in the back or elsewhere • Poor self-rated general health • Kinesophobia • Belief that pain is uncontrollable, report of extremely high intensity of pain, e.g., above 10, on a 0–10 VAS • Belief that pain is harmful resulting in fear-avoidance behavior • Belief that all pain must be abolished before attempting to return to work or normal activity • Catastrophizing, thinking the worst, misinterpreting bodily symptoms • Passive attitude to treatment, excessive reliance on use of drugs, surgery, aids, or appliances • Health professional sanctioning disability • Experience of conflicting diagnoses or explanations for back pain, • Dramatization of back pain by health professional • Numerous consultations, numerous different health professionals, lack of satisfaction with previous treatment • Overprotective partner/spouse, emphasizing fear of harm or encouraging catastrophizing • Familiar or social "reward" from being sick • Socially punitive responses from spouse • Lack of support person to talk to about problems	• Clinical depression • Major personality disorders • Posttraumatic stress disorders • Drug and alcohol abuse/addictions Other possible red flags that require attention: • Cauda Equina Features • Younger age (< 20) • History of drug abuse or immunodeficiency • History of inflammatory disease • Unexplained weight loss • Nonmechanical pain • Fever, chills, night sweats • Thoracic pain • General malaise • Deformity • Neurological symptoms • Recent infection or procedure causing bacteremia	• Belief that work is harmful; that it will do damage or be dangerous • Skepticism about the further management of work tasks and about return to work at all • Previous experience of ineffective management of injuries/sickness • Work history, including frequent job changes, stress at work, job dissatisfaction, lack of vocation • Unsupportive or unhappy work environment, low appreciation of efforts • Low educational background, low socioeconomic status • Low personal control of job conditions • History of extended time off work due to injury or other pain problem • History of previous back pain, with a previous claim(s) and time off work	*Category I* • Adverse sickness policy • Ongoing disability claim • Unemployment • National/regional legal aspects and insurance system • Lack of financial incentive to return to work • Delay/dispute in accessing income support and treatment cost • Absence of interest from employer *Category II* • High biomechanical job demands • Job involves shift work or working unsociable hours • Minimal availability of selected duties and graduated return to work pathways

Abbreviations: ADL, activities of daily living; VAS, visual analogue scale.

two red flags (age > 50 years and urinary retention) were each associated with both cancer and fracture; thus, 22 red flags were identified overall.

Two high-quality diagnostic reviews from the Cochrane Collaboration systematically addressed the evidence on the usefulness of red flag assessment to specifically screen for vertebral fracture[9] and malignancy[13] in patients presenting with LBP. In the first review, the available evidence did not support the use of many red flags to specifically screen for vertebral fracture in patients presenting with LBP. When combinations of red flags were used, the screening performance appeared to improve. Authors of the second review concluded that there was insufficient evidence to provide recommendations regarding their diagnostic accuracy or usefulness for detecting spinal malignancy, and that indications should not be based on the results of a single red flag question. Because spinal malignancy is a rather rare finding in LBP patients (less than 1% in primary care studies as compared with 3 to 11% for fractures[9,13]), it probably reduces the possibility of reaching statistically relevant and homogeneous conclusions until larger amounts of data are collected.

Despite these unsatisfactory evidence reviews, I believe it is still a good idea to assess for red flags when examining a new patient with LBP, and reassess them periodically, especially if the condition is not self-limiting, as occurs in most cases. Most of these items are part of a common medical anamnesis anyway, and may help in getting to know the patient and establishing a good physician–patient alliance. It should be noted, however, that many red flags have high false-positive rates, and if used without any critical clinical judgment, the result could be the referral for many inappropriate examinations with consequences for the cost of management and the outcomes of patients with LBP. The choice of an age to be considered at risk (over 50, 64, 70, 74?) largely influences sensitivity and specificity, and should be considered with caution, as not all 70-year-old people are similar. Probably a combination of a limited number of factors (osteoporosis, history of trauma, corticosteroid use, older age, and female gender) with a threshold of at least two positive findings is the best choice at present when screening for a vertebral fracture, whereas a history of cancer (possibly combined with age) is the most important item to assess when screening for malignancy. A history of infection or immunodeficiency and inflammatory disease can help to diagnose some otherwise unexplained nonmechanical back pain, but this does not necessarily mean a different (and more expensive) pathway in stable patients with an established diagnosis who experience a "normal" mechanical LPB. Clinical features of cauda equina syndrome (saddle anesthesia, sphincteric dysfunctions) should also be investigated when neurologic involvement is suspected.

More generally, positivity of findings should not necessarily prompt a referral for expensive diagnostic testing, but they may indicate the need to ask further questions, even using some of the discarded red flags (e.g., unexplained weight loss, nonmechanical pain, etc.) to confirm or exclude suspects, or to search for "reassurance" in other possible sources of a mechanical back pain (workload changes, new mattresses, recent increase in household duties, etc.). Finally, clinicians should remember that the clinical examination is a powerful and rather inexpensive way to confirm some of the red flag suspicions, and all elements should be taken into account before proceeding to the prescription of expensive diagnostic imaging and laboratory tests.

Yellow Flags and Orange Flags

Having excluded specific causes of LBP with red flags, the vast majority of patients with aspecific LBP still remain to be assessed, and in some cases treated or helped to find a way back to their usual activities without pain or disability. This occurs in most cases, even without any treatment, but in some people the pain lasts longer, and may become a frequent or constant presence, affecting quality of life and return to work. The introduction of the biopsychosocial model in LBP opened new perspectives in recognizing patients at risk of heading toward less favorable outcomes. In their appendix to the New Zealand Acute Low Back Pain Guide, Kendall et al[5] started from the assumption that most of the known risk factors for long-term disability, inactivity, and work loss are psychosocial, and they proposed a long list of factors (yellow flags) that increase the risk of these problems developing, so that health professionals could subsequently act to prevent these problems, starting in the early stages of management. After this first formulation, other guidelines have proposed their own lists, and other theoretical models described the development and prolongation of LBP with different mechanisms. This led to a great number of psychosocial yellow flags to be assessed. Even after the distinction of work-related blue and black flags (see below), the list of potential influencing factor became long, but the evidence is sparse.

Can yellow flags influence outcomes in people with acute or subacute LBP? Can yellow flags be targeted in interventions to produce better outcomes? Systematic reviews yielded conflicting results, and have even been criticized from a methodological standpoint.[14] There might also be a geographic or culturally determined variation in the influence of some factors. For example, fear avoidance beliefs have been shown not to influence the disability and quality of life of Spanish LBP patients.[15] A randomized controlled trial comparing the assessment and modification of psychosocial prognostic factors with standard care in the treatment of (sub)acute LBP in general practice found no evidence that general practitioners should adopt a treatment strategy aimed at psychosocial prognostic factors in these patients.[16] In an interesting systematic review of risk and prognostic factors for nonspecific musculoskeletal pain classified into International Classification of Functioning (ICF) dimensions, the authors found that for LBP, there is high evidence that fear avoidance and poor social support at work are not prognostic factors for LBP, and that poor social support at work and poor job content are not risk factors for LBP.[17] The authors suggested that fear-avoidance beliefs and poor social support at work perhaps should be removed as yellow flags.

More recently, another color has been added to the flag system: orange.[7] Orange flags indicate the presence of psychopathology, that is, more severe mental health and psychological problems than those indicated by yellow flags, alerting the clinician to serious psychiatric problems that could require referral to a mental health specialist or psychiatrist, rather than following the normal course of management for mild mental health conditions such as anxiety. Orange flags can indicate excessively high levels of distress, major personality disorders, posttraumatic stress disorders, drug and alcohol abuse/addictions, or clinical depression. It has been recommended that all practitioners should screen for the presence of orange flags, particularly in patients who have been off from work due to illness for more than 4 weeks. At this stage, there is only experts' opinion on this subject, and orange flags have been defined only insofar as they may be mistaken for yellow flags, and they have not been well studied. However, it does seem to be common sense that clinicians suspecting a previously undiagnosed psychiatric problem should triage patients to a mental health specialist. This does not imply that these patients' back problem should be left untreated in the end, and reassessment after specialist treatment should be recommended, at least.

Thus, similarly to what has been said about red flags, taking into account yellow flags, particularly when they are at high levels, does seem a better idea than either ignoring them or providing interventions to people regardless of psychological risk factors. This does not necessarily imply a recommendation to use a formal set of items, which would be done in a comprehensive clinical evaluation. In general, practitioners should not expect that a strict protocol and a "cookbook" solution will simply help them avoiding patients with a bad prognosis, but they could use some of these factors to try to assemble a more complete picture and to help establish a good physician–patient relationship. In more specialized settings, with more severe patients, assessment of yellow flags is probably part of the treatment itself anyway, as some of the multidisciplinary interventions specifically address psychological issues.

Blue Flags and Black Flags

It is well known that LBP continues to have a great impact on sick leave and work disability in the industrialized world. Although most working-age adults are able to recover from acute back pain or manage to cope with a recurrent or chronic condition with few work absences, others experience significant periods of work disability or even need to change their job or professional path.

Because there seems to be no anatomic or physiopathological feature that can help identify those at risk of having a poor work-related outcome, a considerable amount of research has been devoted to study nonmedical prognostic factors that could predict such an unfavorable evolution. We have already discussed the importance of psychosocial factors in the discussion about yellow flags. Blue flags have been subsequently defined to help clinician address specific workplace factors that might influence outcomes in LBP patients.[6] Originally many of these factors were considered as yellow flags, because they implied a *subjective* perception about work issues, such as negative expectations of return to work, job dissatisfaction, stress at work, work-related fear-avoidance beliefs (i.e., belief that work is harmful or fear of reinjury), perceptions of physical job demands, and poor colleague or supervisor relationships. On the other side, to balance these subjective factors, black flags indicate actual *objective* workplace conditions that can affect disability, including on one side employer and insurance system organizational characteristics (category I) and on the other side measures of physical workload and job features (category II).[18]

Systematic reviews have addressed several blue or black flags as prognostic factors, with negative (job stress), conflicting (job dissatisfaction, work fear avoidance), or at least wavering and inconsistent (recovery expectations, physical job demands, low social support at work) findings. Several review authors recommend that standardized, psychometrically robust instruments should be used in future studies to enable deriving reproducible measurements; however, a systematic review of these instruments for the assessment of blue flags in individuals with nonspecific LBP found that none of the identified instruments, in their current stage of development, could be recommended as blue flag assessment tools.[19]

Consequently, we have even less robust data on the usefulness of blue flags and black flags in clinical decision making, and these measures have seen limited dissemination in clinical practice, not only because the predictive performance of some tools has not been sufficiently demonstrated, but more importantly, because screening results have rarely been linked to appropriate early intervention strategies.

As stated by the authors of the "Decade of the Flags" Working Group,[18] other problems include errors in classifying patients, the time and effort required to administer and score assessment measures and discuss results with patients, and limited treatment options (or effective power) for addressing workplace and psychosocial concerns. Some providers may feel reluctant or unprepared to explore these nonmedical domains, despite their prominence in published medical guidelines for the treatment of LBP.

Despite these limitations, many guidelines still recommend assessing all flags in aspecific LBP patients. Although this probably reflects the attitude of guideline working groups to rely more on anecdotal evidence or expert opinion when making recommendations on issues different from therapeutic interventions, some degree of clinical common sense still advises us to at least consider the possibility of investigating blue flags and black flags in clinical practice.

Questions on physical activities at work or at leisure should be part of the initial assessment, and patients very often introduce the issues addressed by blue flags and black flags themselves, when asked about their job in the context of a medical examination. Clinicians should not ignore the explicit or implicit requests in their patients' answers; trying to improve pain or disability outcomes in a person who is only (or mainly) there to obtain a certification of temporary or permanent inability to work might prove to be a daunting task. At the same time, despite all the laws on workplace preventive interventions, many workers and employers, especially in small businesses, still ignore some basic steps that can produce good results without requiring expensive structural changes. For those interested in a more formal assessment, while we wait for a valid international standardized recommendation, the 55 questions of the Obstacles to Return To Work Questionnaire (ORTWQ), which was the only instrument that showed adequate psychometric properties even though it is not considered clinically feasible in its present format, according to the previously mentioned systematic review,[19] could be a good starting point to identify items that might be relevant for clinical practice and future research.

Decision Algorithms

Having critically reviewed the literature on the flag system, and having noted the lack of evidence to inform clinical practice, other than a generic recommendation to consider the respective issues as suggested by the different colors, readers will understand our skepticism toward the extensive use, especially in practice guidelines, of decision algorithms (and the underlying classification systems), which reflect in most cases the expert panel's personal views rather than an extensive review of the evidence. Although promising to be an easy-to-use guide throughout the decision-making process of complex clinical conditions, these tools instead promote the idea of cookbook medicine, which is the opposite of what the founders of evidence-based medicine had in mind. A systematic review of articles that specifically described a clinical classification system for chronic LBP reported on the reliability of a classification system, or evaluated the effectiveness of classification-specific interventions,[20] and identified 28 classification systems that met inclusion criteria: 16 diagnostic systems, seven prognostic systems, and five treatment-based systems. All the systems were directed at nonoperative management. The authors recommend that none of these classification systems should be adopted for all purposes, and that future efforts in developing a classification system should take into account multidisciplinary (invasive and noninvasive) treatments. A brief screening tool (Keele STarT Back Screening Tool—SBST) designed to identify subgroups of patients to guide the provision of early secondary prevention in primary care, including items that built a psychosocial subscale, has been proposed and subsequently tested in a RCT. The results showed that, at 12 months, stratified care was associated with a mean increase in generic health benefit and cost savings. The SBST (also available online and as an App) stratifies patients into low, medium or high risk categories and for each category there is a matched treatment package.[21] More recently, the Nijmegen Decision Tool for Chronic Low Back Pain was presented as the first clinical decision tool based on current scientific evidence and formal multidisciplinary consensus that helps in referring the patient for consultation to a spine surgeon or a nonsurgical spine care specialist.[22] Despite the extensive preparatory work based on a systematic review of the available evidence and the appropriate methodology applied to reach consensus within a multidisciplinary panel, only a first version of the decision tool was developed, consisting of a Web-based screening questionnaire and a provisional decision algorithm. This decision tool will require further development and testing before it can be widely recommended.

Chapter Summary

The first catalogue of red flags for back pain appeared in the literature in the early 1980s, and since then numerous lists have been compiled. The term *yellow flag* was introduced in 1997 to cover psychological, social, and environmental risk factors (in contrast to red flags for physical risk factors). Subsequently, in 2002, workplace factors that were originally considered as yellow flags were classified in two separate categories: black flags for workplace objective conditions, and blue flags for subjective perceptions about work issues. In 2005, orange flags that identify signs of a serious mental disorder were added. Two Cochrane reviews evaluated the usefulness of red flag assessment to specifically screen for vertebral fracture and malignancy, respectively, and did not support the use of many red flags to specifically screen for vertebral fracture in patients presenting for LBP, and concluded that there was insufficient evidence to recommend their use when searching for spinal malignancy, whereas some combination of these might prove to have some value. The evidence about other flags is even more inconclusive. Despite these limitations, many guidelines still recommend in favor of assessing all flags in aspecific LBP patients, but the risk is to overemphasize the use of subsequent diagnostic testing. Decision algorithms have even less data to support their use, and very often reflect simply the panel members' opinion. It is probably a good idea to assess a limited set of flags in the examination of a new LBP patient, and reassess them periodically especially if the condition is not self-limiting. When used critically and with clinical good sense, most of the flag items are part of a common medical anamnesis anyway, and may help getting to know the patient and establishing a good physician–patient alliance.

Pearls

- Red flags assess physical risk factors for a serious underlying pathology.
- Yellow flags assess psychological, social, and environmental risk factors.
- Black flags assess workplace objective conditions.
- Blue flags assess subjective perceptions about work issues.
- Orange flags identify signs of a serious mental disorder.
- Evidence from many systematic reviews including two Cochrane reviews is insufficient to recommend the widespread uncritical use of flags.
- Decision algorithms have even less data to support their use, and very often reflect simply the panel members' opinion.
- Clinical good sense advises in favor of an anamnestic assessment of some of the flag items as a way to get a general picture, not as a simple checklist to guide the prescription diagnostic test.

Pitfalls

- Use of red flags without any critical clinical judgment could result in referring the patient for many inappropriate examinations, with consequences for the cost of management and the outcomes of patients with LBP.
- Use of flags should not be intended as a way to avoid a problematic patient, but as an aid in identifying sources of problems and maximizing treatment outcomes.
- Clinicians should not assume that others have already excluded the presence of relevant risk factors, because even the most skilled practitioner can miss them, and clinical situations might change over time.

References

Five Must-Read References

1. https://en.wikipedia.org/wiki/Red_flag_(idiom)
2. Welch E. Red flags in medical practice. Clin Med (Lond) 2011;11:251–253
3. Waddell G, McCulloch JA, Kummel E, Venner RM. Nonorganic physical signs in low-back pain. Spine 1980;5:117–125
4. Waddell G. 1987 Volvo award in clinical sciences. A new clinical model for the treatment of low-back pain. Spine 1987;12:632–644
5. Kendall NA, Linton SJ, Main CJ. Guide to Assessing Psychosocial Yellow Flags in Acute Low Back Pain: Risk Factors for Long-Term Disability and Work Loss. Wellington, New Zealand: Accident Rehabilitation and Compensation Insurance Corporation of New Zealand and the National Health Committee; 1997
6. Main CJ. Concepts of treatment and prevention in musculo-skeletal disorders. In: Linton SJ, ed. New Avenues for the Prevention of Chronic Musculoskeletal Pain and Disability. Pain Research and Clinical Management, vol 12. New York: Elsevier; 2002: 47–63
7. Main CJ, Phillips CJ, Watson PJ. Secondary prevention in health-care and occupational settings in musculoskeletal conditions focusing on low back pain. In: Schultz IZ, Gatchel RJ, eds. Handbook of Complex Occupational Disability Claims: Early Risk Identifica-

tion, Intervention and Prevention. New York: Kluwer Academic/Plenum; 2005:387–404

8. Airaksinen O, Brox JI, Cedraschi C, et al; COST B13 Working Group on Guidelines for Chronic Low Back Pain. European guidelines for the management of chronic nonspecific low back pain. Eur Spine J 2006;15(Suppl 2):S192–S300
9. Williams CM, Henschke N, Maher CG, et al. Red flags to screen for vertebral fracture in patients presenting with low-back pain. Cochrane Database Syst Rev 2013;1:CD008643
10. Leerar PJ, Boissonnault W, Domholdt E, Roddey T. Documentation of red flags by physical therapists for patients with low back pain. J Manual Manip Ther 2007;15:42–49
11. Zanoli G, Romanini E, Tucci G, et al. Mal di schiena Banca dati comparativa tra linee guida e analisi critica delle raccomandazioni. GIOT 2011;37:113–130
12. Dagenais S, Tricco AC, Haldeman S. Synthesis of recommendations for the assessment and management of low back pain from recent clinical practice guidelines. Spine J 2010;10:514–529
13. Henschke N, Maher CG, Ostelo RW, de Vet HC, Macaskill P, Irwig L. Red flags to screen for malignancy in patients with low-back pain. Cochrane Database Syst Rev 2013;2:CD008686
14. Hayden JA, Chou R, Hogg-Johnson S, Bombardier C. Systematic reviews of low back pain prognosis had variable methods and results: guidance for future prognosis reviews. J Clin Epidemiol 2009;62:781–796.e1
15. Kovacs FM, Muriel A, Abriaira V, Medina JM, Castillo Sanchez MD, Olabe J; Spanish Back Pain Research Network. The influence of fear avoidance beliefs on disability and quality of life is sparse in Spanish low back pain patients. Spine 2005;30:E676–E682
16. Jellema P, van der Windt DA, van der Horst HE, Twisk JW, Stalman WA, Bouter LM. Should treatment of (sub)acute low back pain be aimed at psychosocial prognostic factors? Cluster randomised clinical trial in general practice. BMJ 2005;331:84
17. Lakke SE, Soer R, Takken T, Reneman MF. Risk and prognostic factors for non-specific musculoskeletal pain: a synthesis of evidence from systematic reviews classified into ICF dimensions. Pain 2009;147:153–164
18. Shaw WS, van der Windt DA, Main CJ, Loisel P, Linton SJ; "Decade of the Flags" Working Group. Early patient screening and intervention to address individual-level occupational factors ("blue flags") in back disability. J Occup Rehabil 2009;19:64–80
19. Gray H, Adefolarin AT, Howe TE. A systematic review of instruments for the assessment of work-related psychosocial factors (blue flags) in individuals with non-specific low back pain. Man Ther 2011;16:531–543
20. Fairbank J, Gwilym SE, France JC, et al. The role of classification of chronic low back pain. Spine 2011; 36(21, Suppl):S19–S42
21. Hill JC, Whitehurst DG, Lewis M, et al. Comparison of stratified primary care management for low back pain with current best practice (STarT Back): a randomised controlled trial. Lancet 2011;378(9802): 1560–1571. doi: 10.1016/S0140-6736(11)60937-9
22. van Hooff ML, van Loon J, van Limbeek J, de Kleuver M. The Nijmegen decision tool for chronic low back pain. Development of a clinical decision tool for secondary or tertiary spine care specialists. PLoS ONE 2014;9:e104226

3 The Supremacy of the Clinical Evaluation

Roberto Chapa Sosa and Neil N. Patel

Introduction

A comprehensive clinical history and physical examination is imperative to enable physicians to thoroughly and accurately assess patient with back pain, a complaint that may be complex and multifactorial. Clinical history should include time of onset of symptoms (acute < 12 weeks vs. chronic ≥ 12 weeks),[1] quality and intensity of pain, aggravating and alleviating factors, and any concerning red flag symptoms (bowel or bladder dysfunction, fevers, night sweats, unexpected weight loss, progressive weakness, etc.). Physical examination should assess for point tenderness and location of pain, aggravation or alleviation with flexion and extension of the lumbar spine, and a complete neurologic exam. The clinical history and physical examination in conjunction with appropriate imaging and possible lab work may help to tease out the true etiology of the patient's back pain.[2]

At times, history and physical examination are not completely performed and advanced imaging tests (computed tomography [CT] or magnetic resonance imaging [MRI]) are ordered early in the diagnostic process. This can be misleading and can incorrectly diagnose the etiology of the patient's symptoms. Boden et al. performed a study that suggested that MRI finding can be highly misleading if used alone.[3] This study prospectively reviewed 67 patients with no lumbar spine symptoms and found a lumbar spine abnormality on MRI in 20% of study subjects less than the age of 60 and 57% of study subjects 60 years or older. This suggests that if the diagnostic process is rushed and treatment is highly reliant on imaging without correlative clinical history and physical exam, the treatment may be misguided and consequently unsuccessful.[4–6]

Clinical History

The diagnostic process begins with a complete clinical history which can help physicians identify the etiology of the patient's symptoms. Especially in the setting of back pain, which can be vague and ambiguous, certain clinical clues can help narrow differential diagnoses. For example, back pain in a slender, postmenopausal woman can prompt a physician to evaluate for osteoporotic compression fractures, especially in the setting of previous osteoporotic fractures, chronic steroid use, or history of osteoporosis. Overall, the clinical history should include specifics regarding onset of symptoms, quality and intensity of pain, aggravating and alleviating factors, and any concerning red flag symptoms (bowel or bladder dysfunction, fevers, night sweats, unexpected weight loss, progressive weakness, etc.). Along with that, the history should include other medical diagnoses, previous surgeries, current and previous medications, social history, psychosocial status, and employment status.

One key aspect of successful management of back pain is analysis of response to previous treatments, which may include anti inflammatory medications, physical therapy, diagnostic and therapeutic injections, chiropractic care, and acupuncture. Specifically, diagnostic and therapeutic injections can be useful to determine the cause of the patient's symptoms, especially if successful response with relief is noted with targeted injections.

As discussed, the location and quality of pain can give clues to its etiology (**Fig. 3.1**). For example, if pain is more paraspinal and cramping, a muscular cause can be inferred. However, if the pain follows a dermatomal distribution and is worse with flexion, a disc related neurologic compression should be high on the differential diagnosis. In an over simplified general manner of thinking, back pain worse with flexion is likely diskogenic, where as back pain worse with extension is likely related to the posterior elements (facet arthropathy, pars fracture, etc.). A thorough understanding of spine anatomy, biomechanics, and load distribution is essential in the diagnostic process.[1]

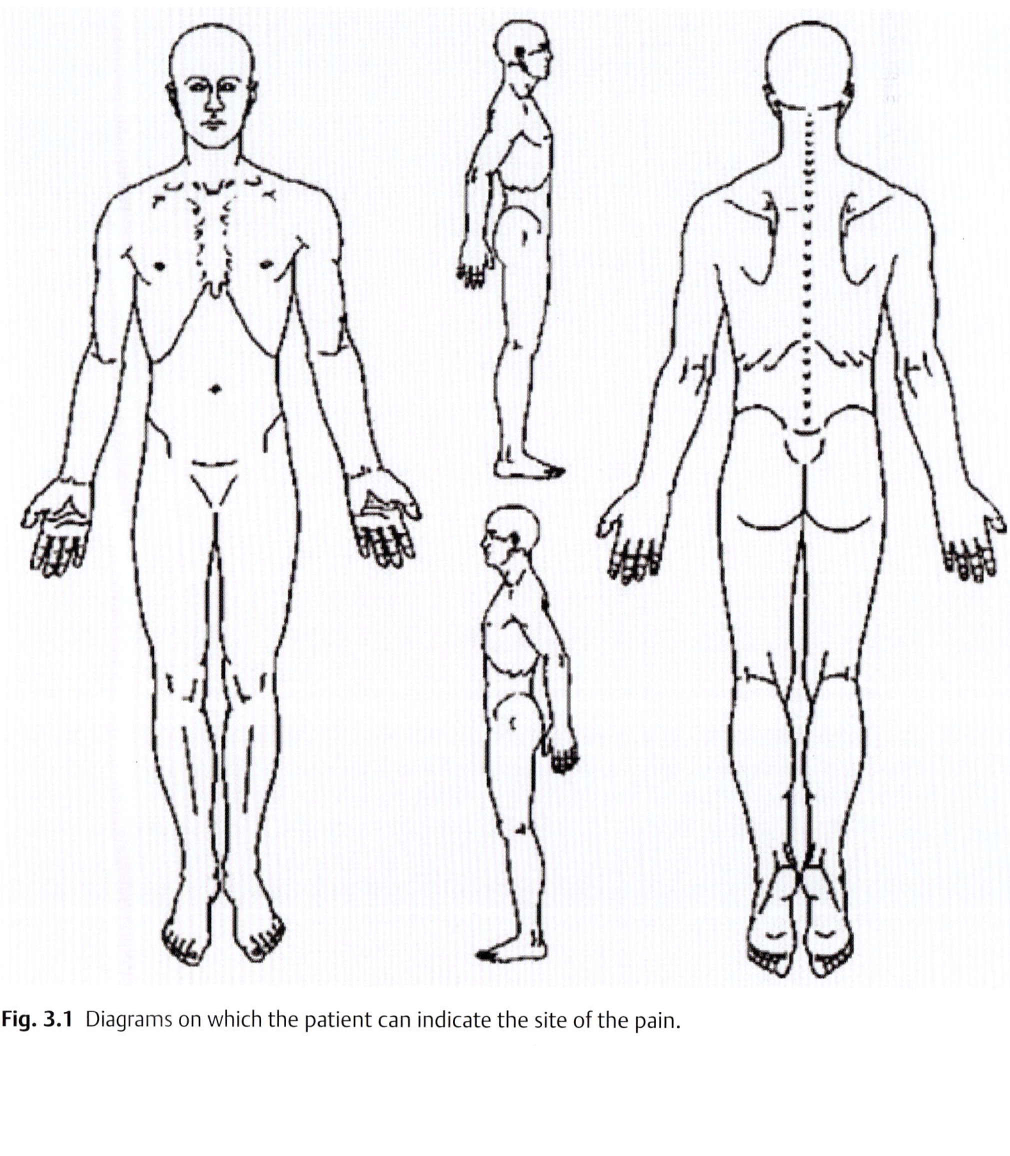

Fig. 3.1 Diagrams on which the patient can indicate the site of the pain.

Box 3.1 Differential Diagnosis of Back Pain

Spine Injury

Structural
- Segmental instability
- Diskogenic pain, annular tears
- Facet arthropathy
- Ligamentous or muscle sprains
- Spondylolisthesis

Spinal Stenosis
- Fractures
- Infections
  - Diskitis
  - Vertebral osteomyelitis
- Inflammatory
  - Ankylosing spondylitis
  - Rheumatoid arthritis
- Tumors
  - Primary
  - Secondary myeloma

Endocrine
- Osteomalacia
  - Osteoporosis
  - Acromegaly

Hematologic
- Sickle disease

Extraspinal Injuries

Visceral
- Renal calculi, urinary tract infections, pyelonephritis
- Duodenal ulcers
- Thoracic or abdominal aortic aneurysms
- Mitral valve disease left atrial growth
- Pancreatitis
- Retroperitoneal neoplasms
- Gallstones

Gynecologic
- Ectopic pregnancy
- Endometriosis
- Sickle disease

Medications
- Corticosteroids as a cause of osteoporosis
- Methysergide products for retroperitoneal fibrosis
- Steroidal anti-inflammatory drugs can be produced peptic ulcer

Musculoskeletal
- Hip diseases
- Sacroiliitis
- Scapulothoracic pain
- Psychogenic

Source: From Fardon DF, Garfine SR, et al, eds. Orthopaedic Knowledge Update: Spine 2. Rosemont, IL: American Academy of Orthopaedic Surgeons; 2002:39–51. Adapted with permission.

Differential Diagnosis

The differential diagnosis for back pain is extensive and is easier to consider if grouped in to intra- and extraspinal etiologies (**Box 3.1**). Several extraspinal neurologic diagnoses should also be considered in the diagnostic process (**Box 3.2**). In order to narrow the potential causes, it is essential to consider all aspects of the history and physical exam.

It is important to ask the patient to assess the degree and intensity of pain on a visual analog scale. Other tests and questionnaires can also help the physician assess the degree of disability and measure the patient's progress once treatment has begun.

Physical examination should not only include a thorough neurologic and spine examination, but include potential organ systems based on clinical clues. For example, a skin examination should be performed if herpes zoster is considered as a cause of back pain. Similarly, costovertebral angle tenderness should be assessed if the clinical history points to pyelonephritis as a potential cause.

Box 3.2 Extraspinal Causes of Sciatic

Intrapelvic Extraneural Compression
- Tumors
- Psoas hematoma
- Endometriosis
- Abscesses
- Aneurysms

Extrapelvic Extraneural Compression
- Aneurysm of the gluteal artery
- Pseudoaneurysms
- Tumors
- Abscesses
- Piriformis syndrome
- Fracture avulsion of the greater trochanter

Intraneural
- Diabetes mellitus
- Neural tumors
- Sciatic nerve fibrosis

Source: From Fardon DF, Garfine SR, et al, eds. Orthopaedic Knowledge Update: Spine 2. Rosemont, IL: American Academy of Orthopaedic Surgeons; 2002:39–51. Adapted with permission.

The complete clinical history should provide the physician with an appropriate picture of the patient's problem, and thus pave the way for performing the physical examination.

Physical Examination

The physical exam is performed to further elucidate the information provided in the clinical history, to help narrow the differential diagnosis, and to determine the cause of the back pain. Particular attention is paid to pathology or other alteration in the hips, knees, and sacroiliac joints, as well as to neurologic or vascular problems that could be associated with the patient's back pain.

The physical exam really begins the moment the patient enters the office. The physician should observe the patient's posture and positioning while walking, standing, and sitting, particularly with regard to the coronal and sagittal planes. The physician should observe if any type of deformity exists, such as kyphosis, scoliosis, or any other alteration in the patient's balance or in the height of the shoulders. The position of the knees, hips, and pelvis, when flexed, could indicate a secondary lumbar kyphosis problem, such as spondylolisthesis[7] (**Fig. 3.2**).

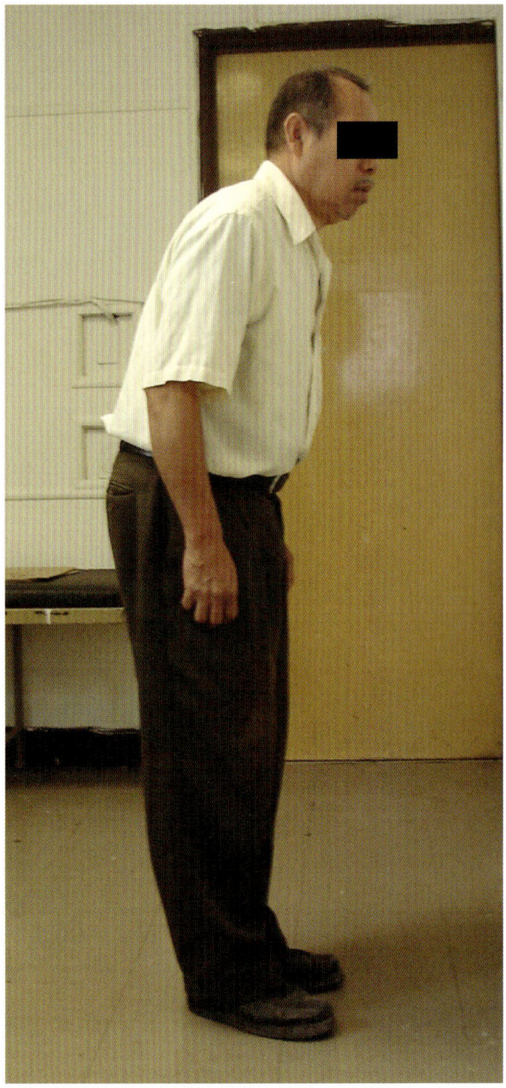

Fig. 3.2 Positive sagittal balance.

Diagnostic Considerations

Skin Examination

The physician should examine any skin changes that could explain the pain, such as herpes zoster. Brown spots could indicate a neurofibromatosis (**Fig. 3.3**).

Gait and Range of Motion

The patient's gait pattern helps the physician determine if the pain is of an antalgic type or if it reflects any neurologic alteration such as asymmetry or pelvic obliquity. The physician should also determine if the standing position aggravates the pain and the sitting position lessens it, or vice versa[8] (**Fig. 3.4**).

Range of movement should also be assessed at the thoracolumbar level and the lumbar spine in flexion and extension. As stated, pain that is worse with flexion is likely diskogenic, whereas back pain that is worse with extension is likely related to the posterior elements (facet arthropathy, pars fracture, etc.).

Alignment Examination (Figs. 3.5 and 3.6)

As stated, the overall spinal alignment examination begins as soon as the patient walks in to the room. Positive sagittal balance should be

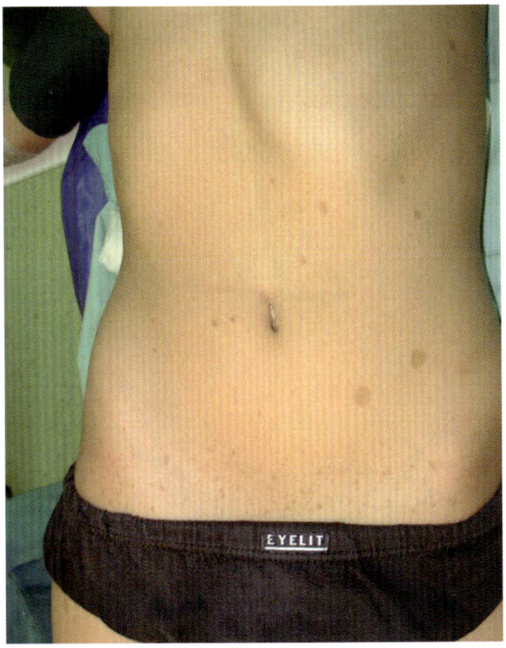

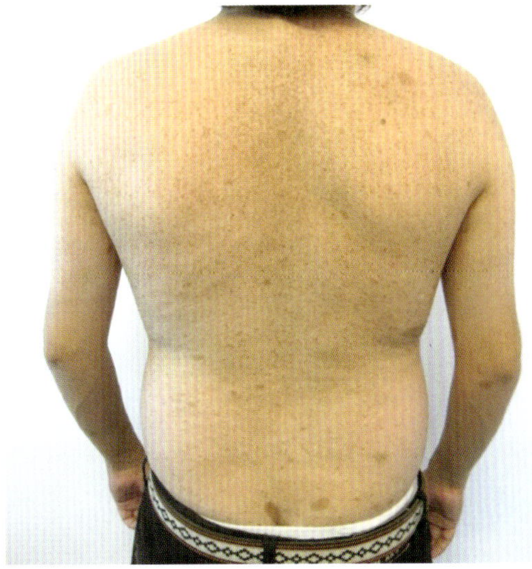

b

Fig. 3.3 Consider neurofibromatosis. **(a,b)** Discolored brown spots on the skin.

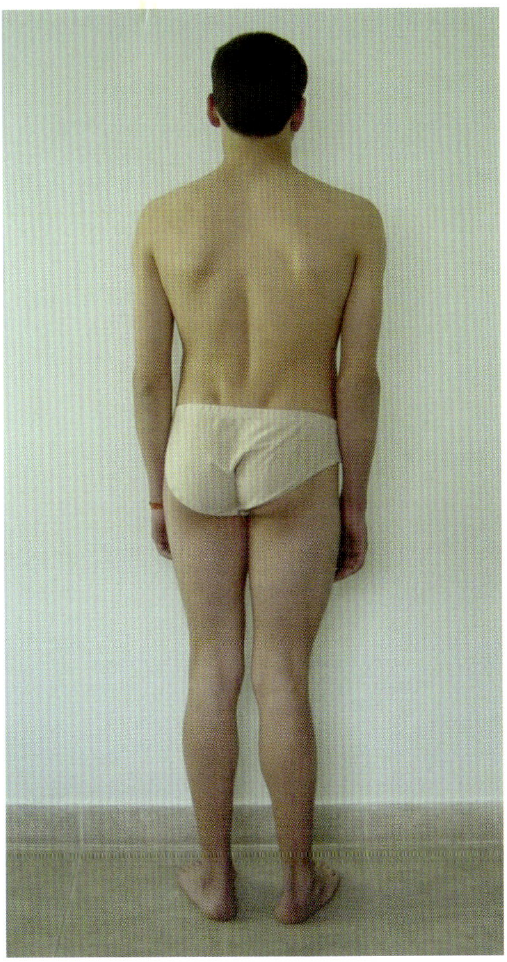

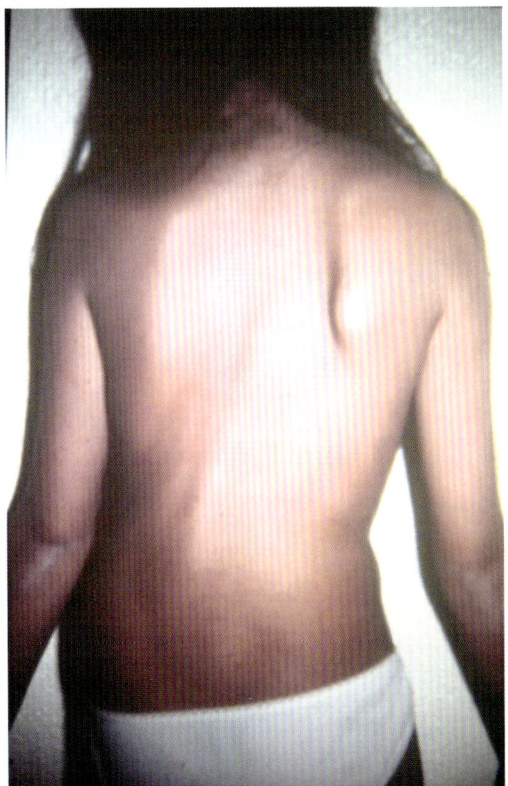

b

Fig. 3.4 (a,b) Coronal imbalance.

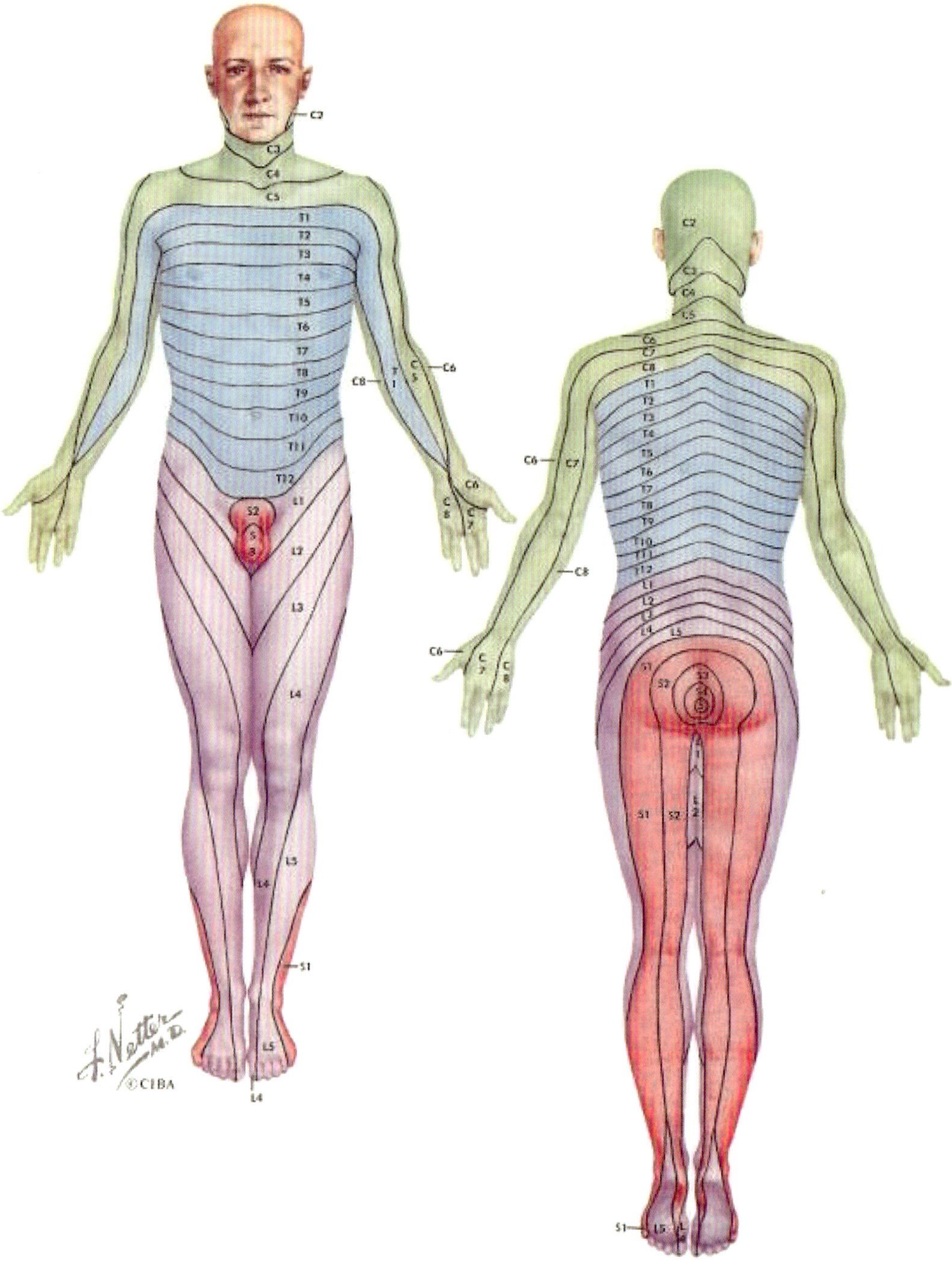

Fig. 3.5 Corporal dermatomes.

noticed, as that could be a contributing factor to the patient's symptoms and can affect management. Posterior standing examination can notice signs of coronal imbalance as well, which include asymmetry in the shoulder blades or rib cage.[9]

Neurologic Examination

Complete sensory and motor examination should be performed with analysis of any deficit (**Fig. 3.5**). Gait examination and reflex tests should be performed on all patients to assess for spinal cord compression (**Fig 3.6**).

Diagnostic Tests (Figs. 3.7, 3.8 and 3.9)

Patrick's Test

Patrick's test is a physical exam maneuver that allows evaluation of sacroiliac joint dysfunction. The patient's knee is flexed on one side, with the thigh abducted and externally rotated and placed in a figure of 4 fashion. Pressure is placed on the knee (**Fig 3.7**). If pain is elicited anteriorly at the hip, hip pathology should be considered. If pain is elicited at the sacroiliac joint, SI pathology should be considered.

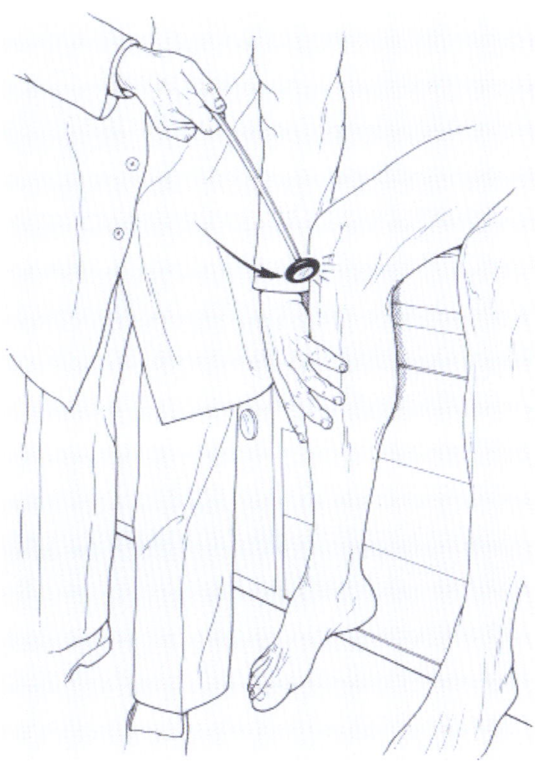

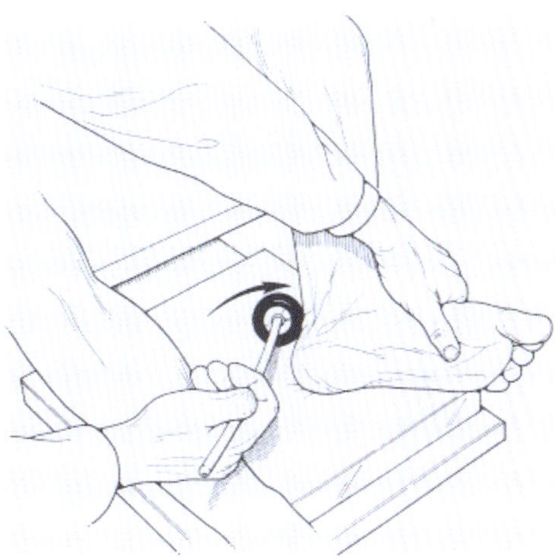

b

Fig. 3.6 Gait examination and reflex tests. **(a)** The knee jerk. **(b)** The ankle jerk. [From Walker HK, Hall WD, Hurst JW, eds. Clinical Methods: The History, Physical, and Laboratory Examinations, 3rd ed. Boston: Butterworths; 1990. Reprinted by permission.]

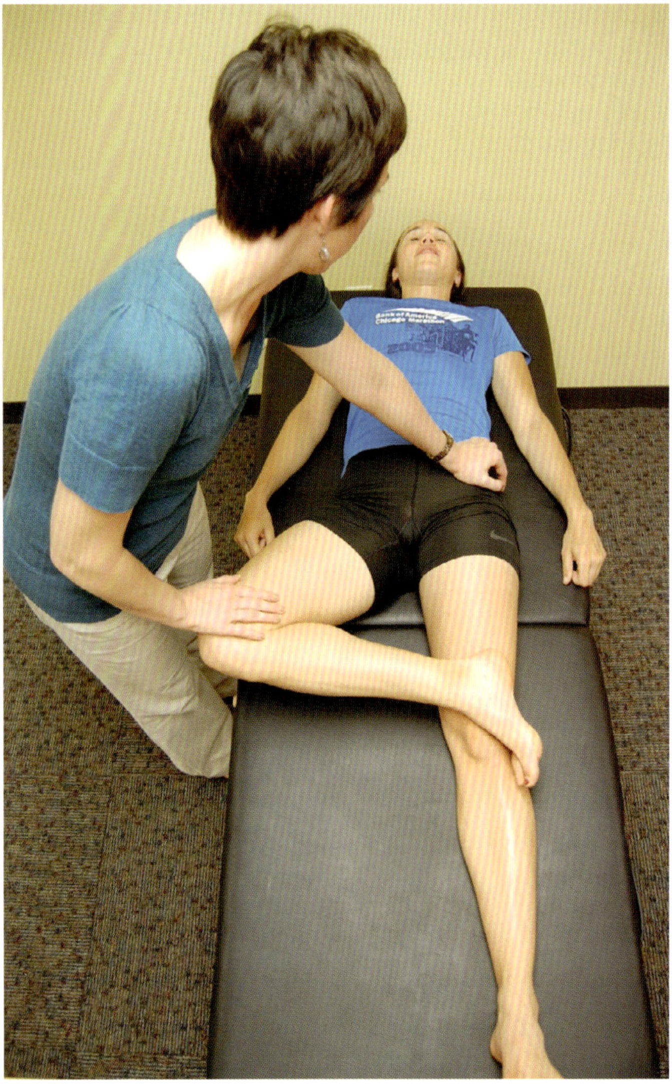

Fig. 3.7 Patrick's test.

Lasègue Sign

Lasègue sign is a physical exam maneuver in which the patient's leg is passively elevated while straight. A positive test would include reproduction of radicular symptoms down the affected extremity between 30 and 70 degrees for flexion. A modification of the test is to passively dorsiflex the ankle to increase the response (**Fig. 3.8**). This test essentially increases tension of the sciatic nerve to reproduce the patient's symptoms and points towards a spinal etiology.

Stinchfield Test

While supine, the patient flexes the hip while keeping the entire lower extremity straight. The examiner places resistance on the extremity during flexion to elicit a response (**Fig. 3.9**). A positive response would elicit hip pain and suggest intra or peri-articular hip pathology

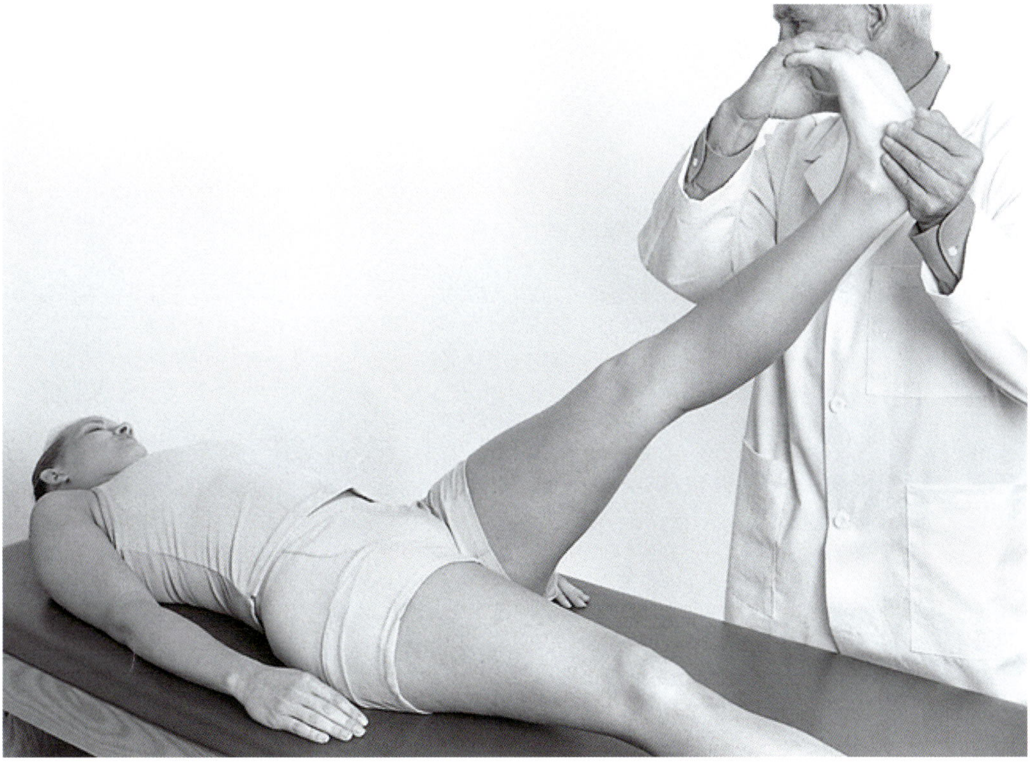

Fig. 3.8 Lasègue sign.

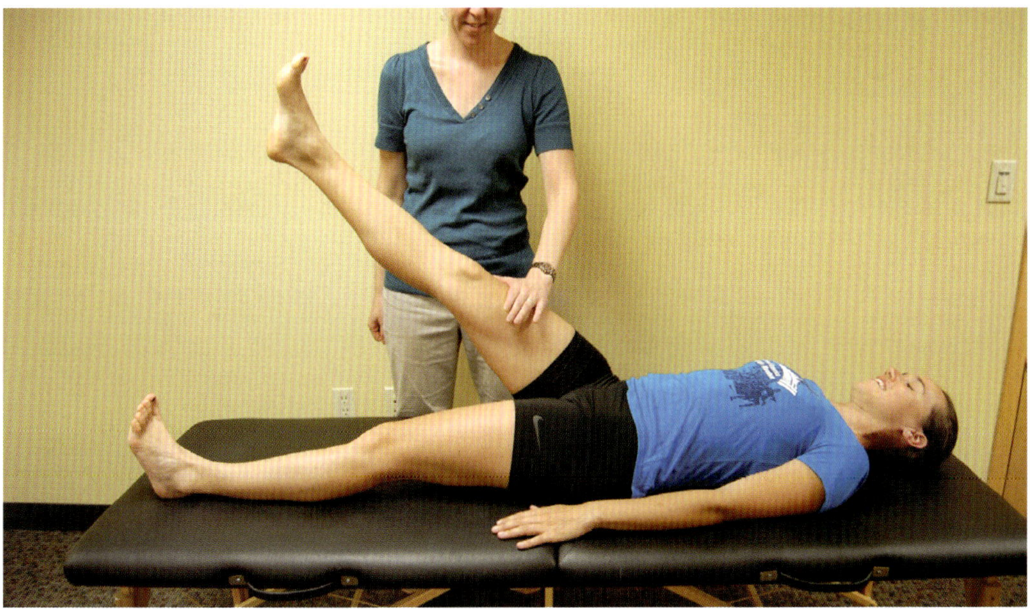

Fig. 3.9 Lift the leg against resistance (Stinchfield test).

as the cause of the patient's symptoms, rather than spinal etiology.

Chapter Summary

The clinical evaluation of a patient with back pain is essential to determine the probable diagnosis. The evaluation includes the clinical history and physical examination. The exam is conducted based on the information derived in the history. The relevant laboratory or imaging studies are ordered based on the findings in the physical exam. Guided treatment based on all of that information should be administered. Rushing the diagnostic process by not completing a thorough history and physical exam and basing treatment on imaging alone, can be misguided and likely unsuccessful.

Pearls

- Always perform a clinical history and physical examination for every patient with back pain.
- Do not make the mistake of ordering imaging studies first to find a quick and simple cause of the pain.
- Analyze the possible differential diagnoses and request relevant studies only based on the results of the clinical evaluation.
- Develop diagrams of the distribution of pain and disability or perform function tests.
- Adhere to the appropriate international guidelines.

Pitfalls

- Failure to recognize the importance of carrying out a clinical evaluation in all patients with spinal problems can lead to inappropriate diagnoses or treatments.
- Establish good communication with the patients, and explain the importance of this assessment and why studies should not be ordered before the examination.

References

Five Must-Read References

1. Deyo RA, Weinstein JN. Low back pain. N Engl J Med 2001;344:363–370
2. Lee KS, Doh JW, Bae HG, Yun IG. Diagnostic criteria for the clinical syndrome of internal disc disruption: are they reliable? Br J Neurosurg 2003;17:19–23
3. Boden SD, Davis DO, Dina TS, et al. Abnormal magnetic-resonance scans of the lumbar spine in asymptomatic subjects. A prospective investigation. J Bone Joint Surg Am 1990;72(3):403–408
4. Koes BW, van Tulder MW, Ostelo R, Kim Burton A, Waddell G. Clinical guidelines for the management of low back pain in primary care: an international comparison. Spine 2001;26:2504–2513, discussion 2513–2514
5. COST B13 Working Group. European guidelines for the management of acute nonspecific low back pain in primary care. 2005. http://www.backpaineurope.org/web/html/wg1_results.html
6. COST B13 Working Group. European guidelines for the management of chronic nonspecific low back pain. 2004. http://www.backpaineurope.org/web/html/wg2_results.html
7. McLain, RF, Dudeney, S. Clinical history and physical examination. In: DE Fardon, SR Garfin (Eds.) Orthopaedic Knowledge Update Spine 2. AAOS, Rosemont, IL; 2002:39–51
8. Zhou Y, Abdi S. Diagnosis and minimally invasive treatment of lumbar discogenic pain—a review of the literature. Clin J Pain 2006;22:468–481
9. Wilson JJ, Furukawa M. Evaluation of the patient with hip pain. Am Fam Physician 2014;89:27–34

The Eye of the Tiger

4

Imaging in Back Pain

Alberto Zerbi

Introduction

Aging, trauma, infections, tumors, and degenerative diseases can all cause low back pain (LBP). Hip arthritis, sacroiliac joint pathologies, and visceral pathologies of the pelvis or of the abdomen can mimic LBP symptomatology. As spine specialists, we have to consider all of the possible causes of LBP symptomatology. Thus, it is mandatory that an accurate clinical examination be performed first, and then, on the basis of this examination, the patient can be referred to a radiologist if necessary. We are, first, doctors in medicine and second, spine superspecialists, so don't be a subspecialist!

In choosing the chapter subtitle "The Eye of the Tiger," I vaguely recalled a romantic quotation from Rudyard Kipling or some other classic author, but instead I found a novel from John Edmund Delezen entitled *Eye of the Tiger: Memoir of a United States Marine, Third Force Recon Company, Vietnam*, a title and subtitle that well describe how radiologists must learn to survive in everyday medicine, being friendly with referring clinicians but using their claws when necessary and looking with the eye of a tiger at the images to comprehend every obvious or subtle aspect of the spine.

Referring a Patient to the Radiologist

When you refer a patient to the radiologist, submit a clinical summary that includes relevant anamnestic data and suspected pathology. Never request "L/S MRI, LBP" without first providing other important information, such as the precise site of pain, if left or right sided; the neurologic impairments, such as sciatica; previous surgery; previous trauma; major pathology, such as a breast cancer; and other relevant information.

If you do not provide the relevant information to the radiologist, he or she will not be able to determine the most appropriate examination protocol for your patient. Radiologists are imaging specialists, not spine specialists, and they need the most appropriate information from you in order to determine the correct diagnosis by using the least biologically invasive and the least costly diagnostic procedure possible.

Clinical Findings Determine the Need for Imaging

When the patient's symptoms, clinical signs, and anamnestic data are not sufficiently specific to determine the pathology, ask first for the most widely available, the least costly, and the most readily obtainable imaging modality—the lumbar spine X-ray.

There are very few situations in which a lumbar spine X-ray should be bypassed as the first imaging modality. One such situation is when the clinical and anamnestic data clearly indicate that a nerve or the cauda is compressed by a disk herniation or by other causes. In this case, a magnetic resonance imaging (MRI) of the lumbar spine can be requested as the first imaging modality. In most other cases, a lumbar spine X-ray is the first imaging to be done.

Reasons for Requesting an X-Ray

The X-ray is a powerful, panoramic, inexpensive, and readily available imaging technique. Unfortunately, due to the difficulty in reading it and its less trendy appeal, it is frequently overlooked in favor of more expensive and more trendy techniques such as MRI or computed tomography (CT).

The difficulties in reading X-rays are mostly due to the fact that everything is shown in one bidimensional plane, so that more skill and experience is needed by the radiologist or the clinician to interpret the images than to interpret the imaging of other tomographic techniques such as CT or MRI. The X-ray, moreover, has several objective limitations compared with the other techniques, such as a lower sensitivity in recognizing lithic lesions of bone, and the inability to directly show soft tissue damages. The image quality of the X-ray is affected by the size and the compliance of the patient and the ability of the technician to obtain a correctly exposed and oriented film.

On the other hand, X-ray is the only technique that can assess the spine as a whole and demonstrate malalignments, deviations of the spine, malformations, and pelvic parameters. It is very helpful in assessing most of the pathologies affecting the spine, from fracture and dislocations, to infections and tumors, to degenerative modifications and metabolic pathologies. Moreover, being panoramic, it can show pathologies of other anatomic structures, for instance, near joints like the sacroiliac joints or hip joints that can frequently mimic symptoms related to the lumbar spine.

Determining the Type of X-Ray to Request

The standard radiological protocol is an anteroposterior (AP) and latero-lateral (LL) view of the lumbar spine obtained with the patient lying on the table. The AP field of view (FOV) is from T11 to the half sacrum and laterally barely includes the vertebral transverse processes. The LL view shows the lumbar spine from T11 to the midsacrum.

This standard X-ray protocol is no longer adequate to the modern clinical concepts about LBP and its origin, and is mostly useless in answering the needs of the spine specialists. This is the reason why the standard AP and LL views should be supplanted by the lumbopelvic views (De Seze view) with the patient in standing position (**Fig. 4.1**). The FOV of these views is wide enough to demonstrate, both in AP and LL, the spine from T11 to the head of the femurs. From these lumbopelvic views, we can obtain information about the lumbar spine, as with the standard protocol, as well as information about the hip and sacroiliac joints and the lumbopelvic parameters. Adapting the imaging protocol to the new clinical criteria, at the same cost, we acquire much more useful infor-

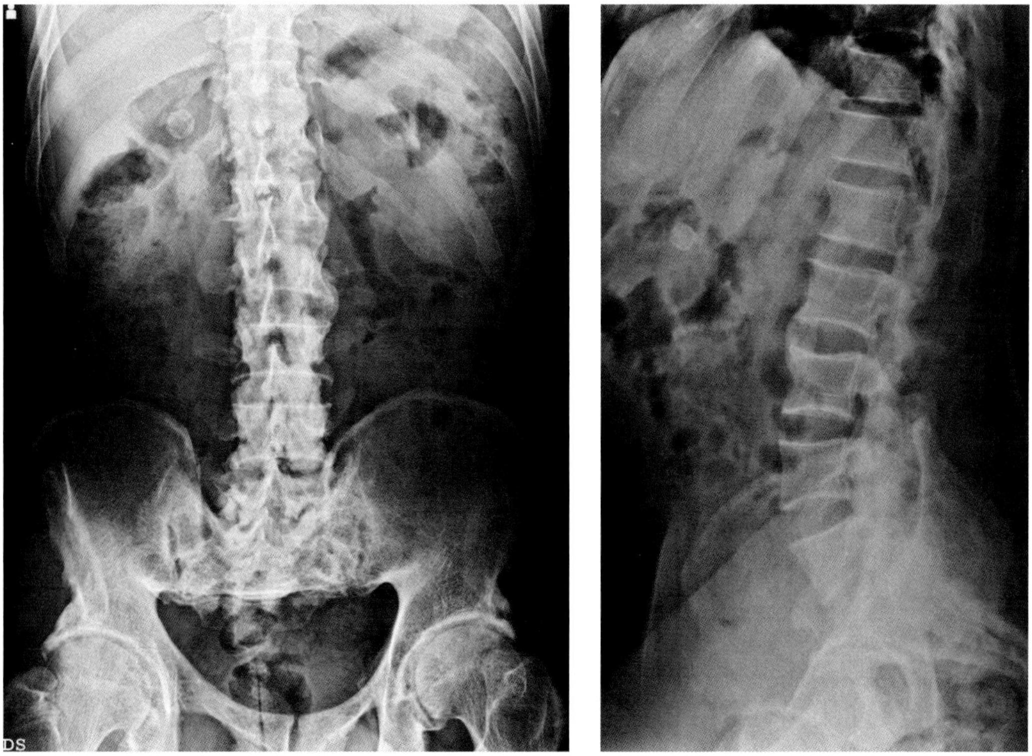

b

Fig. 4.1 Lumbopelvic X-ray: De Seze view in a 62-year-old patient with long-standing low back pain (LBP). Note hip and sacroiliac joints arthritis with subchondral sclerosis and osteophytes. **(a)** Anteroposterior (AP) view. **(b)** Latero-lateral (LL) view.

mation to better understand the causes of the patient's back pain.

Flexion-extension views can be added to demonstrate reciprocal dynamic modifications of the vertebral bodies and of the disks. It is not yet established if this imaging should be done with the patient in the standing, sitting, or lying positions. It may be difficult for aging or ailing patients to perform maximum range of motion while sitting or standing without holding on to a device, impairing the results of the examination. Moreover, muscular function can impair the reciprocal movement of the vertebrae. For these reasons, it is more appropriate to obtain the dynamic, flexion-extension views with patients lying on their side.

There are few indications for obtaining oblique views because the information about the apophyseal joints and pars are more easily available with other techniques such as MRI or CT. However, oblique views are preferable to CT in young patients because of concerns about the radiation dose.

Whole spine imaging is necessary when the alignment of the spine, the sagittal and frontal balance, and pelvic parameters need to be assessed. The protocol for this imaging must be carefully followed. The patient must be standing in a comfortable, unforced position on both feet. The technician must pay maximum attention in checking the position of the pelvis in AP to avoid rotation. The patient's hands must be on the collarbones or on the forehead. If a holding device is necessary, or a step for the patient to stand on, this must be communicated by the technician and described by the radiologist. The FOV suggested is in AP from C3 to the femoral head, wide enough to show the iliac crests, and in LL from the acoustic foramina to the first 15 cm of the femurs.

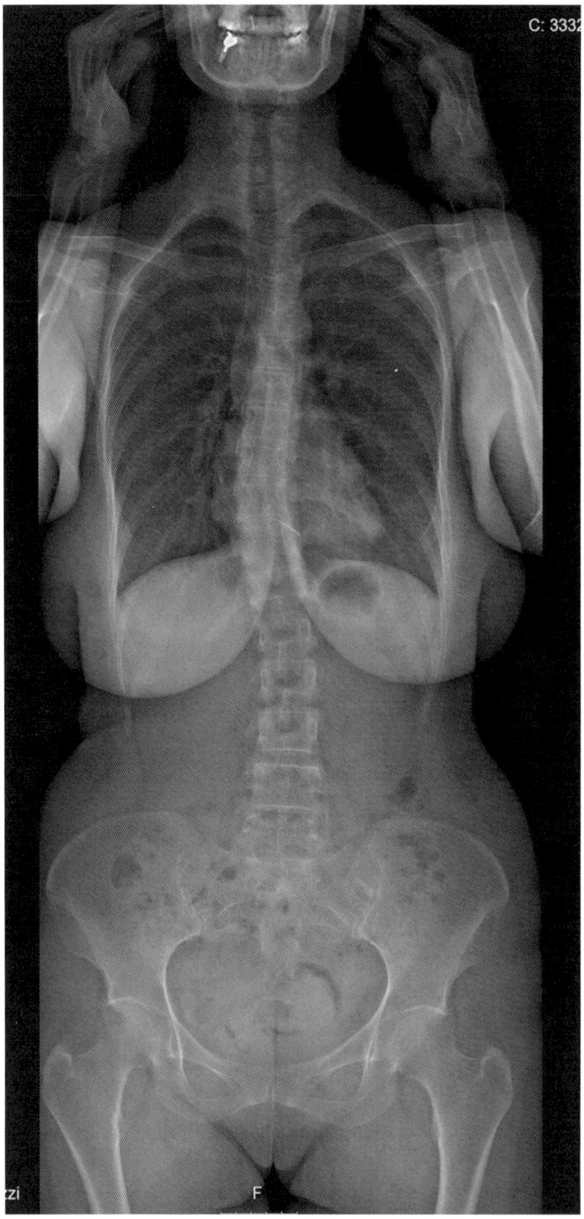

a

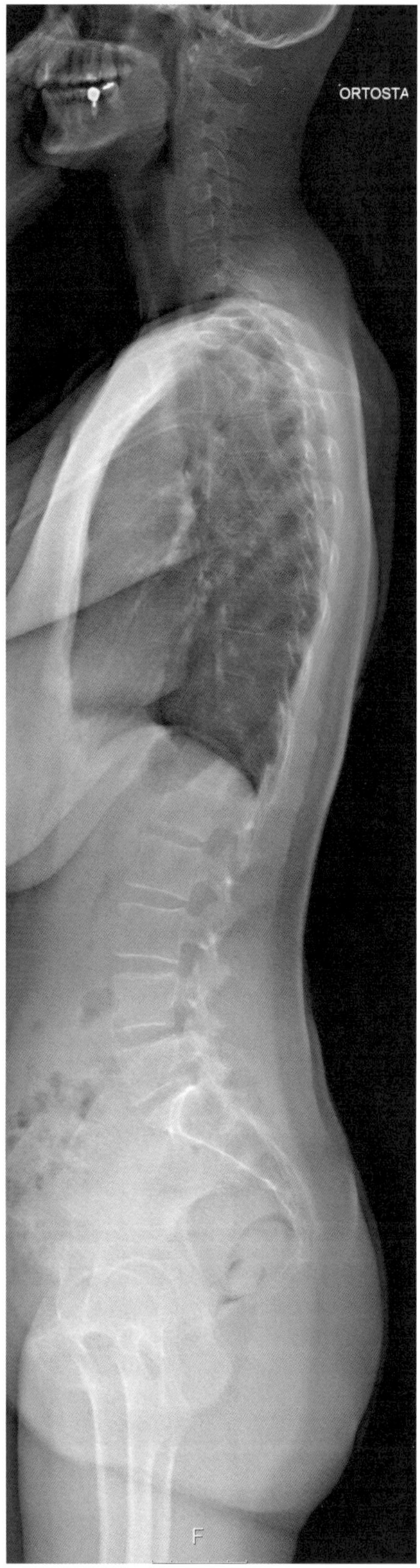

Fig. 4.2 A standing X-ray of spine with the EOS® method in a 39-year-old patient who presents with LBP due to scoliosis. EOS uses two perpendicular X-ray beams collimated in two very thin, horizontal, fan-shaped beams along with two detectors. This enables obtaining **(a)** frontal and **(b)** lateral X-rays of a patient simultaneously.

To avoid excessive irradiation of the patient, the technician must pay maximum attention to precisely aiming the FOV and checking the position of the patient so that repetitions of the exposure are avoided. The EOS® system (EOS Imaging Inc., Cambridge, MA) is a revolutionary X-ray machine that enables the simultaneous exposure of the body in anterolateral (AP) and LL standing view (**Fig. 4.2**). For this reason, a three-dimensional (3D) reformation of the spine can be postprocessed to provide important information about the position of the spine and of the pelvis. Moreover, due to its revolutionary detectors, for which the inventor Georges Charpak won the Nobel Prize in Physics in 1992, the EOS machine gives one-tenth the radiation dose compared with standard modern X-ray machines. [1,2,3,4]

When to Request an MRI

An MRI should be the second imaging modality requested unless the findings of the physical examination clearly indicate a root impingement pathology by disk herniation, thus precluding the need for X-ray and further imaging. But this rarely happens; when it does, it is based on the clinical skill of the clinician, who notes the typical pattern of the specific pathology of a disk herniation.

The MRI is the most powerful imaging modality for diagnosing inflammatory, degenerative, neoplastic, or traumatic lesions of the lumbar spine. Its ability to detect both bone and soft structures with anatomic and tissue quality precision is invaluable.

The quality of the imaging of the spine is affected by several factors with which the clinician may not be familiar but that are well studied by the radiologist doing the examination. The factor most affecting the MRI image quality is the magnet field strength, with 1.5 tesla (T) being the current gold standard, but with 3T rising in quality. With 1T or less powerful magnet units, the examination must be performed with time-consuming skill so that the image quality can come close to that of the most powerful units. Other factors affecting the quality of the image are the coil quality, the patient's compliance (staying still during the examination), the choice of the sequences for the single magnet unit, and the knowledge of the suspected pathology, so that the protocol of examination can be aimed at the specific pathology. Other local problems can affect the image quality, such as the presence of foreign bodies like postsurgical devices (screws, hooks, bars, cages, etc.) and metal dust from surgical instruments. In these cases, artifacts cannot be completely avoided, but an imaging strategy to reduce these artifacts can be adopted. A two-point strategy is used in these cases: (1) the radiologist must be informed of the presence of such devices and be provided with an X-ray of the lumbar spine; (2) the radiologist uses a protocol for metal artifact reduction called the metal artifacts reduction sequence (MARS) that is adapted for each specific MRI unit.

Standard and Special Protocols and Sequences, and the Use of Gadolinium

The standard study protocol of the lumbar spine is based on at least three sequences. The choice of the sequences is the responsibility of the radiologist and it is based on the characteristics of the MRI unit. Two sagittal sequences (usually spin echo T1 and T2) and an axial T2 complete the examination.

The sagittal views must show the entire lumbar spine from the inferior half of T11 to S2 or S3, depending on the sacral inclination. The slices laterally must include not only the vertebral body but also the complete lateral foramina. That means that a 70-mm-wide volume must be studied with at least 15 slices of 4-mm thickness with a 0.6-mm gap in between.

The axial slice thickness is usually 3 or 4 mm with a 10% gap in between. The slices must be oriented parallel to the upper end plate of the lower vertebra of each disk space that must be completely studied from the pedicle of the upper vertebra to the pedicle of the lower one.

The FOV must be wide enough to include the whole vertebra and the transverse and spinous processes. At the lumbosacral junction, a wider FOV must be used to demonstrate at least the upper part of the sacroiliac joint and the sacral wings.

To this standard study protocol other views and sequences can be added, depending on the appearance of the standard study or the clinical question to be answered.

Schematically, if a scoliosis is noted or a malformation or a far lateral herniation or a cord or roots lesion is seen or suspected, a coronal T2 or T1 sequence should be added, whereas if a deformation of a vertebral body with or without signal intensity alteration is seen, a fat-suppressed sequences (FAT SAT or STIR) must be added to facilitate the diagnosis of a fracture, a tumor, or an inflammatory process. Diffusion-weighted images can help distinguish between pathological and osteoporotic fractures (**Fig. 4.3**).

Endovenous (EV) injection of contrast medium (gadolinium) is generally used for a more complete diagnosis when a discitis or neoplastic lesion is suspected. In the postoperative spine, gadolinium is generally indicated as the gold standard for a differential diagnosis between scar tissue and disk herniation recurrence.[5] Gadolinium is an expensive pharmaceutical with rare but well-known side effects; thus, it must be used by knowledgeable technicians. It can be suggested or proposed by the clinician but it cannot be ordered. In fact, its use is strictly the choice and responsibility of the radiologist, who, knowing the clinical question and checking the standard images, will decide whether or not to inject the drug in the patient, after considering the risks of administration (**Fig. 4.4**).

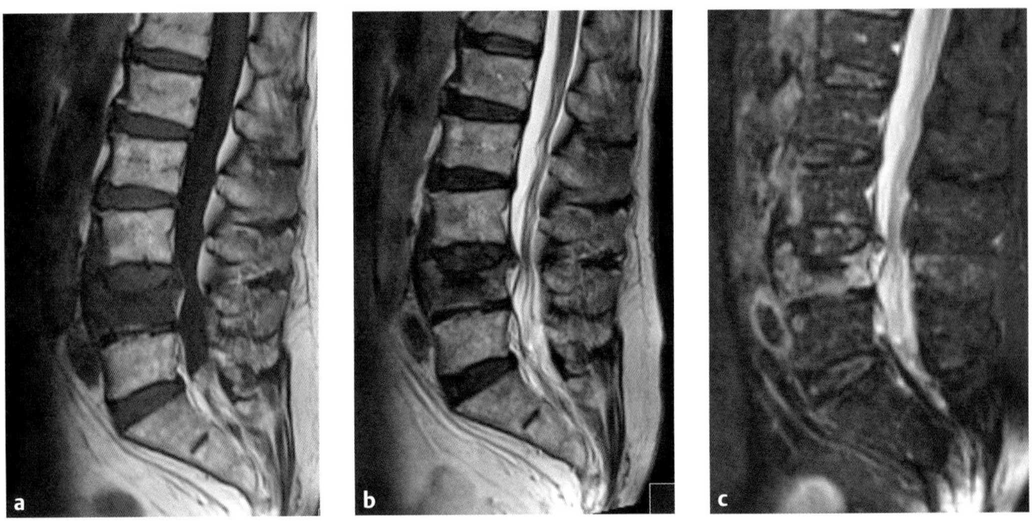

Fig. 4.3 Two patients with same level lesion: the first has a compression fracture, the second has metatstatic vertebral lesions. **(a–c)** Imaging of a 65-year-old man with a traumatic L4 fracture. **(a)** T1-weighted MRI sequence shows compression fractures of L4 with normal residual bone marrow signal intensity in the vertebral body. Retropulsion of a bone fragment is present at the posterior portions of the vertebral body. **(b)** T2-weighted sequence shows that the collapsed vertebral body is relatively isointense to adjacent vertebrae. **(c)** Sagittal short tau inversion recovery (STIR) sequence show high signal of collapsed vertebra.

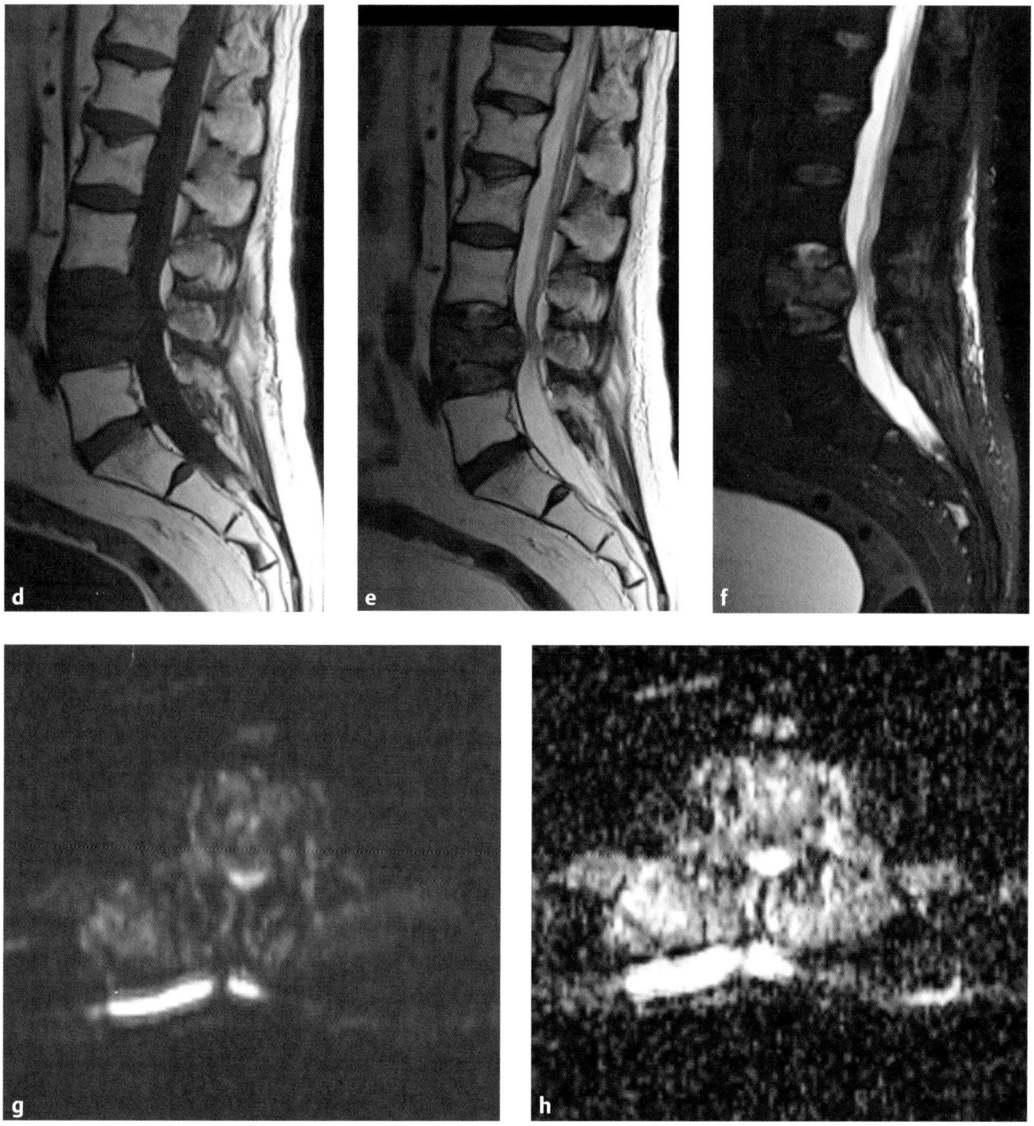

Fig. 4.3 (*continued*) **(d–h)** Imaging of a 61-year-old man with a pathological fracture of L4 due to metastasis from prostatic cancer, with a second small localization in L3. **(d)** T1-weighted sequence shows a compression fracture with complete replacement of the normal bone marrow of the L4 vertebral body. There is a rounded metastatic focus within an adjacent noncollapsed vertebral segment at the level above the compression fracture. **(e)** T2-weighted shows that the L4 vertebral body is heterogeneously hypointense. **(f)** STIR sequence shows homogeneous enhancement of the L4 vertebral body. The L4 vertebral body demonstrated heterogeneous enhancement on other sections. Note the enhancement of the metastatic focus at the vertebral level above the compression fracture. **(g)** Axial diffusion-weighted imaging (DWI) at the same level (L4) showing high intensity signal at b1000, suggestive of neoplastic infiltration. **(h)** Apparent diffusion coefficient (ADC) map at the same level.

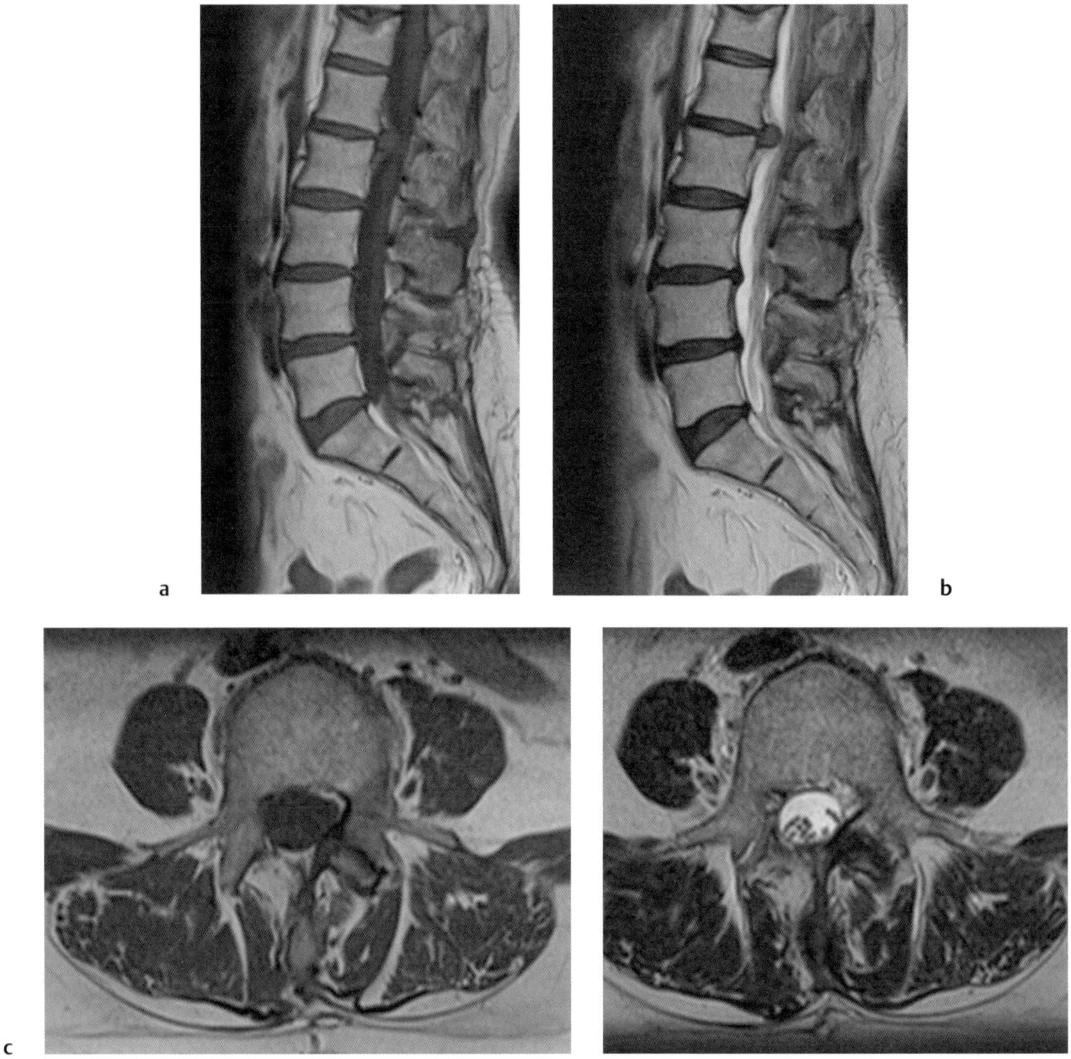

Fig. 4.4 Case 1: L4–L5 right, 1 year postlaminectomy: sagittal images. **(a)** Spin echo T1-weighted (SET1W) sequence. **(b)** SET2W sequence. **(c)** Axial T1 and **(d)** T2 sequences showing no disk herniation recurrence or scar tissue in the canal. Note the huge disk herniation in L1–L2. Case 2: L5-S1 right, 2 months post-laminectomy.

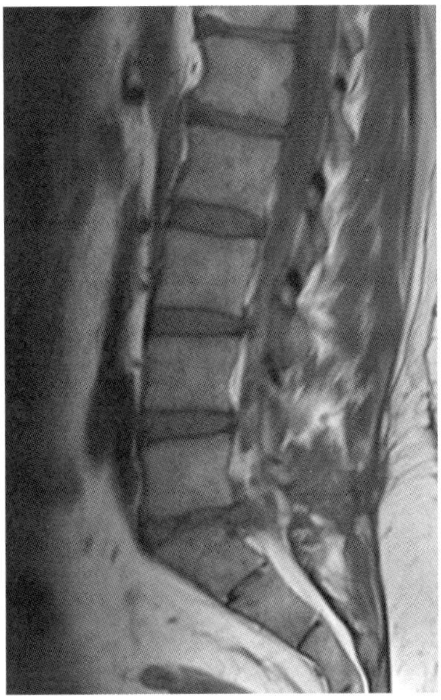
e

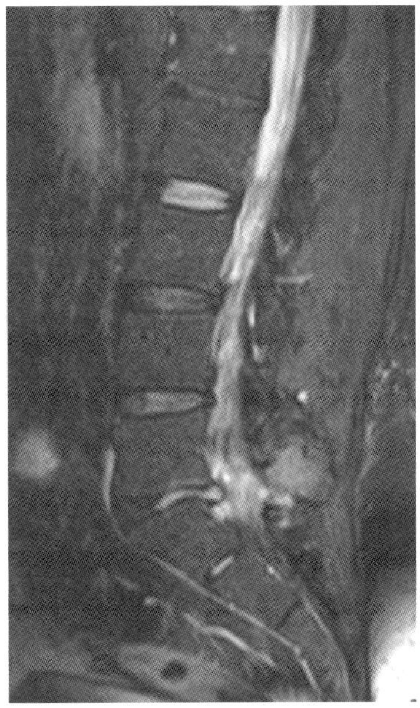
f

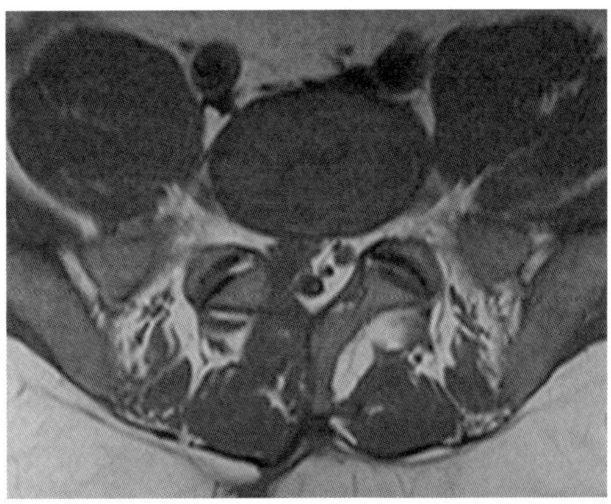
g

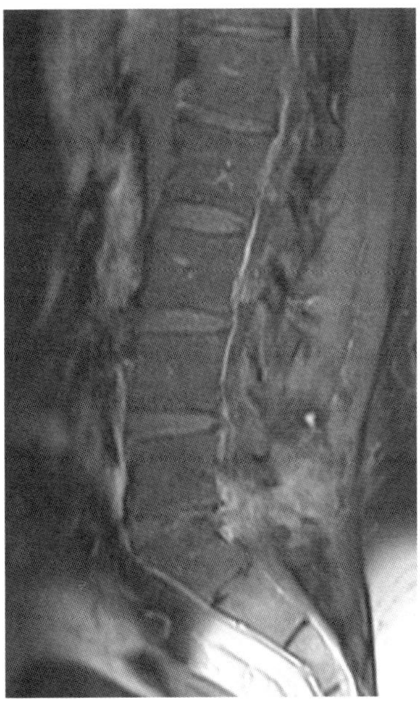
h

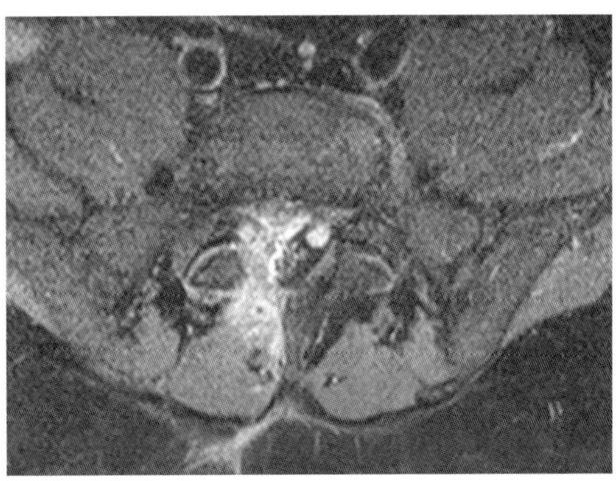
i

Fig. 4.4 (*continued*) **(e)** Sagittal SET1W, **(f)** STIR, **(g)** axial SETW1, **(h)** sagittal spin echo T1 fat saturated (SET1FS), and **(i)** axial SET1FS postcontrast of disk herniation recurrence and gadolinium-enhanced right posterior scar tissue.

Standing and Positional MRI

A standard MRI is performed with the patient lying on his or her back. This position is obligatory in the traditional MRI units, has many technical advantages due to the architecture of the MRI units and of the coils, and allows the patient to be comfortable and to lie still during the examination.

The disadvantages of this positioning are that the patient is examined in a position that usually entails no pain, and this position is the opposite of the position of the patient in the operating room.

Red flags are used to identify patients who can have a metameric instability. These signs are basically linked to the degenerative cascade of the spine unit and include disk degeneration (Pfirrmann grades 3 and 4), the thickening of the flava ligaments, apophyseal joint arthritis with joint effusion, and the crowded and serpiginous aspect of the roots of the cauda. If one or more of these red flag signs are present, a dynamic flexion-extension and standing study is indicated to check if a spine unit instability is present. This result is usually achieved by dynamic flexion-extension or lateral bending X-ray of the spine, but an MRI standing and positional study can also be done. There are, in fact, MRI units in which the patient can be studied in a sitting or standing position. These MRIs are very useful because the patient can be studied in the position in which the referred pain is experienced, which facilitates analyzing the interference of the soft tissues, disks, ligaments, cauda, and roots with the bony part of the spine while the patient is standing, bending, sitting, or twisting.[6,7,8] The most important limitations of these devices are due to the medium strength (0.5, 0.6T) of the magnetic field and to purely technical factors that affect the image quality. However, these MRIs are very useful in particular cases when a functional diagnosis is needed.

Contraindications to MRI

There are important contraindications to using the MRI—factors that can harm the patient's life or physical integrity. Pacemakers, acoustic devices, and heart valves are considered absolute contraindications, where others, such as metal implants in the body (e.g., screws, plates, joint prostheses, surgical clips, electronic devices, etc.) are considered relative contraindications. Managing these contraindications is the duty of the radiologist, who must check the compatibility of the devices in the MR environment and judge the risk/usefulness ratio of the examination based on the clinical expectation. The spine specialist must highlight the presence of these devices when submitting the request for MRI.

When and How to Request a CT

Computed tomography has limited indications in the study of the lumbar spine, and due to its significant radiation dose, it should be utilized as a last resort in the assessment of the lumbar spine pathologies. As a general rule, a CT should never be performed if an MRI is possible, but when indicated it should be done strictly for a specific aim. For this reason, the clinician requesting a CT must specify exactly the indications for the examination and submit a precise question so that the radiologist can aim the study at the problem, reducing as much as possible the radiation dose. The best way to reduce the dose is to keep the volume examined as small as possible for the clinical question.

In general practice, no more than a couple of vertebra should be studied with CT, and when a wider study is needed (e.g., to assess the position of pedicle screws) a dose-reduction strategy must be adopted by the radiologist.

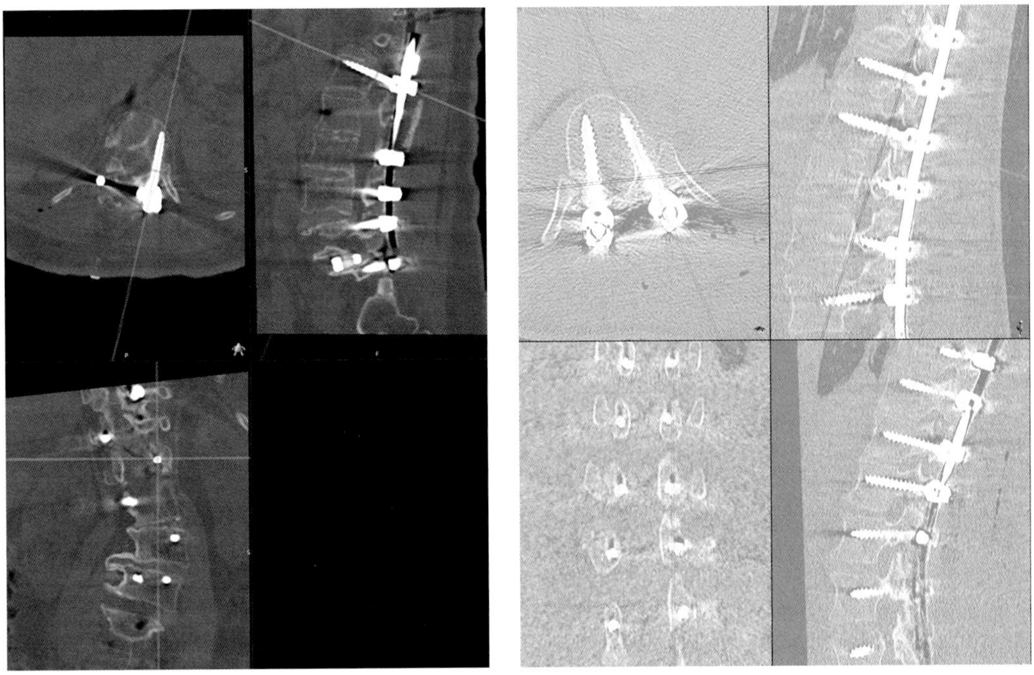

b

Fig. 4.5 (a) Standard and **(b)** low-dose computed tomography (CT) reformatted images showing pedicular screw position. Reformations are done on the screw true axis. CT is effective in showing the position of the screws within the pedicles.

CT can be performed with several different parameters that can affect the image quality and the radiation dose. The aim of the radiologist is to keep the dose at the minimum level achievable following the basic "ALARA" principle: *a*s *l*ow *a*s *r*easonably *a*chievable.[9]

Indications for CT are basically the study of the vertebral bone for facet joints arthritis, the bony component of a central or lateral stenosis, the assessment of a vertebral fracture, the postoperative follow-up of vertebral fixation devices (e.g., screws, bars, hooks, cages), small focal bone lesions (e.g., osteoid osteoma), and neoplastic assessment. CT should never been utilized to assess disk, cauda, or root pathologies.

Modern CT technology enables the radiologist to image a given volume of the body that is then postprocessed with different reformation 2D and 3D views and different imaging algorithms.

Usually the images are shown in axial, sagittal, and coronal reformations with bone and soft tissue algorithms. The volume can be reformatted in any oblique plane when necessary. Typically when the position of a pedicle screw must be verified, oblique sagittal, oblique coronal, and oblique axial reformations are obtained, aimed at each single screw (**Fig. 4.5**).

Due to the appropriateness rule, the radiologist always has the last word in how to proceed with a CT examination or other imaging techniques such the MRI, based on the clinical question submitted by the clinician.

Postsurgery Imaging

Postsurgery imaging can encompass all of these imaging techniques, but the metallic hardware that has been implanted causes important artifacts.

The postsurgical imaging follow-up is based on immediate postoperative imaging controls and follow-up controls. The schedule of imaging follow-up is based on a standard protocol for each type of surgery.

The immediate postoperative imaging control is usually based on a standard X-ray lumbar spine with AP and LL views. On these views it may be difficult to accurately check the position of the screws, hooks, bars, and cages, but these views are useful for determining that the general surgical plan has been followed properly.

A more precise diagnosis is needed when there is a clinical suspicion that something went wrong and when the standard X-rays provide doubtful results.

If the position of the screws, hooks, and cages must be checked, a CT aimed at the site of the suspected malpositioned hardware should be done. When a more complex clinical outcome entails neurologic impairments that can be due to a suspected lesion of the cord or of the cauda, an MRI is necessary. Both of these imaging techniques may be very difficult to perform due to the patient's postoperative condition; the patients frequently are unconscious and remain under general anesthesia, and the implanted hardware presents its own technical problems. The goal is to obtain the best MRI possible in the given situation of metallic hardware being present at the site of a suspected and sometimes subtle pathology. In these cases, the amount of artifacts can only be reduced, not eliminated, adopting metal artifact reduction imaging procedures.

During follow-up, the controls consist of a series of X-rays (AP and LL views) in which the evolution of the imaging situation can be followed. There are several signs that must be checked at the site of the surgery: signs of loosening or mobilization of the devices, or signs of bone bridge formation at the site of the arthrodesis. Moreover, the adjacent sites to the surgery must be controlled; these sites can frequently degenerate quicker than expected in a nonsurgery spine, leading to the so-called adjacent-level pathology. In these cases, the X-ray may be enough to control the evolution of the pathology, but an MRI can be added to check more precisely the situation of the disks and the eventual impingement in disk material, nerve roots, and other factors.

When a mobilization of the hardware is suspected, a control CT must be performed at the entire site of surgery to check every single screw, hook, or cage for signs of mobilization, such as loosening around screws and hooks or subsidence of the cages in the end plates.

A CT scan is particularly useful to verify that the fusion has been obtained or to determine if a nonunion is present. In these cases, a very accurate postprocessing analysis must be performed directly by the radiologist with multiplanar reformation (MPR) or maximum intensity projection (*MIP*) postprocessing tools to check for the continuity of the fusion or its interruption, the grade of homogeneity of the transplanted bone and grafts, and the fusion with the host bone.

Chapter Summary

Imaging can be complex and very expensive for both the patient and the health service, but it can provide information that was unavailable even as recently as 25 years ago. The imaging techniques are continuously evolving, with new hardware and more effective software. While the imaging specialist who is interested in spine pathology cannot keep up with the rapid evolution of clinical medicine and therapeutic improvements in spine treatment, similarly the spine clinician cannot keep up with the rapid evolution in imaging techniques and imaging possibilities. For these reasons, spine specialists and spine radiologists must work together in both standard and complex cases to obtain the maximum diagnostic results with the minimum biological and financial costs.

Pearls

- Before requesting imaging, do a proper clinical evaluation of your patient.
- Include your clinical suspicion in the request for imaging, together with any relevant clinical data.
- Respect the enormous diagnostic impact of the simple X-ray.
- Inform the radiologist of your clinical and diagnostic doubts.
- Refer to the radiologist for a more rational diagnostic pathway for a specific clinical suspicion.
- Carefully consider the possible differential diagnosis for spine patients.
- If there is a mismatch between the clinical and the imaging picture, discuss your concerns with the radiologist. We are playing on the same team.

Pitfalls

- Do not review an imaging examination without reading the radiological report.
- Do not requesting imaging techniques at random.
- Do not look at an MRI as if it were a CT. The information provided by these techniques differs significantly.

References

Five Must-Read References

1. Charpak G. La detection des particules. Recherche 1981;128:1384–1396
2. Dubousset J, Charpak G, Dorion I, et al. [A new 2D and 3D imaging approach to musculoskeletal physiology and pathology with low-dose radiation and the standing position: the EOS system]. Bull Acad Natl Med 2005;189(2):287–297, discussion 297–300
3. Kalifa G, Charpak Y, Maccia C, et al. Evaluation of a new low-dose digital x-ray device: first dosimetric and clinical results in children. Pediatr Radiol 1998; 28(7):557–561
4. Melhem E, Assi A, El Rachkidi R, Ghanem I. EOS(®) biplanar X-ray imaging: concept, developments, benefits, and limitations. J Child Orthop 2016;10(1): 1–14
5. Wilkinson LS, Elson E, Saifuddin A, Ransford AO. Defining the use of gadolinium enhanced MRI in the assessment of the postoperative lumbar spine. Clin Radiol 1997;52(7):530–534
6. Smith FW. Patient friendly positional MRI improves diagnosis. Imaging Management 2004;4(3):36–37
7. Elsig JPJ, Kaech DL. Dynamic imaging of the spine with an open upright MRI: present results and future perspectives of fmri. Eur J Orthop Surg Traumatol 2007;17:119–124
8. Smith F, et al. Dynamic MRI using the upright or positional MRI scanner. In:Gunzburg R, Szpalski M, eds. Spondylolysis, Spondylolisthesis, and Degenerative Spondylolisthesis. Lippincott, Williams & Wilkins; 2005:67-78
9. Richards PJ, George J, Metelko M, Brown M. Spine computed tomography doses and cancer induction. Spine 2010;35(4):430–433

5

Myth and Reality of Sacroiliac Joint Pathology

Kristen E. Jones and David W. Polly, Jr.

Introduction

Sacroiliac (SI) joint dysfunction is a significant source of disability that is an often-overlooked cause of low back pain, buttock pain, and leg pain.[1–3] The burden of SI joint pain is higher than many commonly disabling medical conditions such as chronic obstructive pulmonary disease (COPD) and angina.[4] Diagnosis of SI joint pain is often difficult because of significant overlap with referred pain from disorders of the lumbar spine and hip. Correct identification of SI joint pain requires dedicated physical examination maneuvers and diagnostic injection sequences, followed by a trial of nonoperative management. However, there are significant annual direct medical costs associated with nonsurgical management of SI joint dysfunction.[5] A recent prospective multicenter randomized controlled trial has shown the superiority of SI joint minimally invasive fusion to nonoperative management at 1-year follow-up.[6]

Spine surgeons and spine care providers must have a thorough understanding of SI joint anatomy and physiology in order to correctly diagnose spinal disorders and to understand the connection between the spine and the SI joint. The complex structural and biomechanical interactions of the SI joint require ongoing attempts to better understand, correctly diagnose, and effectively treat this difficult pathology.

Anatomy and Biomechanics

As the largest axial joint in the human body, the SI joint functions to transmit loads from the trunk and spine to the lower extremities. The SI joint provides some flexible adaptation of the bony pelvis via articulation with the sacral aspect of the spine. Each SI joint is diarthrodial, with sinusoidal, auricular-shaped surfaces containing both fibrocartilage and hyaline cartilage.[7,8] The SI joint surface forms an angle oblique to the sagittal plane and is typically present between sacral segments S1, S2, and S3 and the ilium.[8] Because the sacrum is triangular in shape, widest and thickest at its superior aspect, it functionally wedges between the iliac wings and resists against vertical forces.[8,9] The intra-articular surfaces exhibit a coarse texture with interdigitating ridges and depressions, a biomechanical adaptation to increase the coefficient of friction across the joint and to help resist shear forces, to which the SI joint is particularly susceptible.[9,10] Strong ligamentous attachments act as stabilizing forces across the joint, including the anterior and posterior SI, sacrospinous, sacrotuberous, interosseous, and iliolumbar ligaments. The gluteus maximus runs perpendicular to the joint surface, and the thoracolumbar fascia additionally acts as a stabilizing structure.[7–9,11]

The SI joint has mechanoreceptors and nociceptors in its articular surfaces for proprioception and pain signal transmission.[12] Considerable debate exists over the pattern of SI joint innervation, with likely significant variation present from person to person. Anatomic studies have shown that a large contribution of joint innervation comes from the dorsal primary rami of the lower lumbar and upper sacral nerve roots.

Although the SI joint is encapsulated, the ventral capsule is thin. Importantly, the lumbosacral plexus lies immediately adjacent to the ventral capsule. Fluoroscopic-guided SI joint arthrography has shown that in 61% of patients with SI joint pain, intra-articular contrast extravasation occurs ventrally adjacent to the lumbosacral plexus, superiorly at the sacral ala adjacent to the L5 nerve root, or posteriorly adjacent to the dorsal sacral foramina.[13] Inflammatory mediators leaking from a pathological SI joint following a similar path could irritate the lumbosacral plexus, representing one hypothesis as to why SI joint pain can cause radicular patterns of irritation in the lower extremity.[12,13]

Iliac motion occurs relative to the sacrum across the SI joints in a transverse axis with concomitant rotation and translation, termed nutation and counternutation, respectively. Nutation occurs with lumbar extension as the sacral base translates anteriorly and inferiorly relative to the ilium. Counternutation is the opposite, occurring with lumbar flexion when the sacral base moves posterior and superior to the ilium.[2] The exact degree of movement is unknown, but a widely accepted average is approximately 3 degrees. Importantly, lumbar spine movement is tied to SI joint movement.[9] Lumbar fusion constructs have been associated with an SI joint radiographic degeneration rate of up to 75% within 5 years postoperatively, presumably from increased loads across the SI joint with lack of lumbar flexion/extension.[14]

Pathophysiology

Sacroiliac joint dysfunction can result from inflammation, pregnancy, and disproportionate load from spinal forces such as occurring after lumbar fusion, traumatic injury, and degeneration.[7,11] Inflammatory spondyloarthropathies such as ankylosing spondylitis commonly result in SI joint pain, and should be ruled out as a contributing factor.

Pregnancy results in hormonal-induced laxity of pelvic ligamentous structures and can contribute to significant SI joint pain.[15] The SI joint exhibits structural as well as functional sexual dimorphism. Females have smaller joint surface area and lack the bony tubercle seen on the sacral aspect of most male SI joints, resulting in a completely concave sacral joint surface with fewer articulations to prevent slipping.[7] For women during childbearing, mobility of the pelvic inlet and outlet is crucial and is accomplished via hormone-induced relaxation of the ligamentous structures of the symphysis pubis and SI joints. SI joint pain incidence increases significantly in pregnancy, and asymmetric laxity of the SI joint ligaments is a prognostic factor for development of pain.[15]

Compared with the lumbar facet joints, the SI joints are significantly more vulnerable to shearing forces, approximately 20 times more susceptible to axial compression failure, and twice as likely to fail upon axial torsion loading.[2]

Common traumatic injury to an SI joint results from asymmetric loading via one lower extremity's impact, such as a misstep into a hole in the ground or a motor vehicle accident with one foot on the brake.[1,2] Shearing injury via lateral pelvic impact is also common. Only the most blatant traumatic disruption is likely to be seen on imaging. Much of traumatic and degenerative pathology of the SI joint is not directly correlated with radiographic features.[2,7] It is important to note that because significant SI joint pathology can be present even with negative radiographic imaging, diagnosis of SI joint dysfunction is commonly overlooked and requires a dedicated approach.

Diagnosis

Low back pain originates in the SI joint in 15 to 30% of patients.[3] Because the SI joint commonly produces low back pain radiating to the buttocks or lower extremity, differentiating SI joint pathology from lumbar spine or hip pathology is often difficult. Patients with SI joint pain may describe a band-like distribution of low back pain, and when asked to point specifically to the painful area, they may further localize it to a region medial and inferior to the posterior superior iliac spine (PSIS), representing a positive Fortin Finger Test.[1–3] After careful history taking, diagnosis of SI joint pain begins with dedicated physical examination maneuvers. Because each maneuver individually lacks sufficient specificity or sensitivity to make the diagnosis, the following combination of examination maneuvers must be completed.[16]

In standing position, the patient is asked to point to the greatest site of pain (Fortin Finger Test). The PSIS is then evaluated for point tenderness to palpation.

A series of six SI joint diagnostic exam maneuvers are then performed, as described elsewhere.[17] Although these exam maneuvers may cause discomfort in multiple areas, it is crucial to ask patients whether each maneuver reproduces the exact type of pain that they typically experience. The patient is placed in the supine position on the examination table and pelvic gapping, flexion/abduction/external rotation, and thigh thrust maneuvers are performed (**Fig. 5.1**). The patient is placed in the lateral position for Gaenslen's maneuver and pelvic compression, performed on each side. Sacral thrust is then performed with the patient prone. A full examination of the lumbosacral spine, lower extremity, and hip is also performed.

A systematic review of the validity of the diagnostic criteria for SI joint pain supports using a threshold of three positive tests that reproduce the patient's pain to indicate that the SI joint is a major source of pain generation.[16]

Nonoperative Treatment

Physical Therapy

In a patient with three or more positive diagnostic maneuvers, conservative therapeutic intervention targeting the SI joint is begun. This consists of specialized SI joint physical therapy that should be performed by a therapist with specific SI joint training, targeting postural control of the joints via core and pelvic stabilization exercises.[1] Pelvic stabilization orthoses, such as SI belts or tape, can be used as adjuncts to rehabilitation therapy and are maximally effective when applied just superior to the greater trochanter to limit SI joint motion.[1] Oral nonsteroidal anti-inflammatory medications are commonly used adjuncts during therapy.

Injections

For patients in whom conservative treatment fails to render significant improvement, the diagnosis of SI joint dysfunction warrants further investigation via diagnostic injection. Although physical exam maneuvers may be positive indicators of SI joint pain, they also invariably place stress on adjacent structures with the potential for pain-generating capacity and they do not differentiate among such structures.[16] Intra-articular injection of local anesthetic can add valuable diagnostic information. Using fluoroscopic guidance, intra-articular SI joint injection of local anesthetic is performed.[18] The capacity of the SI joint is ~ 1 mL.[1] Selective infiltration of the intra-articular portion of the joint is the goal, and care must be taken not to allow undue extravasation of medication into structures adjacent to the joint, which will muddle the diagnostic capacity of the injection. Two separate diagnostic injections provide pain relief for SI joint dysfunction in 10 to 19% of patients with suspected SI joint pathology.[1,18] Following successful diagnostic injection to confirm SI joint pain, patients may be treated with an injection of a combination of steroid and local anesthetic medication. Long-term data on this treatment are not available, and thus it is unclear which patients may benefit from repeated injection, but in general we consider a patient to have failed control with injection therapy if an injection of steroid and local anesthetic fails to provide at least 50% pain relief for 1 month, or if a patient requires more than three injections within 12 months.

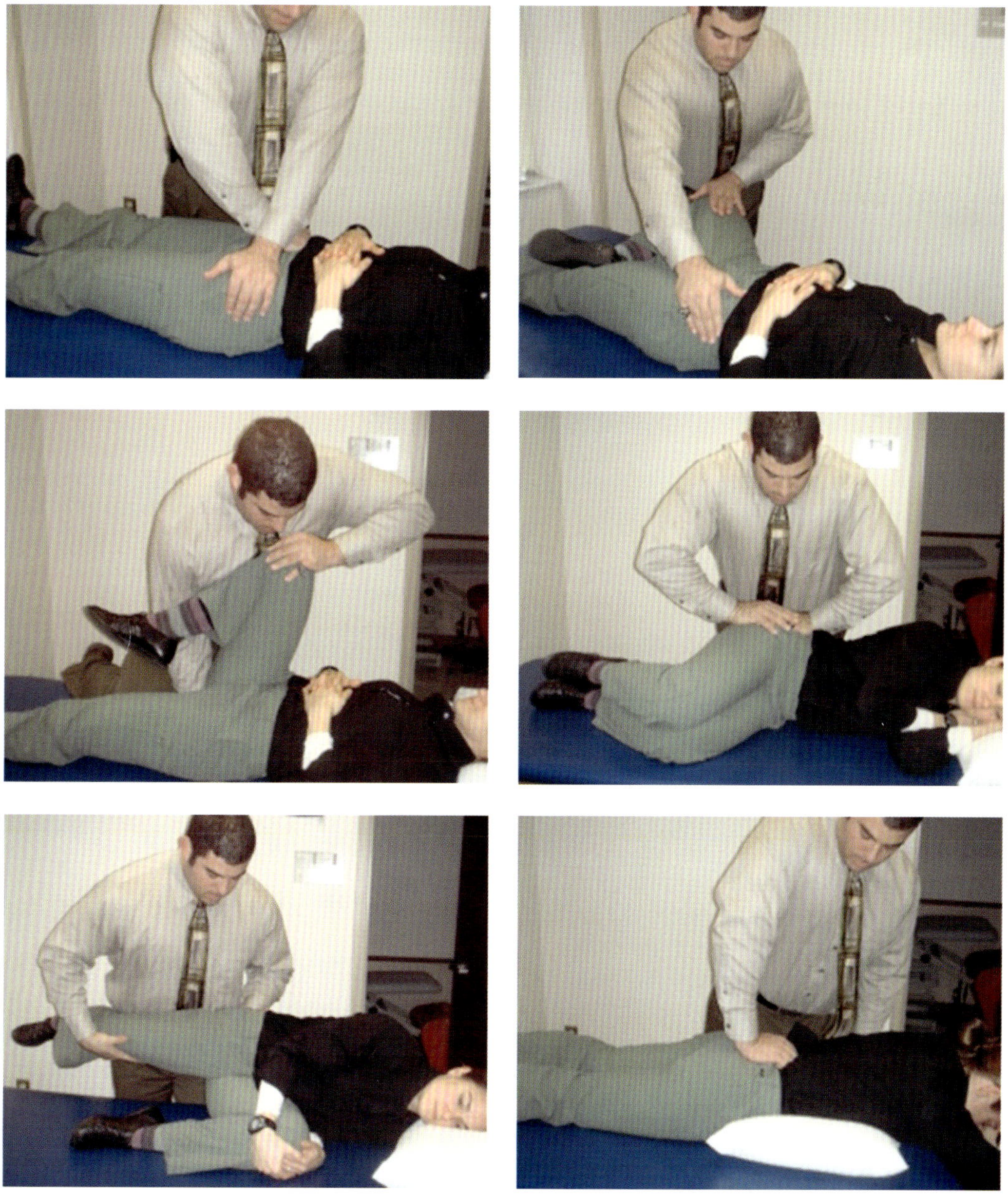

b

d

f

Fig. 5.1 Sacroiliac (SI) joint provocative physical exam maneuvers. **(a)** Pelvic gapping. **(b)** *F*lexion, *ab*duction, *e*xternal *r*otation (FABER/Patrick's test). **(c)** Thigh thrust. **(d)** Compression. **(e)** Gaenslen's maneuver. **(f)** Sacral thrust.

Despite the care taken to perform isolated intra-articular injection, considerable contrast reflux has been demonstrated along the lumbar plexus, indicating the significant contribution of lumbosacral nerves to SI joint innervation and potentially explaining radicular patterns of referred pain from SI joint dysfunction.[13]

Radiofrequency Ablation

Patients with a good but transient response to SI joint injection are candidates for radiofrequency ablation (RFA). Because of individual variations in joint innervation, RFA of the SI joint has widely reported clinical efficacy.[19] Diligent attention to dorsal root contributions of the lumbosacral nerves likely yields the greatest potential for significant pain relief, but it is often accompanied by buttock skin anesthesia.[19] Prolotherapy and cryotherapy have also been used for refractory SI joint pain, but there is insufficient evidence of their efficacy.

Surgical Treatment

Because the SI joint is a mobile structure that can generate pain, intuitively it follows that immobilizing the joint via fusion is a treatment option for SI joint dysfunction refractory to conservative management.

Sacroiliac joint fusion can be performed via open anterior, open posterior, or minimally invasive lateral approaches. Despite several modifications to technique, the open approaches for SI joint fusion have been typically associated with substantial pain, blood loss, and prolonged recovery periods due to extensive soft tissue dissection as well as nonunion rates varying from 9 to 41% and significant complication rates as high as 13%.[20] Minimally invasive SI joint fusion can have consistent and durable results at 5 years. Compared with open SI joint fusion, minimally invasive SI joint fusion has a higher rate of clinical success, does not entail bone graft harvesting, enables faster postoperative mobilization and a shorter hospital stay, and entails fewer complications.[20] Minimally invasive SI joint fusion can be performed as an outpatient procedure in appropriately selected patients.

Minimally invasive SI joint fusion leads to clinically and statistically significant improvement in back pain, function, and health-related quality of life with high patient satisfaction and a low complication rate. Level 1 evidence has demonstrated the safety and effectiveness of minimally invasive SI joint fusion.[6] A multicenter prospective randomized controlled trial has shown the superiority of minimally invasive SI joint fusion to nonsurgical management in relieving pain and improving function and quality of life at 6 and 12 months of follow-up.[6] Cost neutrality is achieved at 6 years between minimally invasive SI joint fusion and nonoperative management.[5]

Preoperative Preparation

Once a patient has exhausted nonoperative management and been deemed a potential surgical candidate, a noncontrast computed tomography (CT) scan of the pelvis is obtained to evaluate the SI anatomy for feasibility of implant placement. The patient attends a preoperative physical therapy teaching session for training in using crutches with toe-touch weight bearing.

Operative Procedure

Minimally Invasive Sacroiliac Joint Fusion

Minimally invasive SI joint fusion is performed under general anesthesia. The patient is positioned prone, with the hips and knees extended on a radiolucent table using either fluoroscopic guidance with anteroposterior (AP) and lateral images, or three-dimensional (3D) computer navigation based on intraoperative CT scan, as described elsewhere.[20] After imaging has helped determine the starting point on the lateral gluteal region (**Fig. 5.2a**), the skin is infiltrated with local anesthetic and a 3- to 5-cm incision is made in the skin and fascia with dissection carried down to the ilium. Using image guidance, a Kirschner wire (K-wire) is placed across the SI joint into the sacrum, exercising vigilance to remain lateral to the neuroforamina.

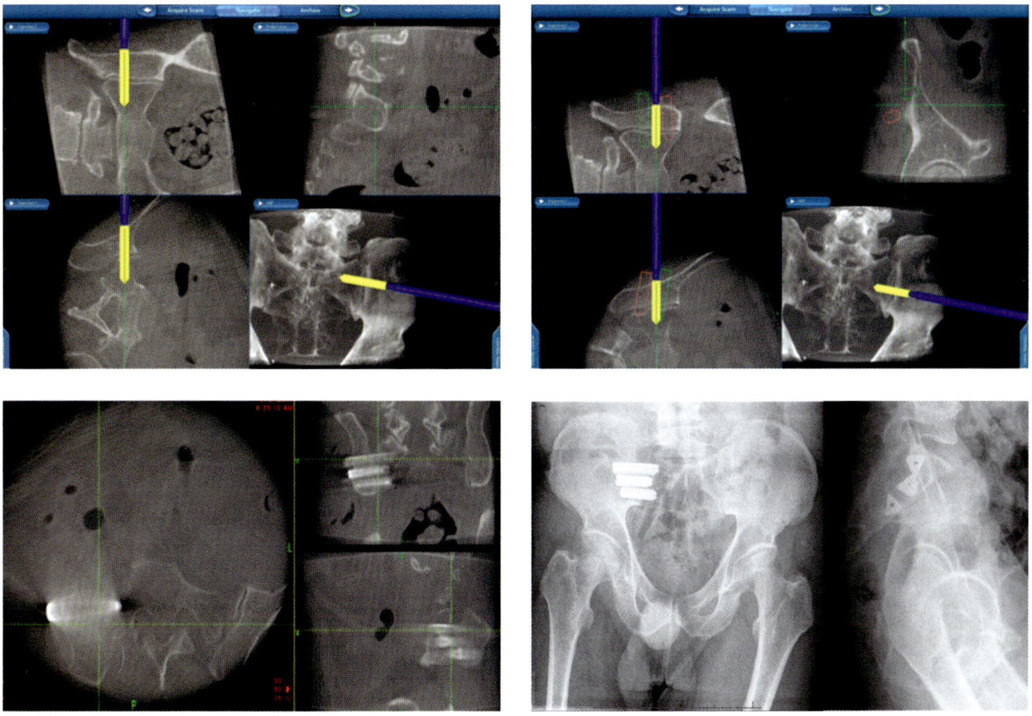

b

d

Fig. 5.2 Minimally-invasive SI joint fusion. **(a)** Intraoperative real-time three-dimensional computed tomography (CT)-based navigation of percutaneous implant placement across the SI joint. **(b)** Intraoperative planning of implant trajectories and subsequent navigated placement. **(c)** Intraoperative CT scan of the SI joint to assess implant placement. **(d)** Postoperative radiographs of the pelvis with three fusion rods across the SI joint.

Fluoroscopy is used to check the location. The implant length is determined. Cannulated serial dilators are used for the soft tissue envelope. After drilling a pilot hole with a cannulated drill bit, a cannulated broach is malleted across the SI joint, taking care not to advance the K-wire (**Fig. 5.2b**). The implant is then manually inserted. Fluoroscopy is used to check the location. This process typically is repeated for a total of three implants. Intraoperative CT scan is used to check the final implant location (**Fig. 5.2c**). The wound is irrigated and closed. Other techniques using screw-in type devices with or without fenestrations are available as well.

Open Anterior Sacroiliac Joint Fusion

Open anterior SI joint fusion is performed under general anesthesia with the patient in the supine position.[20] An ilioinguinal incision ~ 20 cm in length is made through the skin and subcutaneous tissue over the symptomatic joint. The external oblique and gluteal fascia are exposed with sharp dissection, and an interval is developed. The iliacus is elevated from the iliac fossa with subperiosteal dissection with monopolar electrocautery. A retractor is placed inside the iliopectineal line of the pelvis until the superior capsule of the SI joint is visualized. The capsule is then removed off the iliac and sacral portion of the SI joint with a 15-blade scalpel. A pointed Homan retractor is inserted on the sacral ala after careful exposure to avoid injuring the L5 nerve root. The SI joint cartilage is resected using a series of curettes and rongeurs, removing all cartilage back to the posterior ligamentous structures. Bone graft is harvested from the inner table of the ilium and then morselized and packed into the SI joint after predrilling both the sacral and the iliac side, creating multiple 2.5-mm drill holes. A three-hole, 4.5-mm reconstruction plate is contoured and fixed with a fully threaded 6.5-mm cancellous screw on the sacral side and with two cortical screws on the iliac side. The plate is inspected to ensure no soft tissue is trapped or placed under tension. A ⅛-inch Hemovac drain is placed into the iliac fossa. Gelfoam is placed into the bone graft harvest site. The external oblique and transversalis fascia are repaired to the gluteal fascia with multiple figure-of-eight sutures, and the wound is closed in layers.

Revision Sacroiliac Joint Fusion

When surgery fails to relieve the patient's pain, and SI joint physical exam maneuvers remain positive, reevaluation is appropriate. Typically we use CT-guided SI joint injection with local anesthetic. If this relieves the patient's pain, then the patient may be a candidate for SI joint revision surgery. There is no single revision strategy that can be applied in all cases, as it is implant-, anatomy-, and patient-specific. Principles of bone grafting and mechanical stabilization guide treatment.

Postoperative Management

Minimally Invasive Sacroiliac Joint Fusion

The procedure is performed on an outpatient basis or with an overnight hospital stay. Prior to discharge, AP/lateral/Ferguson plain radiographs are obtained (**Fig. 5.2d**) and a physical therapy evaluation is performed to ensure that the patient has been properly instructed in toe-touch weight bearing on the operative side using crutches or a front-wheeled walker. Toe-touch weight-bearing is continued for 3 weeks postoperatively, and then the patient is progressively increased to full ambulation. Beginning 2 weeks postoperatively, the patient undergoes individualized physical therapy twice a week for 6 weeks. Postoperative X-rays are repeated at 6 and 12 weeks to ensure that implant loosening/halo formation has not occurred.

Open Anterior Sacroiliac Joint Fusion

The patient is admitted to hospital until pain control is adequate and flatus returns. AP/lateral/Ferguson plain radiographs are obtained prior to discharge (**Fig. 5.3**). The patients is evaluated by a physical therapist to ensure that the patient has been properly instructed in toe-touch weight bearing on the operative side using crutches or a front-wheeled walker, which is continued for 6 weeks postoperatively. At 6 weeks, the patient begins pool therapy and continues with progressive weight bearing for 4 more weeks. This is followed by 8 weeks of land-based physical therapy focusing on core body strengthening. Postoperative X-rays are repeated at 6 and 12 weeks.

a

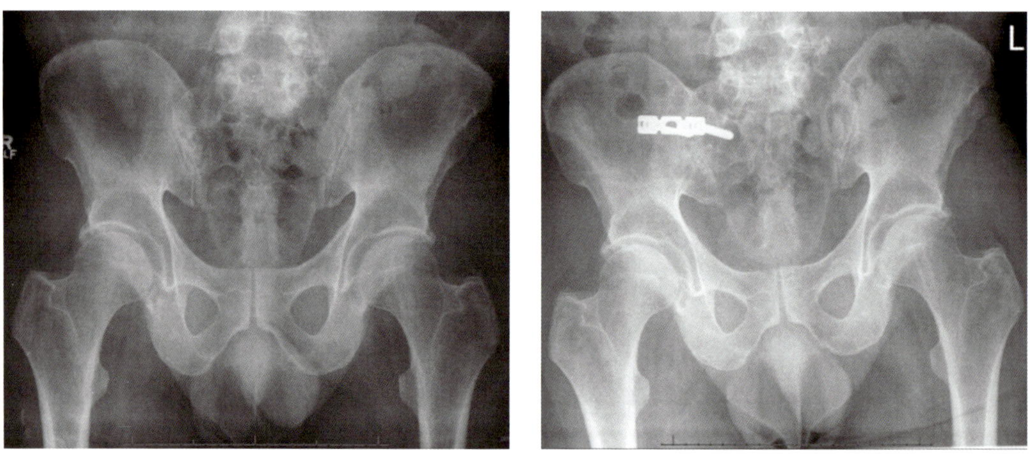

Fig. 5.3 Open anterior SI joint fusion. **(a)** Preoperative radiograph of the pelvis. **(b)** Postoperative radiograph of the pelvis with a three-hole reconstruction plate spanning the sacroiliac joint.

Chapter Summary

The paired SI joints are the largest axial joints in the human body. The SI joints are a significant source of pain that is difficult to diagnose due to widely variable presentation. SI joint pathology can closely mimic both lumbosacral spine and hip pathology, manifesting as low back pain, buttock pain, groin pain, or pain radiating to the lower extremity. Proper diagnosis necessitates clinical suspicion followed by a targeted SI joint physical exam with six specific maneuvers, diagnostic injections, and radiographic evaluation to exclude other pathology. SI joint pathology is often not accompanied by any abnormal radiographic findings. Nonoperative management for SI joint pathology includes physical therapy and injections as well as postural stabilization orthoses. Patients failing nonoperative management are candidates for SI joint fusion, which can be performed via open or a minimally invasive technique. Minimally invasive SI joint fusion entails a lower estimated blood loss, a shorter hospital stay, a lower complication rate, and a faster recovery time than does open SI joint fusion. A multicenter prospective randomized controlled trial has demonstrated the safety and effectiveness of minimally invasive SI joint fusion compared with nonoperative management for SI joint pathology.

Pearls

- Sacroiliac joint pain occurs in a wide array of referral patterns, including low back, buttock, and lower extremity pain.
- Perform a thorough SI joint physical examination with pelvic gapping, flexion/abduction/external rotation, thigh thrust, Gaenslen's maneuver, pelvic compression, and sacral thrust maneuver.
- Fluoroscopy-guided diagnostic intra-articular SI joint injection with local anesthetic can assist in diagnosing SI joint pain for patients with three or more positive exam maneuvers and failure to improve with physical therapy.
- After nonoperative management has been exhausted, level 1 evidence indicates that properly selected patients have significant, durable benefit from SI joint fusion.

Pitfalls

- Do not rule out SI joint pathology based on the absence of radiographic pathology.
- Do not rule out SI joint pathology based on the presence of radicular pain in the lower extremity.

References

Five Must-Read References

1. Forst SL, Wheeler MT, Fortin JD, Vilensky JA. The sacroiliac joint: anatomy, physiology and clinical significance. Pain Physician 2006;9:61–67
2. Fortin JD. Sacroiliac joint dysfunction: a new perspective. J Back Musculoskeletal Rehabil 1993;3: 31–43
3. Sembrano JN, Polly DW Jr. How often is low back pain not coming from the back? Spine 2009;34:E27–E32
4. Cher D, Polly D, Berven S. Sacroiliac joint pain: burden of disease. Med Devices (Auckl) 2014;7:73–81
5. Ackerman SJ, Polly DW Jr, Knight T, Schneider K, Holt T, Cummings J Jr. Comparison of the costs of nonoperative care to minimally invasive surgery for sacroiliac joint disruption and degenerative sacroiliitis in a United States commercial payer population: potential economic implications of a new minimally invasive technology. Clinicoecon Outcomes Res 2014;6: 283–296
6. Polly DW, Cher DJ, Wine KD, et al; INSITE Study Group. Randomized controlled trial of minimally invasive sacroiliac joint fusion using triangular titanium implants vs nonsurgical management for sacroiliac joint dysfunction: 12-month outcomes. Neurosurgery 2015;77:674–690, discussion 690–691
7. Vleeming A, Schuenke MD, Masi AT, Carreiro JE, Danneels L, Willard FH. The sacroiliac joint: an overview of its anatomy, function and potential clinical implications. J Anat 2012;221:537–567
8. Vleeming A, Stoeckart R, Volkers AC, Snijders CJ. Relation between form and function in the sacroiliac joint. Part I: clinical anatomical aspects. Spine 1990;15:130–132
9. Snijders CJ, Vleeming A, Stoeckart R. Transfer of lumbosacral load to iliac bones and legs. Part 1: biomechanics of self-bracing of the sacroiliac joints and its significance for treatment and exercise. Clin Biomech (Bristol, Avon) 1993;8:285–294

10. Vleeming A, Volkers AC, Snijders CJ, Stoeckart R. Relation between form and function in the sacroiliac joint. Part II: biomechanical aspects. Spine 1990;15: 133–136
11. Snijders CJ, Vleeming A, Stoeckart R. Transfer of lumbosacral load to iliac bones and legs. Part 2: loading of the sacroiliac joints when lifting in a stooped posture. Clin Biomech (Bristol, Avon) 1993;8:295–301
12. Fortin JD, Kissling RO, O'Connor BL, Vilensky JA. Sacroiliac joint innervation and pain. Am J Orthop 1999;28:687–690
13. Fortin JD, Washington WJ, Falco FJ. Three pathways between the sacroiliac joint and neural structures. AJNR Am J Neuroradiol 1999;20:1429–1434
14. Ha KY, Lee JS, Kim KW. Degeneration of sacroiliac joint after instrumented lumbar or lumbosacral fusion: a prospective cohort study over five-year follow-up. Spine 2008;33:1192–1198
15. Damen L, Buyruk HM, Güler-Uysal F, Lotgering FK, Snijders CJ, Stam HJ. The prognostic value of asymmetric laxity of the sacroiliac joints in pregnancy-related pelvic pain. Spine 2002;27:2820–2824
16. Szadek KM, van der Wurff P, van Tulder MW, Zuurmond WW, Perez RS. Diagnostic validity of criteria for sacroiliac joint pain: a systematic review. J Pain 2009;10:354–368
17. Laslett M, Young SB, Aprill CN, McDonald B. Diagnosing painful sacroiliac joints: A validity study of a McKenzie evaluation and sacroiliac provocation tests. Aust J Physiother 2003;49:89–97
18. Maigne JY, Aivaliklis A, Pfefer F. Results of sacroiliac joint double block and value of sacroiliac pain provocation tests in 54 patients with low back pain. Spine 1996;21:1889–1892
19. Rupert MP, Lee M, Manchikanti L, Datta S, Cohen SP. Evaluation of sacroiliac joint interventions: a systematic appraisal of the literature. Pain Physician 2009;12:399–418
20. Ledonio CG, Polly DW Jr, Swiontkowski MF. Minimally invasive versus open sacroiliac joint fusion: are they similarly safe and effective? Clin Orthop Relat Res 2014;472:1831–1838

6

Biology, Mechanics, and Genetics of the Disk: State of the Art

Mauro Alini, Sibylle Grad, Hans-Joachim Wilke, Fabio Galbusera, and Alessandra Colombini

Introduction

The human spine has a challenging mechanical role in the musculoskeletal system. Being located in the center of the human body and articulated with the head and the four limbs, the spine is subjected to high loads in all anatomic planes. At the same time, it must ensure a certain degree of flexibility to enable physiological movement and it must adequately protect the spinal cord. One of the key elements to fulfill these mechanical functions are the intervertebral disks (IVD), which account for 15 to 20% of the total length of the human spine, depending on age, degeneration, work load, and diurnal variation. Each IVD acts like a soft pad connecting adjacent vertebral bodies and homogeneously distributing the stresses on the vertebral end plates. Furthermore, together with the spinal ligaments, it governs spine flexibility by enabling sufficient mobility to perform physiological tasks but avoiding excessive movement that would put the spinal cord at risk. These capabilities are made possible by its highly optimized structure, both macroscopically and microscopically.

To fulfill these functions as a joint connecting the vertebral bodies, the IVD is composed of three morphologically distinct tissues (**Fig. 6.1**). The central part, the nucleus pulposus (NP), is a highly hydrated tissue containing proteoglycan (PG)-rich extracellular matrix (ECM). The NP core is circumferentially constrained by the annulus fibrosus (AF), a fibrous tissue consisting of collagen fibrils arranged in concentric lamellae. In the transition zone or the inner AF, a gradual change in ECM composition ensures the proper integration of the tissues. Located cranially and caudally from the disk, thin layers of hyaline cartilage, the cartilaginous end plates (EPs), function to prevent NP bulging into the vertebrae and to enable the nutrition of the disk cells. The adult human IVD is an avascular organ, with blood capillaries terminating at the outer surface of the AF and the vertebral bodies; diffusion and fluid flow are thus essential for transport of nutrients and waste products into and out of the tissues.

The complex regulation of cellular and extracellular components in the IVD can be disturbed as a consequence of aging, genetic predisposition, and epigenetic or environmental factors. The degenerative cascade, which involves cell senescence, eventually cell death, matrix breakdown, tissue dehydration, and fibrosis, leads to a loss of function of the disk and spinal instability.[1] Fissures and tears in the AF, bulging or herniation of the NP, inflammatory processes, and pathological ingrowth of nerves and blood vessels can cause debilitating pain and a severe reduction in quality of life. Genetic and hereditary factors are considered to play a central role as susceptibility factors

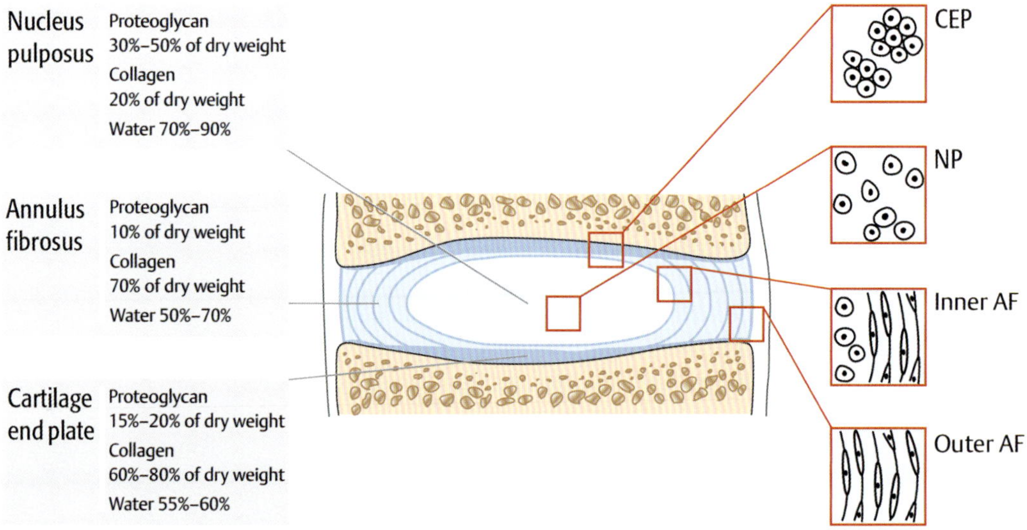

Fig. 6.1 Schematic illustration of the mature intervertebral disk. Midsagittal cross section shows the anatomic regions with matrix composition and representative cell types. CEP, cartilaginous end plate; NP, nucleus pulposus; AF, annulus fibrosus.

for developing disk degeneration and back pain. This chapter discusses the fundamentals of intervertebral disk biology and mechanics, the changes occurring during disk degeneration, and the genetic variants that may be involved in the initiation and progression of the degenerative process.

Biology of the Intervertebral Disk

The template for the development of the spinal segments is provided by the notochord. The early notochord is a rod-like axial structure derived from the mesoderm. Cells within the notochord synthesize PGs that increase the osmotic pressure within cell vacuoles, raising the pressure within the notochord and causing it to elongate and straighten. This forms the basis of the vertebral column. Sclerotome-derived mesenchymal cells condense to a perinotochordal sheath to give rise to the AF. Noncondensed regions of the sheath form the cartilaginous primordial of the vertebrae and the cartilaginous end plate; finally the retained notochord begins to condense to form the NP.[2]

Nucleus Pulposus

The ECM of the NP primarily consists of PGs, in particular aggrecan and versican, which are large aggregating PGs that contain high numbers of negatively charged glycosaminoglycan (GAG) side chains.[3] Specifically, aggrecan contains chondroitin sulfate and keratan sulfate side chains and binds to hyaluronan, forming large molecules entrapped in a collagen network. The high concentration of fixed negative charge provides the NP with a substantial osmotic potential that, by pulling in water, confers the high hydration of the NP. In a young healthy disk, the water content reaches 90%, whereas this proportion generally drops to 70% in older adults. Besides aggrecan and versican, smaller PGs are also found in the NP, including biglycan, decorin, and fibromodulin that function to organize the ECM structure, facilitate cell signaling, and bind growth factors. About 20% of the ECM in the NP consists of collagenous molecules, primarily collagen type II, although collagen types III, V, VI, IX, and XI are also present. Different from articular cartilage, the collagen fibrils appear distributed in a random way, and the ratio of PG to collagens, measured as GAG to hydroxyproline, has been documented as 27:1 in the young NP, as compared with 2:1 in hyaline cartilage end plate.[4]

The cell population of the early postnatal NP mainly consists of large (30–40 μm) notochordal cells that contain intracellular vacuoles and are commonly arranged in clusters. In humans, notochordal cells are lost within the first decade of life and are replaced by mature NP cells. Although the cells of the mature NP have originally been described as chondrocyte-like due to their similar morphology and ECM synthesis, large-scale gene expression studies have provided more in-depth insight into their phenotype.[5] Phenotypical features of mature NP cells that may distinguish them from other cell types reflect their adaptation to the hypoxic, acidic, nutrition-deprived microenvironment, such as expression of hypoxia inducible factor (HIF)-1α , carbonic anhydrase 12, and glucose transporter proteins, their development from the notochord, such as expression of brachyury, cytokeratins 8, 18, and 19, and PGs; and their secretion of a specific ECM molecule composition with a high PG/collagen ratio. In addition, CD24 has been suggested as a marker of mature NP cells.[6]

Both the density (around 4,000 cells/mm^3) and the metabolic activity of NP cells are low compared with other cartilaginous tissues,[7] which may be one reason for the limited regenerative potential of the NP. However, several recent reports have described the presence of cells with stem or progenitor characteristics in the human adult NP.[8] These cells were shown to express typical surface markers of mesenchymal stem cells and to have the ability to differentiate into osteogenic, chondrogenic, and adipogenic lineages. In particular, a progenitor cell population positive for the angiopoietin receptor Tie2 and disialoganglioside 2 (GD2) has been identified in the NP.[9] These cells form spheroid colonies, are clonally multipotent, and maintain their growth and differentiation potential after in vivo transplantation. A significant decrease in the number of these NP progenitor cells was observed with aging and degeneration of the human disk, indicating impaired capacity for regeneration.

Annulus Fibrosus

During intervertebral development, while the notochord differentiates to generate the NP, it pushes against the surrounding annular condensations, thereby inducing the formation of the inner and outer AF. The outer AF is composed of dense concentric lamellae with type I collagen fibers lying parallel within lamellae, whereas the inner part of the AF is made of more widely spaced layers with higher amounts of type II collagen and PG. A network of elastin fibers is also present between the layers. The large aggregating PGs aggrecan and versican, and the small interstitial PGs decorin, biglycan, fibromodulin, and lumican compose 10 to 20% of the AF dry weight.[5] Similar to the NP, the roles of the GAG substituted PGs are tissue hydration enabling rapid reversible deformation, whereas binding of PG to collagens, growth factors, and other matrix components plays a role in the ECM assembly and in repair processes.

With ~ 9,000 cells/mm^3, the cellularity of the human AF is higher compared with the NP.[7] AF cells appear fibroblast-like with spindle-shaped morphology,[10] although spatial variations exist depending on the local mechanical situation. Similarly, regional differences exist with respect to the AF cell phenotype.[5] Outer AF cells primarily synthesize type I collagen, whereas the more chondrocyte-like cells toward the inner AF increasingly produce type II collagen. Without distinguishing regional variations, the GAG-to-hydroxyproline ratio in human lumbar disk AF is around 1.6:1, with little variation by age or by extent of degeneration.[4]

Expression ratios of matrix proteins are effective to distinguish between cellular phenotypes in IVD and cartilage tissues. Collagen II/aggrecan and collagen II/collagen I ratios have been reported highest in cartilage, with collagen II/aggrecan higher in AF than in NP, and collagen II/collagen I higher in NP than in

AF cells. In addition, the greatest expression of collagen V was found in AF cells, suggesting that this collagen might be considered as an AF cell marker. Microarray studies have revealed expression profiles of AF cells (reviewed by Pattappa et al[5] and Guterl et al[11]), although challenges remain to characterize the AF phenotype due to high local and species-dependent variations. Ten genes with AF/NP intensity ratios ≥ 10, including the PG decorin, were reported in rat cells. In canine, 77 genes with a NP/AF signal log ratio of ≤ -1 were recognized, among which were collagen XIV, cell adhesion molecules, and integrin precursors. Tenomodulin, a member of the small PG family, was found to be increased in bovine and human AF compared with NP and cartilage cells. Yet the difficulty of determining clear cutoffs between AF and NP cells has given rise to the assignment of certain molecules as general IVD markers.

The presence of cells with stem or progenitor cell characteristics has also been described in the AF of different species, including human healthy and degenerative tissue.[8] Although this finding confirms the general intrinsic healing potential, different circumstances may limit the effectiveness of a repair response. These factors include the decline in the number of progenitor cells and increased cell senescence with aging, potential traumatic lesions, systemic diseases, and genetic associations.[8]

Cartilaginous End Plate

The end plate consists of a thin layer of hyaline cartilage that has its maximal thickness at birth and becomes thinner with age. In the adult, the EP width is 0.5 to 1 mm. Different functions can be assigned to this cartilaginous structure; it is a mechanical barrier that prevents the IVD from applying pressure directly onto the bone, contributes to load distribution toward the vertebrae, and plays a role in preserving the nutrition and vitality of the NP cells. As with articular cartilage, the main component is water (close to 80% at birth, < 70% in adults), and the chondrocytic cells are embedded in an aggrecan and type II collagen-rich ECM.[5] The cell density is around 15,000 per mm^3, and the PG to collagen (expressed as GAG to hydroxyproline) ratio has been measured as 2:1,[4] which also approximates the levels of articular cartilage. The EP transitions into bone through a region of calcified cartilage.

The EP represents the main route by which nutrients diffuse into the NP. The exchange of solutes is ensured by capillaries present in the calcified part of the EP. It has been reported that the central region enables the highest diffusion of small molecules, whereas at the tissue periphery the cartilage is less permeable. However, the molecule size and charge play an important role, such that small molecules like glucose and oxygen can migrate through the disk more easily than large molecules (e.g., proteins).[7,12]

Cells with stem cell characteristics similar to bone marrow stromal cells were also identified in the end plate of degenerative human disks. In addition, stem cell niches have been described in tissues surrounding the IVD.[8] In particular, populations of slow cycling cells were detected in the AF border to ligament zone and the perichondrium of rabbit, porcine, and human IVDs; moreover, cell migration routes from these niches toward the IVD were described.[8,13]

Intervertebral Disk Microenvironment

One striking aspect of IVD biology is that the cells of the NP and the inner part of the AF are removed from the vascular system. Capillaries of blood vessels supplying the vertebral bone terminate at the end plate, traversing just its superficial region. Similarly, only small numbers of capillaries are found at the very outer surface of the AF.[14] As a consequence, biochemical analyses and modeling studies have reported that the oxygen tension within the IVD is substantially reduced, and the cell metabolism is essentially anaerobic. It has been found that disk cells adapt to this hypoxic environment by limiting the consumption of oxygen and by consecutive stabilization of the transcription factor HIF-1α.[15] The anaerobic metabolism also brings elevated lactic acid and low pH conditions, posing further challenges for cell survival.

Another important feature that characterizes the disk specific environment is the increased osmolarity. The high osmotic pressure, reaching values up to 200 mOsm/kg above the norm, is important to resist the axial loads acting on the spine. Specific factors, such as the transcription factor tonicity enhancer binding protein (TonEBP), are expressed by the disk cells to regulate the levels of nonionic osmolytes for the maintenance of the osmotic properties of the cytosol, which is critical for cell survival.[16] Due to the avascular nature of the IVD, residual fragments of the ECM turnover tend to accumulate in the disk matrix rather than diffusing into the circulation.[17] With aging, the levels of these fragments gradually increase. However, in the case of aggrecan fragments, the negatively charged GAG chains continue to contribute to the swelling pressure as long as they are retained in the NP.

Degenerative Processes

Intervertebral disk degeneration (IDD) is a complex multifactorial process that is determined by the interaction of genetic and environmental factors. Hallmarks include altered matrix composition, overall degradation of matrix components, and changes in cell numbers, cell phenotype, and metabolic activity. Although similar changes are observed during the normal aging process, their pathological acceleration and augmentation can lead to painful debilitating conditions. Morphologically, degenerative changes are evident as a reduction in disk height, disk bulging, and loss of NP/AF demarcation. These changes result from an increased collagen I/collagen II synthesis ratio of the NP cells, loss of sulfated GAGs, subsequent dehydration of the NP, and disruption of collagen orientation in the AF. There is also an increase in collagen cross-linking, rendering the tissue stiffer and more prone to rupture.[11] The PG composition is changing, showing an overall loss of aggrecan, combined with a shift toward versican, biglycan, and decorin production. An increase in nonenzymatic glycosylation can lead to the production of advanced glycation end products (AGEs) that can cause further tissue stiffness. Enhanced fibronectin production and fibronectin fragment accumulation has also been described during degeneration, further accelerating matrix breakdown.[1,3,18]

Matrix degradation is primarily mediated by a variety of proteolytic enzymes, in particular members of the matrix metalloproteinase (MMP) and a disintegrin and metalloprotease with thrombospondin motifs (ADAMTS) families.[18] Several MMPs, such as MMP1, 3, 7, and 13, have been shown to be upregulated in degenerative disk tissue. Similarly, the expression of the aggrecanases ADAMTS1, 4, 5, 9, and 15 is increased with degeneration. In addition, cathepsins and high temperature requirement serine protease A1 (HTRA1) are involved in IVD matrix turnover. All these enzymes are regulated by soluble mediators, such as anabolic, catabolic, and inflammatory factors, and by tissue inhibitors of metalloproteinases (TIMPs), which function to inhibit MMPs and ADAMTSs.

Both nerve and vessel ingrowths into the IVD occur during the degenerative process. This innervation and vascularization may be triggered by the loss of PG, annular clefts and tears, or soluble angiogenic and neurotrophic factors, such as pleiotrophin, vascular endothelial growth factor (VEGF), nerve growth factor (NGF), and brain-derived neurotrophic factor (BDGF), which have been identified in degenerative and painful disks.[19]

A range of proinflammatory factors are induced or upregulated during disk degeneration.[20] These include interleukins (ILs) (predominantly IL-1), tumor necrosis factor-α (TNF-α), prostaglandin E_2 (PGE_2), nitric oxide, and interferon-γ (IFN-γ), although other pathways such as IFN-α signaling may also contribute to the process. Inflammatory mediators can trigger the expression of the above-described proteases, angiogenic and neurogenic molecules, thereby accelerating the degradation. In addition, chemotactic and anabolic factors may induce cell attraction and differentiation, initiating a repair response. However, the diminished capacity renders this response insufficient in the adult IVD.[8]

Mechanics of the Intervertebral Disk

The combination of the three anatomic structures, the NP, the AF, and the vertebral end plates, determines a highly uniform stress distribution inside the disk and vertebral bodies, thus minimizing the risk of failures and disruptions even under the action of high loads. The disk nucleus is a gel-like material with high water content, ranging up to 90% in the lumbar spine. Its PG content gives it the capability to attract water molecules and therefore to create an osmotic pressure gradient with respect to the external environment. Previous studies found that the intradiskal pressure is almost hydrostatic, that is, it acts with equal magnitude in all directions,[21] and is therefore orthogonally and homogeneously transmitted to the inner surface of the AF. The annulus has also a rather high water content (50–70% in the lumbar spine), but mainly differs from the nucleus in its highly organized network of collagen fibers rather than the unstructured, jelly appearance of the NP. Similar to fiber-reinforced tanks designed to contain fluids under pressure, the concentric layers of collagen fibers of the annulus limit the nucleus bulging that would result from the intradiskal pressure. In addition, the criss-cross pattern of the fibers in combination with a complex three-dimensional network connecting the adjacent fiber layers enable a certain degree of disk bending without risking excessive local strains and possible disruptions. Finally, the vertebral end plates ensure a strong yet elastic connection between the intervertebral disk and the adjacent vertebral bodies. End plates consist of a thin layer of hyaline cartilage adjacent to a layer of semiporous subchondral bone, which exhibits several small marrow contact holes enabling nutrient supply and waste removal.[22]

Structural Integration of the Nucleus, Annulus, and End Plates

A recent series of reports highlighted a complex structural integration between the components of the intervertebral disk. Indeed, a complex three-dimensional fiber network exists both at the nucleus–annulus interface[23] as well as at the frontier between the disk and the vertebral end plates.[24,25] Microstructural analyses of ovine specimens found that the nucleus has a distinct fibrosity, mostly vertically oriented, which extends into the inner annulus and is connected to its collagen fiber structure.[25] This fibrosity is capable of sustaining nonnegligible tensile loads (up to 30 N for the whole nucleus) and covers the whole structure, from end plate to end plate. Despite its disordered appearance, mechanical tests revealed that the nucleus fibrosity is highly structured. Fibers appear highly convoluted and folded in the physiological state, and progressively unfold with increasing tensile load. In addition to the vertical fibrosity integrating the nucleus with the end plate, horizontally aligned fibers connecting the nucleus with the inner annulus were also revealed by microstructural analysis and mechanical testing.[23]

The integration between the annular fibers and the end plates was also found to exhibit a high degree of complexity.[24] To withstand high loads, both axial and shear ones, and taking into account the thinness of the cartilage end-plate layer and therefore the difficulties in achieving a strong connection, fiber bundles branch into multiple sub-bundles, named “leaves” by the authors, which have the function of increasing the area of interaction between the annular fibers and the end plate. By exploiting this optimized structure, the annulus–end-plate interface proved to be able to sustain loads with magnitude comparable to those that may disrupt the annular fibers themselves.

Spinal Loads

The organized and optimized structure of the intervertebral disk evolved as a strategy to minimize the risk of mechanical failure while supporting the high loads acting in the spine. As a matter of fact, the exact magnitudes and directions of the loads active in the spine are technically challenging to measure and remain only limitedly known. In vitro and computational studies hypothesized a compressive load ranging from 400 to 500 N acting in the lumbar spine in the standing posture. The load was supposed to be aligned with the longitudinal axis of the spine and to follow its curvature, and was therefore defined as a follower load. This hypothesis was tested by means of numerical simulations and proved to be a simple but rather reliable estimation of the spinal loads in standing.[26] However, more sophisticated computational studies explicitly simulating the action of the trunk muscles, predicted a more complex loading environment even for the standing posture, in which shear loads and bending moments should not be neglected especially in the lower lumbar spine.[27]

Higher loads are acting in the spine in other postures and movements, such as in forward bending, and are aggravated if external loads are also present, for example by lifting a weight. By combining in vitro tests and measurements conducted on patients implanted with telemeterized spinal fixators, Wilke et al[28] estimated a force generated by the erector spinae of 520 N for a forward flexion of 30 degrees, and of 130 N for an extension of 15 degrees. Regarding axial rotation, the best match with in vivo data was predicted for a compressive load of 720 N combined with a moment of 5.5 Nm (newton meters).[29] As a matter of fact, the loads mentioned above are for the most part sustained by the intervertebral disk. Despite spinal ligaments and facet joints also being subjected to remarkable loads, it was found that 80 to 90% of the compressive load acting in standing is supported by the intervertebral disk. In vitro studies based on stepwise reduction of a lumbar functional spine unit demonstrated that the disk is the structure responsible for most of the motion restriction also in flexion-extension and axial rotation,[30] thus arguably supporting for the most part the spinal loads also in other postures and during daily activities.

Stresses in the Intervertebral Disk

In vivo evaluation of the stresses acting in the intervertebral disks has been performed by means of pressure transducers implanted in living subjects (**Table 6.1**). The technique was pioneered by Nachemson and coworkers[21,31,32] and used in several later studies.[33–35] Wilke et al[34] analyzed the intradiskal pressures in the lumbar spine during a wide range of daily activities and physical exercises (**Fig. 6.2**). High values up to 2.3 MPa (megapascals) were recorded during physically demanding tasks such as weight lifting. Similar results were obtained using the same measuring technique in the thoracic spine.[35]

Adams and coworkers[36] measured the stress profile in cadaveric spine specimens subjected to various loads by means of linear transducer elements mounted on thin needles. With this technique, the whole stress profile in the direction of the needle can be estimated, thus

Table 6.1 In Vivo Intradiskal Pressure Measurements in the Lumbar Spine

Author	Disk	Population	Posture	Pressure (MPa)
Nachemson and Morris[31]	L3-L4 and L4-L5	16 healthy subjects	Standing	0.72–1.07
Nachemson and Elfström[32]	L3-L4	9 healthy subjects	Standing	0.58–0.95
			30 degrees of flexion	1.12–1.47
Sato et al[33]	L4-L5	8 healthy subjects and 28 patients with low back pain	Standing	0.54 ± 0.18 (sensor vertical)
				0.53 ± 0.18 (sensor horizontal)
Wilke et al[34]	L4-L5	1 healthy subject	Standing	0.5
			36 degrees of flexion	1.08
			19 degrees of extension	0.6

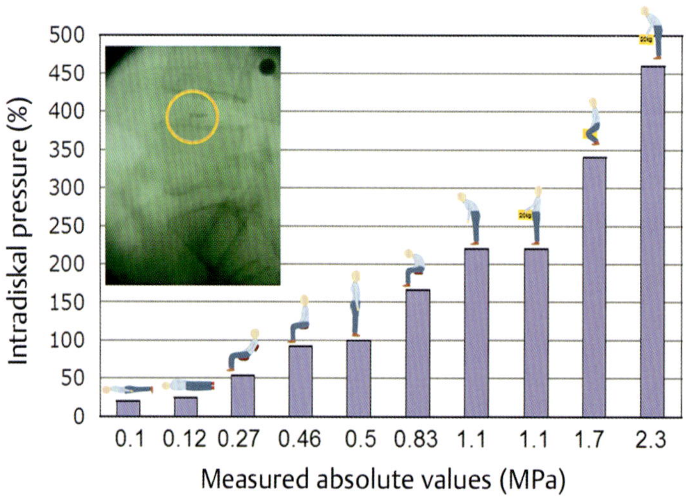

Fig. 6.2 Intradiskal pressure was measured in vivo with a special transducer in disks L4–L5 for different postures or activities. (Adapted from Wilke HJ, Neef P, Caimi M, Hoogland T, Claes LE. New in vivo measurements of pressures in the intervertebral disc in daily life. Spine 1999; 24:755–762.)

providing richer data with respect to the punctual measurements obtained with traditional pressure transducers. Stress profilometry conducted on specimens with no signs of disk degeneration revealed a uniform distribution of the stresses in the whole disk, and confirmed the hydrostatic nature of the stress in the NP.

Fluid Flow and Disk Nutrition

The intervertebral disk exhibits a time-dependent mechanical behavior that has been attributed to its permeable and fluid-rich nature. When subjected to a compressive load, the water content of the disk progressively decreases together with its height and volume, as the fluid is drained through the vertebral end plates and the outer surface of the AF, thus exhibiting a creep behavior (**Fig. 6.3**). If the disk is then left unloaded, water is re-imbibed due to the osmotic gradient, and the disk height and volume are progressively restored. Studies have highlighted the difficulties and technical limitations of the use of in vitro models for the investigation of fluid flow in the intervertebral disk,[37] which therefore remains an open research question.

This topic is especially relevant because of its possible link with the nutrition of the cells of the intervertebral disk. Being that the disk is an avascular structure, nutrient supply and waste removal rely for the most part on convection-diffusion processes, especially through the end plates. Therefore, a restriction of fluid flow due to end-plate sclerosis and consequent decrease of their permeability could in principle be responsible for insufficient nutrition.

Mechanical Alterations Due to Disk Aging and Degeneration

The aging intervertebral disks exhibit several changes compared with young, healthy disks, regarding both morphological and composition aspects. Due to a progressive loss of PG content and the consequent decrease of the osmotic pressure gradient, the fluid content vanishes and water is increasingly replaced by fibrotic tissue.[38] Some intervertebral disks undergo structural failure, showing tears and clefts in both the nucleus and the annulus, and are therefore commonly classified as degenerated disks.[1] Indeed, structural failure of the disk is often correlated with a restriction of the health-related quality of life, because disruptions are a common source of pain.[38]

The aging and degenerative alterations of the disk tissue have a direct impact on the spine biomechanics. The loss of the osmotic pressure gradient and the consequent decrease in intradiskal pressure limit the capability of the disk to uniformly distribute the stresses on the

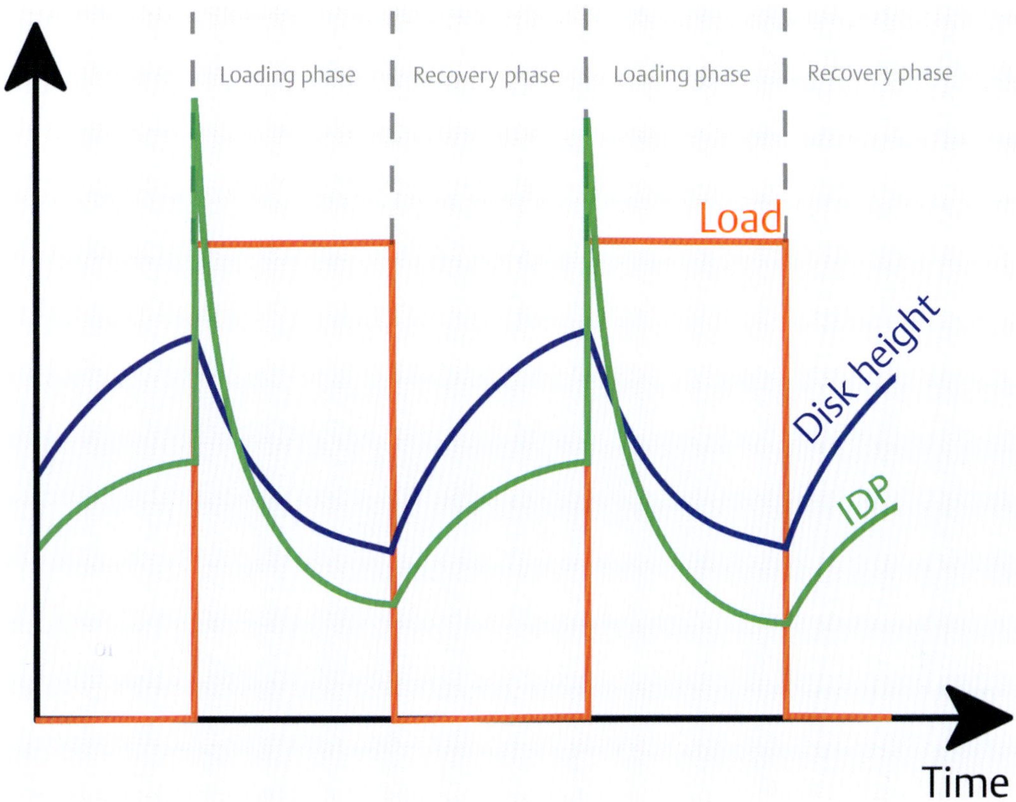

Fig. 6.3 Schematic representation of the mechanical response of the intervertebral disk under a cyclic compressive load *(red line)*. During the loading phases, the disk height decreases due to the reduction of the fluid content *(blue line)*, whereas the intradiskal pressure (IDP) exhibits a peak followed by a fast pressure decrease *(green line)*. During the recovery phases, both disk height and pressure gradually increase due to fluid re-imbibition.

vertebral end plates, as revealed by stress profilometry conducted on degenerated specimens. The resulting local stress concentrations may be responsible of diskogenic pain,[39] in particular for specific postures and movement. Furthermore, the changes in the disk composition together with the presence of tears and clefts may determine a decrease of the spinal stability, which has been proved in experimental studies.[40,41] Despite other in vitro studies that restricted the possible clinical relevance of spinal instability as a consequence of disk degeneration,[42,43] this concept still has a conspicuous relevance to the clinical management of disk degeneration and diskogenic pain.

Genetics

Intervertebral disk degeneration is a multifactorial disease, affected by genetic background and epigenetic processes, with both playing a significant role in its complex etiology and evolution and interacting with environmental, biochemical, and biomechanical factors.[44,45] Different research approaches were used to search for genetic variants potentially involved in IDD. The most common approaches in the past were association studies analyzing single nucleotide polymorphisms (SNPs) in candidate genes. Recently, genome-wide approaches and noncoding sequences have become increasingly used. Genetic information may help first to understand the pathophysiology of the IDD and second to predict a patient's risk for IDD development, enabling preventing or slowing the degenerative process rather than the consequent disability.[44]

SNPs in Candidate Genes Associated with IDD

Candidate gene study using a case-control design was the most common approach for evaluating the association of a few SNPs in preselected genes with IDD. Mayer et al[44] reviewed a large list of genes (20 SNPs) highlighting their functional role in the pathogenesis of the disease. The variants are involved in the preservation of the structural and functional integrity of the disk and in the regulation of inflammatory processes. Of the 20 genes analyzed, SNPs in aggrecan (*ACAN*), type IX collagen (*COL9*), asporin (*ASPN*), matrix metalloproteinase 3 (*MMP3*), interleukins (*IL1*, *IL6*) and vitamin D receptor (*VDR*) are the most promising as functional variants associated with IDD. They have been validated in more than one ethnic population and have biological influence.

SNPs in Structural Genes: *ACAN*, *COL9*, and *ASPN*

The matrix of the inner part of the disk, the NP, is rich in PGs, mainly aggrecan. A region of the *ACAN* encoding for chondroitin sulfate domain (CS1) exhibits a variable number of tandem repeats (VNTRs). Individuals with fewer repeats may have a lower number of CS chains, leading to reduced tissue hydration and swelling pressure and to premature disk degeneration. Associations between VNTR polymorphism in *ACAN* and lumbar IDD were found in Japanese,[46] Korean,[47] and Finnish patients.[48] Two certain *ACAN* polymorphisms (rs1042631 and rs1516797) were associated with signal intensity/disk bulging and with disk height narrowing, respectively, in Finnish males.[49]

Type IX collagen is a heterotrimer of three alpha chains encoded by *COL9A1*, *COL9A2*, and *COL9A3;* this structural protein provides mechanical support to the disk. Two SNPs, Trp2 (Gln326Trp) and Trp3 (Arg103Trp), found in *COL9A2* and *COL9A3*, respectively, have been studied in relation to human IDD. The addition of a hydrophobic tryptophan may affect the type IX collagen structure and the interaction with other matrix molecules, causing the disruption of the triple helix and weakening the disk resistance to compression. The Trp associations are among the most strongly correlated relationships with IDD, with replicated associations in more than two different ethnic populations. An association between the Trp2 allele and IDD was observed in Finnish,[50] Chinese,[51] and Japanese patients.[52] The Trp3 allele was associated with IDD in a Finnish population. Solovieva et al[53] confirmed this association in a Finnish population with the Trp3 allele without the *IL1β* polymorphism (rs1143634). A *COL9A1* polymorphism (rs696990) was strongly associated with the disk intensity and bulging, and a *COL9A2* polymorphism (rs7533552) was associated with the disk intensity in Finnish males.[49]

ASPN encodes a small leucine-rich protein able to provide functional support and regulate signaling molecules. A typical allelic product has 13 aspartic acid repeats at the N-terminus, but a polymorphic allele can contain a variable number of repeats from 9 to 20. Through inhibition of transforming growth factor-β (TGF-β) signaling, this protein inhibited in vitro chondrogenesis and expression of type II collagen and aggrecan, with a stronger inhibitory effect for asporin with 14 aspartate repeats (D14) over others. An allele D14 repeat was associated with IDD in Chinese and Japanese patients.[54]

SNPs in Catabolic and Inflammatory Genes: *MMP3*, *IL1*, and *IL6*

The MMPs are proteins involved in the maintenance of the homeostasis of the disk ECM. A polymorphism in the promoter region of *MMP3* produces alleles with five (5A) or six (6A) repeats of adenine: the 5A allele had twice the promoter activity in comparison with the 6A allele, resulting in more protein produced and potentially in increased degeneration.[55] The 5A allele was associated with IDD in elderly Japanese patients,[55] in English women,[56] and in Chinese patients.[57]

In the disk the synthesis of matrix degrading enzymes and the production of their inhibitors can be regulated by proinflammatory cytokines, particularly IL-1. This cytokine leads to decreased levels of matrix components such as aggrecan, type I and II collagen. An association between the presence of the T allele (rs1800587) in the *IL1α*, causing an increased transcription of IL-1α, and an increased risk of IDD was observed in young Danish girls[58] and Finnish males.[59] Another *IL1α* polymorphism (rs2071375) was found to be associated with the changes in disk signal intensity in Finnish males.[49] Finally, a genetic interaction between the SNP in *IL1β* (rs1143634) and the Trp3 allele of *COL9A3* was shown to determine the risk of IDD.[53]

Enhanced levels of IL-1 can result in an increased expression of IL-6. This is a potent proinflammatory cytokine that also has anti-inflammatory properties counteracting the catabolic effects of IL-1. Many *IL6* polymorphisms have been associated with IDD: rs1800797, rs1800796, rs1800795, and rs13006435. A Finnish study found that the risk allele (A allele) in an *IL6* SNP (rs13006435) was significantly associated with IDD, that the GGGA haplotype from all four cited SNPs was significantly associated with the degeneration, and that the presence of at least one of these alleles increased the risk of degeneration.[60] In another study analyzing the other three SNPs (rs1800797, rs1800796, and rs1800795), the GCG haplotype was associated with an early IDD in Danish girls.[58]

SNPs in Metabolic Genes: *VDR*

Vitamin D is involved in bony and cartilaginous metabolisms. Several SNPs have been identified in the *VDR* sequence, the best known and studied are FokI (rs2228570) and *Taq*I (rs731236). FokI is a C/T transition polymorphic site present in the *VDR* start codon. The allelic variants of this SNP code for structurally different proteins and have a different ability to induce the transcription of vitamin D–dependent genes. *Taq*I is a synonymous SNP located near the 3′ terminus of the gene and does not determine any change in the encoded protein. This SNP is likely in linkage disequilibrium with other nearby functional SNPs in genes, such as *COL2A1*, which could be responsible for the observed associations with several pathological phenotypes. The association between *VDR* variants and IDD has been validated in Italian (FokI),[61] Australian (*Taq*I),[62] British (*Taq*I),[56] Chinese (*Taq*I),[63] Japanese (*Taq*I),[64] and Finnish (FokI, *Taq*I) patients.[65]

Meta-Analysis of Candidate Gene Studies

Eskola et al[66] evaluated the reliability of 52 previously published association variants in a large meta-analysis of candidate gene studies, with the main phenotype considered being disk herniation as characterized by sciatica. Only six genes involved in disk development, composition, and matrix degradation showed a moderate level of association with the pathology. The first group of genes comprises growth differentiation factor 5 (*GDF5*), rs143383, in northern European patients,[67] which plays a role in ligament and tendon development and *KIAA1217* or *SKT*, rs16924573, in Japanese and Finnish patients,[68] which is probably required for normal growth of the NP. The second group of genes comprises collagen type XI alpha 1 (*COL11A1*) and *ASPN*. *COL11A1* is a minor component of the lumbar disk, having an important function in the interplay of collagens and PGs. The rs1676486 SNP has been reported to result in decreased synthesis and stability of *COL11A1* messenger RNA (mRNA), suggesting functional importance in disk degeneration in Japanese patients.[69] *ASPN*, D14 repeat, was associated with disk degeneration in Japanese and Chinese patients.[58] The third group of genes comprises thrombospondin 2 (*THBS2*), rs9406328, which regulates the effective levels of catabolic proteins (MMP2 and MMP9) in the ECM and *MMP9*, rs17576, in Japanese patients.[70]

Genome-Wide Research Approaches

In complex diseases such as IDD, powerful tools are represented by genome-wide association studies (GWASs), in which hundreds of thousands of SNPs are studied throughout the genome and when large cohorts with thousands of subjects are analyzed. A meta-analysis of genome-wide association studies involving 4,600 Europeans and addressing IDD, particularly disk height and osteophyte measures, was published in 2012. The SNPs associated with the condition were as follows: two in the human leukocyte antigen (HLA) region (rs2187689 and rs17034687), indicating immunologic function; and one SNP (rs926849) in the *PARK2*, which plays a role in proteosomal degradation, cell division, and cell growth.[71]

Another genome-wide study conducted in 2013 analyzed 58 SNPs in 35 candidate genes related to specific phenotype for IDD in Indians. Associations with annular tears were observed with rs1042631 of *ACAN*, rs467691 of a disintegrin and metallopeptidase with thrombospondin type 1 motif 5 (*ADAMTS5*), rs4076018 of nerve growth factor-β (*NGFB*), rs1143633 of *IL1β*, rs1420100 of interleukin-18 receptor accessory protein (*IL18RAP*), and rs11225422 of *MMP10*. The SNP of *NGFB* and rs2292657 of *GLI1* were correlated with disk degeneration. The rs2252070 of *MMP13* showed an association with end-plate damage. The validity of all the associations was found to be phenotype dependent.[72] Genetic findings in the field of IDD are summarized in **Table 6.2**.

MicroRNA in Intervertebral Disk Degeneration

Epigenetics has recently been applied to complex diseases. MicroRNAs have been recognized as important posttranscriptional regulatory elements having considerable potential for prevention and treatment of IDD, especially for targeting NP cell proliferation (miR-10b, miR-21), apoptosis (miR-155, miR-27a), and ECM remodeling (miR-155, miR-377).[45]

Phenotype Influence, Racial Differences, Sample Size, and Selection

The lack of a universally accepted definition of IDD and its related phenotype has meant that patient symptoms or various radiological features were often used to define phenotypes in genetic association studies. SNP associations completely change when different phenotypes of disk degeneration are studied. The standardization, using a well-defined phenotype for correlation, will enable achieving sufficient power for studies with smaller cohorts of subjects.[72,73] Other pitfalls in association gene studies leading to inconsistent findings are the small sample sizes and the wide variation in the racial groups and in the selection criteria for the study populations. Replication studies using large cohorts (thousands of individuals) will enable observing true associations. The use of statistical methods to reduce the impact of population stratification and of confounding variables has been developed especially in large GWASs and will reduce genetic heterogeneity and false-positive findings.[44,73]

Table 6.2 Genetic Association Studies Related to Intervertebral Disk Degeneration

	Candidate Gene Studies	Meta-Analysis	Genome-Wide Association Studies
Development		***GDF5*** rs143383 Europeans[67] ***KIAA1217/SKT*** rs16924573 Finnish[68] Japanese[68]	
Structure	***ACAN*** rs1042631 Finnish[49] rs1516797 Finnish[49] VNTR Finnish[48] Japanese[46] Koreans[47] ***COL9A1*** rs696990 Finnish[49] ***COL9A2*** Trp2 Finnish[50] Japanese[52] Chinese[51] rs7533552 Finnish[49] ***COL9A3*** Trp3 Finnish[53] ***ASPN*** D14 repeat Japanese, Chinese[54]	***COL11A1*** rs1676486 Japanese[69] ***ASPN*** D14 repeat Japanese[58] Chinese[58]	***ACAN*** rs1042631 Indians[72]
Catabolism	***MMP3*** 5A repeat Japanese[55] Chinese[57] British[56]	***MMP9*** Rs17576 Japanese[70] ***THBS2*** Rs9406328 Japanese[70]	***MMP10*** rs11225422 Indians[72] ***MMP13*** rs2252070 Indians[72] ***ADAMTS5*** rs467691 Indians[72]
Inflammation	***IL1α*** rs1800587 Finnish[59] Danish[58] rs2071375 Finnish[49] ***IL1β*** rs1143634 Finnish[53] ***IL6*** rs13006435 Finnish[60] rs1800795 Danish[58] rs1800796 Danish[58] rs1800797 Danish[58]		***IL1β*** rs1143633 Indians[72] ***IL18RAP*** rs1420100 Indians[72]
Other	***VDR*** rs2228570 Finnish[65] Italians[61] rs731236 Finnish[65] Japanese[64] Chinese[63] British[56] Australians[62]		***NGFB*** rs4076018 Indians[72] ***GLI1*** rs2292657 Indians[72] ***PARK2*** rs926849 Europeans[71] **HLA region** rs2187689 Europeans[71] rs17034687 Europeans[71]

Chapter Summary

The IVD is a complex organ that functions to distribute stresses acting on the spine and to enable controlled flexibility during spinal movements. These challenges are met by the interaction among the central PG-rich NP, the surrounding fibrocartilaginous AF, and the cartilage end plates, which connect the IVD to the vertebral bone. Due to its avascular nature, the IVD niche is hypoxic and characterized by low pH, nutrition, and cellularity, whereas the large amount of glycosaminoglycan in the nucleus confers a high osmotic pressure. Nutrient supply and removal of metabolites rely on convection-diffusion processes. Disk cells are adapted to this challenging environment; progenitor cells are present in the IVD, although their number and repair potential is deficient. The IVD is subjected to a complex loading environment even during standing posture, involving shear loads and bending movements in addition to the axial compressive load. Intradiskal pressure measurements reported values of up to 2.3 MPa in the human spine during demanding physical exercise. The hydrostatic nature of the stresses in the nucleus enables a uniform stress distribution profile.

Disk degeneration is cell mediated, and characterized by matrix breakdown, tissue dehydration, fibrosis, inflammatory processes, innervation, and neovascularization. Loss of the osmotic pressure gradient leads to disk height reduction, instability, bulging of the annulus, and diminished fluid exchange, impairing cellular function. Painful back, neck, and leg symptoms can occur due to spinal instability and sensitization of nociceptive receptors as a consequence of processes initiated by the degenerative cascade. Genetic background plays a role in the onset and progression of degeneration. SNPs in various candidate genes that regulate disk structure, degradation, and metabolism have been associated with evidence of disk degeneration and pain; genome-wide studies provide comprehensive profiles from larger cohorts. Genetic information may improve our understanding of the pathophysiology, predict the individual risk for a degeneration phenotype, and facilitate personalized treatment.

Pearls

- The IVD is composed of the NP, AF, and cartilage end plate, all containing water, collagen, and PGs in different proportions.
- The interaction of these tissues enables the IVD to transmit loads while enabling a constrained flexibility within the spine.
- The osmotic pressure is important for load transmission and structural stability.
- The IVD niche is avascular and hypoxic.
- The phenotype of the disk cells reflects their adaptation to survive within a mechanically and nutritionally challenging environment.
- Structures of the motion segment guarantee a highly uniform stress distribution inside the healthy disk and vertebral bodies
- Structural organization of the annular fibers and their integration into end plates and nucleus is very complex.
- Intradiskal pressure is roughly 0.1 MPa in the lying position, 0.5 MPa in the standing and sitting positions, and can increase to more than 2.3 MPa.
- Disk degeneration is a multifactorial process in which the disk cells play a central role.
- Degeneration changes stresses in all structures and usually leads to decreased range of motion.
- Evidence exists for the role of seven genes (*COL11A1, THBS2, ASPN, SKT, GDF5, MMP9, PARK2*) and two SNPs in HLA region, affecting disk structure, cellular functions, and inflammatory pathways in IDD.
- Genome-wide studies sequence the exome and the whole genome.
- Epigenetics is an emerging area of research for IDD pathogenesis.
- It is critical to reduce the influence of confounding variables.
- Standardization of specific and well-defined phenotypes is necessary.
- Replication studies in large cohorts are required.
- Statistical methods are essential to reduce the impact of population stratification.

Pitfalls

- Proteoglycan concentration values per se do not enable drawing relevant conclusions about the integrity of the disk tissue; their type, size distribution, and relation to collagen has to be considered.
- Total collagen concentration values are also of limited relevance; the type of collagen is essential.
- The presence of collagen and PGs per se do not indicate the expression of a disk cell phenotype.
- In vitro studies with isolated disk cells commonly do not take into account the niche conditions.
- Most animal models are inappropriate to study human disk degeneration; only specific scientific questions can be addressed.
- Measuring spinal loads in vivo directly is not possible.
- Intradiskal pressure measurements cannot be performed in degenerated disks.
- Mild disk degeneration does not create instability in the motion segment.
- To focus on single SNPs of few candidate genes is inconclusive.
- To study varying phenotypes is inappropriate (SNP associations completely change when different phenotypes are studied).
- Symptoms are not necessarily associated with IDD.
- To compare different racial groups is inconclusive.

References

Five Must-Read References

1. Adams MA, Roughley PJ. What is intervertebral disc degeneration, and what causes it? Spine(Phila Pa 1976) 2006;31:2151–2161
2. Cox MK, Serra R. Development of the intervertebral disc. In: Shapiro IM, Risbud MV, eds. The Intervertebral Disc: Molecular and Structural Studies of the Disc in Health and Disease. Vienna: Springer; 2014: 33–52
3. Roughley PJ. Biology of intervertebral disc aging and degeneration: involvement of the extracellular matrix. Spine(Phila Pa 1976) 2004;29:2691–2699
4. Mwale F, Roughley P, Antoniou J. Distinction between the extracellular matrix of the nucleus pulposus and hyaline cartilage: a requisite for tissue engineering of intervertebral disc. Eur Cell Mater 2004;8:58–63, discussion 63–64
5. Pattappa G, Li Z, Peroglio M, Wismer N, Alini M, Grad S. Diversity of intervertebral disc cells: phenotype and function. J Anat 2012;221:480–496
6. Risbud MV, Schoepflin ZR, Mwale F, et al. Defining the phenotype of young healthy nucleus pulposus cells: recommendations of the Spine Research Interest Group at the 2014 annual ORS meeting. J Orthop Res 2015;33:283–293
7. Maroudas A, Stockwell RA, Nachemson A, Urban J. Factors involved in the nutrition of the human lumbar intervertebral disc: cellularity and diffusion of glucose in vitro. J Anat 1975;120(Pt 1):113–130
8. Li Z, Peroglio M, Alini M, Grad S. Potential and limitations of intervertebral disc endogenous repair. Curr Stem Cell Res Ther 2015;10:329–338
9. Sakai D, Nakamura Y, Nakai T, et al. Exhaustion of nucleus pulposus progenitor cells with ageing and degeneration of the intervertebral disc. Nat Commun 2012;3:1264
10. Roberts S, Evans H, Trivedi J, Menage J. Histology and pathology of the human intervertebral disc. J Bone Joint Surg Am 2006;88(Suppl 2):10–14
11. Guterl CC, See EY, Blanquer SB, et al. Challenges and strategies in the repair of ruptured annulus fibrosus. Eur Cell Mater 2013;25:1–21
12. Urban JP, Smith S, Fairbank JC. Nutrition of the intervertebral disc. Spine(Phila Pa 1976) 2004;29:2700–2709
13. Henriksson H, Thornemo M, Karlsson C, et al. Identification of cell proliferation zones, progenitor cells and a potential stem cell niche in the intervertebral disc region: a study in four species. Spine(Phila Pa 1976) 2009;34:2278–2287
14. Nerlich AG, Schaaf R, Wälchli B, Boos N. Temporospatial distribution of blood vessels in human lumbar intervertebral discs. Eur Spine J 2007;16:547–555
15. Agrawal A, Guttapalli A, Narayan S, Albert TJ, Shapiro IM, Risbud MV. Normoxic stabilization of HIF-1alpha drives glycolytic metabolism and regulates aggrecan gene expression in nucleus pulposus cells of the rat

intervertebral disk. Am J Physiol Cell Physiol 2007; 293:C621–C631
16. Tsai TT, Danielson KG, Guttapalli A, et al. TonEBP/OREBP is a regulator of nucleus pulposus cell function and survival in the intervertebral disc. J Biol Chem 2006;281:25416–25424
17. Roughley PJ, Alini M, Antoniou J. The role of proteoglycans in aging, degeneration and repair of the intervertebral disc. Biochem Soc Trans 2002;30(Pt 6):869–874
18. Sivan SS, Hayes AJ, Wachtel E, et al. Biochemical composition and turnover of the extracellular matrix of the normal and degenerate intervertebral disc. Eur Spine J 2014;23(Suppl 3):S344–S353
19. Krock E, Rosenzweig DH, Chabot-Doré AJ, et al. Painful, degenerating intervertebral discs up-regulate neurite sprouting and CGRP through nociceptive factors. J Cell Mol Med 2014;18:1213–1225
20. Wuertz K, Haglund L. Inflammatory mediators in intervertebral disk degeneration and discogenic pain. Global Spine J 2013;3:175–184
21. Nachemson A. Measurement of intradiscal pressure. Acta Orthop Scand 1959;28:269–289
22. Benneker LM, Heini PF, Alini M, Anderson SE, Ito K. 2004 Young Investigator Award Winner: vertebral endplate marrow contact channel occlusions and intervertebral disc degeneration. Spine 2005;30:167–173
23. Wade KR, Robertson PA, Broom ND. On the extent and nature of nucleus-annulus integration. Spine 2012;37:1826–1833
24. Rodrigues SA, Thambyah A, Broom ND. A multiscale structural investigation of the annulus-endplate anchorage system and its mechanisms of failure. Spine J 2015;15:405–416
25. Wade KR, Robertson PA, Broom ND. A fresh look at the nucleus-endplate region: new evidence for significant structural integration. Eur Spine J 2011;20:1225–1232
26. Patwardhan AG, Havey RM, Meade KP, Lee B, Dunlap B. A follower load increases the load-carrying capacity of the lumbar spine in compression. Spine 1999;24:1003–1009
27. Shirazi-Adl A, El-Rich M, Pop DG, Parnianpour M. Spinal muscle forces, internal loads and stability in standing under various postures and loads—application of kinematics-based algorithm. Eur Spine J 2005;14:381–392
28. Wilke HJ, Rohlmann A, Neller S, Graichen F, Claes L, Bergmann G. ISSLS prize winner: A novel approach to determine trunk muscle forces during flexion and extension: a comparison of data from an in vitro experiment and in vivo measurements. Spine 2003;28:2585–2593
29. Dreischarf M, Rohlmann A, Bergmann G, Zander T. Optimised loads for the simulation of axial rotation in the lumbar spine. J Biomech 2011;44:2323–2327
30. Schmidt H, Heuer F, Simon U, et al. Application of a new calibration method for a three-dimensional finite element model of a human lumbar annulus fibrosus. Clin Biomech (Bristol, Avon) 2006;21:337–344
31. Nachemson A, Morris JM. In vivo measurements of intradiscal pressure. Discometry, a method for the determination of pressure in the lower lumbar discs. J Bone Joint Surg Am 1964;46:1077–1092
32. Nachemson A, Elfström G. Intravital dynamic pressure measurements in lumbar discs. A study of common movements, maneuvers and exercises. Scand J Rehabil Med Suppl 1970;1:1–40
33. Sato K, Kikuchi S, Yonezawa T. In vivo intradiscal pressure measurement in healthy individuals and in patients with ongoing back problems. Spine 1999;24:2468–2474
34. Wilke HJ, Neef P, Caimi M, Hoogland T, Claes LE. New in vivo measurements of pressures in the intervertebral disc in daily life. Spine 1999;24:755–762
35. Polga DJ, Beaubien BP, Kallemeier PM, et al. Measurement of in vivo intradiscal pressure in healthy thoracic intervertebral discs. Spine 2004;29:1320–1324
36. Adams MA, McMillan DW, Green TP, Dolan P. Sustained loading generates stress concentrations in lumbar intervertebral discs. Spine 1996;21:434–438
37. van der Veen AJ, van Dieën JH, Nadort A, Stam B, Smit TH. Intervertebral disc recovery after dynamic or static loading in vitro: is there a role for the endplate? J Biomech 2007;40:2230–2235
38. Boos N, Weissbach S, Rohrbach H, Weiler C, Spratt KF, Nerlich AG. Classification of age-related changes in lumbar intervertebral discs: 2002 Volvo Award in basic science. Spine 2002;27:2631–2644
39. Adams MA, McNally DS, Dolan P. "Stress" distributions inside intervertebral discs. The effects of age and degeneration. J Bone Joint Surg Br 1996;78:965–972
40. Kirkaldy-Willis WH, Farfan HF. Instability of the lumbar spine. Clin Orthop Relat Res 1982;165:110–123
41. Tanaka N, An HS, Lim TH, Fujiwara A, Jeon CH, Haughton VM. The relationship between disc degeneration and flexibility of the lumbar spine. Spine J 2001;1:47–56
42. Kettler A, Rohlmann F, Ring C, Mack C, Wilke HJ. Do early stages of lumbar intervertebral disc degeneration really cause instability? Evaluation of an in vitro database. Eur Spine J 2011;20:578–584
43. Mimura M, Panjabi MM, Oxland TR, Crisco JJ, Yamamoto I, Vasavada A. Disc degeneration affects the multidirectional flexibility of the lumbar spine. Spine 1994;19:1371–1380

44. Mayer JE, Iatridis JC, Chan D, Qureshi SA, Gottesman O, Hecht AC. Genetic polymorphisms associated with intervertebral disc degeneration. Spine J 2013;13: 299–317
45. Li Z, Yu X, Shen J, Chan MT, Wu WK. MicroRNA in intervertebral disc degeneration. Cell Prolif 2015;48: 278–283
46. Kawaguchi Y, Osada R, Kanamori M, et al. Association between an aggrecan gene polymorphism and lumbar disc degeneration. Spine 1999;24:2456–2460
47. Kim NK, Shin DA, Han IB, Yoo EH, Kim SH, Chung SS. The association of aggrecan gene polymorphism with the risk of intervertebral disc degeneration. Acta Neurochir (Wien) 2011;153:129–133
48. Solovieva S, Noponen N, Männikkö M, et al. Association between the aggrecan gene variable number of tandem repeats polymorphism and intervertebral disc degeneration. Spine 2007;32:1700–1705
49. Videman T, Saarela J, Kaprio J, et al. Associations of 25 structural, degradative, and inflammatory candidate genes with lumbar disc desiccation, bulging, and height narrowing. Arthritis Rheum 2009;60:470–481
50. Annunen S, Paassilta P, Lohiniva J, et al. An allele of COL9A2 associated with intervertebral disc disease. Science 1999;285:409–412
51. Jim JJ, Noponen-Hietala N, Cheung KM, et al. The TRP2 allele of COL9A2 is an age-dependent risk factor for the development and severity of intervertebral disc degeneration. Spine 2005;30:2735–2742
52. Higashino K, Matsui Y, Yagi S, et al. The alpha2 type IX collagen tryptophan polymorphism is associated with the severity of disc degeneration in younger patients with herniated nucleus pulposus of the lumbar spine. Int Orthop 2007;31:107–111
53. Solovieva S, Lohiniva J, Leino-Arjas P, et al. Intervertebral disc degeneration in relation to the COL9A3 and the IL-1ss gene polymorphisms. Eur Spine J 2006;15: 613–619
54. Song YQ, Cheung KM, Ho DW, et al. Association of the asporin D14 allele with lumbar-disc degeneration in Asians. Am J Hum Genet 2008;82:744–747
55. Takahashi M, Haro H, Wakabayashi Y, Kawa-uchi T, Komori H, Shinomiya K. The association of degeneration of the intervertebral disc with 5a/6a polymorphism in the promoter of the human matrix metalloproteinase-3 gene. J Bone Joint Surg Br 2001; 83:491–495
56. Valdes AM, Hassett G, Hart DJ, Spector TD. Radiographic progression of lumbar spine disc degeneration is influenced by variation at inflammatory genes: a candidate SNP association study in the Chingford cohort. Spine 2005;30:2445–2451
57. Yuan HY, Tang Y, Liang YX, et al. Matrix metalloproteinase-3 and vitamin d receptor genetic polymorphisms, and their interactions with occupational exposure in lumbar disc degeneration. J Occup Health 2010;52:23–30
58. Eskola PJ, Kjaer P, Daavittila IM, et al. Genetic risk factors of disc degeneration among 12-14-year-old Danish children: a population study. Int J Mol Epidemiol Genet 2010;1:158–165
59. Solovieva S, Kouhia S, Leino-Arjas P, et al. Interleukin 1 polymorphisms and intervertebral disc degeneration. Epidemiology 2004;15:626–633
60. Noponen-Hietala N, Virtanen I, Karttunen R, et al. Genetic variations in IL6 associate with intervertebral disc disease characterized by sciatica. Pain 2005; 114:186–194
61. Colombini A, Brayda-Bruno M, Lombardi G, et al. FokI polymorphism in the vitamin D receptor gene (VDR) and its association with lumbar spine pathologies in the Italian population: a case-control study. PLoS ONE 2014;9:e97027
62. Jones G, White C, Sambrook P, Eisman J. Allelic variation in the vitamin D receptor, lifestyle factors and lumbar spinal degenerative disease. Ann Rheum Dis 1998;57:94–99
63. Cheung KM, Chan D, Karppinen J, et al. Association of the Taq I allele in vitamin D receptor with degenerative disc disease and disc bulge in a Chinese population. Spine 2006;31:1143–1148
64. Kawaguchi Y, Kanamori M, Ishihara H, Ohmori K, Matsui H, Kimura T. The association of lumbar disc disease with vitamin-D receptor gene polymorphism. J Bone Joint Surg Am 2002;84-A:2022–2028
65. Videman T, Leppävuori J, Kaprio J, et al. Intragenic polymorphisms of the vitamin D receptor gene associated with intervertebral disc degeneration. Spine 1998;23:2477–2485
66. Eskola PJ, Lemmelä S, Kjaer P, et al. Genetic association studies in lumbar disc degeneration: a systematic review. PLoS ONE 2012;7:e49995
67. Williams FM, Popham M, Hart DJ, et al. GDF5 single-nucleotide polymorphism rs143383 is associated with lumbar disc degeneration in Northern European women. Arthritis Rheum 2011;63:708–712
68. Karasugi T, Semba K, Hirose Y, et al. Association of the tag SNPs in the human SKT gene (KIAA1217) with lumbar disc herniation. J Bone Miner Res 2009;24: 1537–1543
69. Mio F, Chiba K, Hirose Y, et al. A functional polymorphism in COL11A1, which encodes the alpha 1 chain of type XI collagen, is associated with susceptibility to lumbar disc herniation. Am J Hum Genet 2007; 81:1271–1277
70. Hirose Y, Chiba K, Karasugi T, et al. A functional polymorphism in THBS2 that affects alternative splicing and MMP binding is associated with lumbar-disc herniation. Am J Hum Genet 2008;82:1122–1129

71. Williams FM, Bansal AT, van Meurs JB, et al. Novel genetic variants associated with lumbar disc degeneration in northern Europeans: a meta-analysis of 4600 subjects. Ann Rheum Dis 2013;72:1141–1148
72. Rajasekaran S, Kanna RM, Senthil N, et al. Phenotype variations affect genetic association studies of degenerative disc disease: conclusions of analysis of genetic association of 58 single nucleotide polymorphisms with highly specific phenotypes for disc degeneration in 332 subjects. Spine J 2013;13:1309–1320
73. Näkki A, Battié MC, Kaprio J. Genetics of disc-related disorders: current findings and lessons from other complex diseases. Eur Spine J 2014;23(Suppl 3): S354–S363

7

Neurologic Back Pain: Myopathies, Neuromuscular Disease, Parkinson, and Dystonia

Asdrubal Falavigna and Carlo Domênico Marrone

Introduction

The International Association for the Study of Pain (IASP)[1] defines pain as a disagreeable sensory and emotional experience associated with real or potential tissue damage. Back pain is a symptom that cannot be validated by an external standard or norm, and it is a multifactorial disorder with many possible etiologies.[2] The annual incidence of chronic or recurring back pain varies from 35 to 79%.[3]

Neuromuscular pathologies trigger clinical signs and symptoms, because they compromise the peripheral nervous system or the skeletal striated muscles. The pathologies can affect the following: (1) lower motor neurons (e.g., amyotrophic lateral sclerosis and spinal muscle atrophy); (2) sensory ganglia (e.g., sensory neuronopathies); (3) nerve roots and peripheral or cranial nerves (e.g., Guillain-Barré syndrome, Charcot–Marie–Tooth disease); (4) nerve plexuses (e.g., Parsonage–Turner syndrome); (5) neuromuscular junction (e.g., myasthenia gravis); and (6) muscle (e.g., muscular dystrophies, inflammatory myopathies, drug-induced myopathies, etc.) (**Table 7.1**). The diseases that compromise the movement usually originate in the central nervous systems and comprise the dystonias and parkinsonian syndromes, the most common of them being Parkinson's disease.

This chapter discusses the influence of the neuromuscular diseases, Parkinson's disease, and dystonia on back pain.

Lower Motor Neuron Diseases

The group of lower motor neuron diseases represents hereditary or acquired etiologies, and is characterized by motor function disturbances that are not accompanied by disorders of reasoning, thinking, consciousness, cognition, preserved sensibility, or behavior, or by movements of the bowel, bladder, or eyes (**Table 7.1**).

Amyotrophic Lateral Sclerosis

Amyotrophic lateral sclerosis (ALS) is a progressive neurodegenerative disorder involving primarily motor neurons of the brain cortex, brainstem, and spinal cord that directly control the muscles and movements. Hence, the primary motor neurons, or the central and secondary or peripheral ones, are compromised. It is believed that there is an interaction of

Table 7.1 General Features of Neuromuscular Diseases

Pathology	Primary Involvement	Clinical Presentation	Diagnosis
Amyotrophic lateral sclerosis	Upper and lower motor neuron	• Atrophy • Weakness • Fasciculation • Spasticity • Difficulty swallowing • Cramps • Preserved sensibility	• Clinical presentation • Neurophysiological exam
Spinal muscular atrophy	Lower motor neuron	• Progressive muscle weakness • Deep myotatic areflexia • Hypotonia • Preserved sensibility	• Clinical presentation • Mild elevation of creatine phosphokinase • Neurophysiological exam • Molecular analysis
Guillain-Barré syndrome	Peripheral nerves	• Paresthesias • Distal and ascending progressive muscle weakness • Dysfunction of cranial nerves and of the innervation respiratory muscles • Autonomic dysfunction	• Clinical presentation • Cerebrospinal fluid exam • Electroneurophysiological exam
Acute and subacute myopathy	Muscle	• Symmetric and proximal muscle weakness without sensory involvement • Swallowing problems	• Clinical presentation • Muscle biopsy • Elevation of creatine phosphokinase • Neurophysiological exam
Chronic myopathy	Muscle	• Symmetric and proximal muscle weakness without sensory involvement • Postural scoliosis	• Clinical presentation • Muscle biopsy • Elevation of creatine phosphokinase • Molecular investigation • Neurophysiological exam
Parkinson's disease	Upper motor neuron and ganglion base	• Tremor • Stiffness • Postural alterations • Nonmotor symptoms of the autonomic, cognitive and postural type • Sleep disorders	• Clinical presentation • Neurophysiological exam

genetic defects increasing a person's susceptibility to the disease.

The clinical presentation is usually nonspecific, as the beginning of the clinical picture depends on the neurologic area that has been primarily affected. The physician should suspect the disease during the history taking and examination of the patient when the following conditions are seen: (1) atrophy (e.g., of the first interosseous muscle of the hand); (2) distal muscle weakness (e.g., drop foot in the absence of root pain); (3) disseminated or focal fasciculation; (4) spasticity and signs that the first motor neuron is compromised; (5) progressive motor loss both for swallowing and for movements of the face and tongue; and (6) complaints of sometimes intense cramps, unrelated to physical effort and at less frequent sites (e.g., the submandibular region).

In one study, 78% of patients with ALS reported that the onset of pain occurred in the 24 hours prior to presenting to the physician, with a mean number of 3 points on the pain severity scale that varies from 0 (no pain) to 10

Table 7.2 Description of the Neuromuscular Diseases and Associated Pain

Pathology	Causes of Pain	Usual Location of Pain	Incidence of Back Pain
Amyotrophic lateral sclerosis	Muscle atrophy with joint overload	Shoulder, hip, and back	50%
Spinal muscular atrophy	Muscle atrophy with joint overload and osteoporotic fractures	Shoulder, hip, and back	92%
Guillain-Barré syndrome	Muscle atrophy with joint overload and inflammatory radiculopathy	Back and lower limbs	55 to 72%
Acute and subacute myopathy	Muscle atrophy with joint overload	Shoulder, hip, and back	50 to 60%
Chronic myopathy	Muscle atrophy with joint overload	Shoulder, hip, and back	66 to 76%
Parkinson's disease	Hypertonia, abnormal posture in flexion, and acceleration of diskopathy	Shoulders, pelvis, knee, and ankle	74%

(pain as bad as you can imagine).[4] Moderate to severe pain was found in 33% of the cases. The frequency and intensity of the pain correlated with a worsened function score and with a longer duration of the disease.[5] Back pain affects 50% of patients, without radicular involvement.[4] Other common places where pain appeared were the area of the shoulder and hip, suggesting as an etiologic factor the overload of joints due to the loss of the protective layer caused by muscle atrophy (**Table 7.2**).[4,5]

Spinal Muscle Atrophy

Spinal muscle atrophy (SMA) is an autosomal recessive genetic disorder of the motor neuron. The patient presents with progressive muscle weakness because of the loss of the lower motor neurons located in the anterior horns of the spinal cord and nuclei of the cranial nerves. As to genetics, the gene of motor neuron survival (MNS) is situated on the long arm of chromosome 5 (Sq11.13.3) that encodes the protein that carries its name. Each normal individual has two MNS genes, *MNS1* and *MNS2;* a mutation, deletion, or rearrangement of *MNS1* causes 95% of SMAs.[6]

There are many types of SMA, which can be classified according to their predominantly proximal or distal location. The proximal presentation is more frequent. SMA can also be classified, based on symptom onset, as severe, Werdnig-Hoffmann (type I); intermediate form (type II) (**Fig. 7.1**); juvenile form, Kugelberg-Wellander (type III); and the adult beginning form (type IV).

The clinical presentation of these forms has in common the following findings: progressive muscle weakness, deep myotatic areflexia, hypotonia, and preserved sensitivity, without the involvement of the central nervous system. In type I, symptoms begin early, such as intrauterus, at birth, or in the first 3 to 6 months of life. In these cases the clinical presentation is alterations in respiration and swallowing, and life expectancy is no longer than 2 years. In type II, symptoms begin at ages 6 to 18 months, and include decreased motor development. These patients are able to sit with or without support, and they may reach the stage of being able to stand, generally with external support, but they are unable to walk, and they demonstrate bulbar weakness and difficulty in swallowing. Over time, among other abnormalities, there are respiratory alterations, deformities, and scoliosis. In type III, symptoms begin after 18 months of age and either before the age of 3 (type IIIa) or at age 3 or older (type IIIb). Type IIIa patients are no longer walking by the age of 20 years, and type IIIb patients are no longer

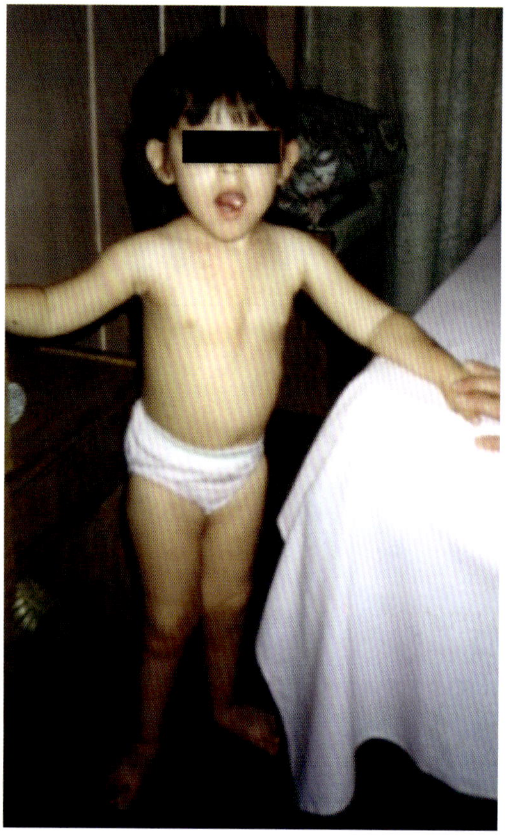

Fig. 7.1 Patient with spinal muscular atrophy type II, standing, with support.

walking at some point after age 20 years, even with difficulty or the help of ortheses. In type IV, symptoms of muscle weakness and areflexia begin between the second and fourth decades of life.

The initial clinical and laboratory picture may be confused with that of other pathologies, especially myopathies due to elevation of creatine phosphokinase (CPK), a muscle marker, to at most five times above the normal value. Electroneuromyography shows a neurogenic pattern. The diagnosis is based on clinical presentation, laboratory findings, electrophysiological results, and molecular analysis showing the absence of exon 7 of the *SMN1* gene.

In one study, 71% of adolescents with SMA type II or III had persistent or recurrent chronic pain in the previous 3 months; of these patients, 92% experienced pain for longer than 3 months.[7] The pain lasted less than 1 hour in 46% of cases and between 1 and 12 hours in 36%. The most common site of pain, in 92% of cases, was the region of the neck or back, and was more severe in the nonambulating patients (**Table 7.2**).

None of the adolescents with SMA type II who were treated with spine surgery ambulated, whereas in SMA type III 57% could ambulate. Despite surgery, a large number still reported back pain and neck pain. A possible cause of this pain was osteoporotic fractures.[7] The pain was exacerbated when the patients were being lifted and transferred (62%), when seated (46%), and during other activities (39%). Pain relief was observed from measures that did not involve drugs. Rest and change of position relieved pain in 62% of the cases, and, in patients who did not ambulate, change of position was the maneuver that gave the most relief.

Polyradiculoneuropathies

Guillain-Barré syndrome (GBS) is an acute inflammatory polyradiculoneuropathy that presents with muscle weakness and reduction or absence of deep myotatic reflexes. It has several subclassifications: acute inflammatory demyelinating polyradiculoneuropathy (AIDP), acute motor axonal neuropathy (AMAN), acute sensorimotor axonal neuropathy (ASMAN), and Miller Fisher syndrome.

Initially it was described as a demyelinating process, but other similar cases were described that affect the axon and the node of Ranvier. The disease is characterized by an immune-mediated disorder, usually preceded by an infection, that induces the production of antibodies that attack components of the nerve root and the nerve, especially components of the myelin sheath, such as gangliosides and glycolipids (e.g., GM1 and GD1b).

The triggering phenomenon may be a mild respiratory or intestinal infection 2 to 4 weeks before the symptoms begin. The clinical presentation generally includes paresthesia, as well as progressive muscle weakness, usually ascending, from the lower limbs to the upper limbs and trunk, and it can evolve within hours or days to dysfunction of the cranial nerves and of the innervation of respiratory muscles. The clinical picture generally reaches its worst point in 30 days, but the abnormalities may take days, months, or years to revert. Normally, 70% of patients recover within 12 months and 82% within 24 months. Unfortunately, some patients may have definitive sequelae or even die as a consequence of respiratory failure and autonomic alterations such as hypotension and cardiac arrhythmia.

The diagnosis is suspected from the clinical picture of paresis/flaccid ascending paralysis, sensory alteration on a smaller scale, and areflexia. The examination of cerebrospinal fluid after about 1 week shows a protein-cytological disproportion, with increase of proteins and normal white cellularity in 80 to 90% of patients. Electroneuromyography shows a demyelinating involvement from the third or fourth day onward, but generally with characteristic signs after the first and especially the second week of onset of the disease. Because myelin is responsible for speed in the transport of information, there is a slowdown in nerve conduction, with or without prolonged latency, as well as temporal dispersion, partial or total conduction blockage (generally motor), and prolonged late waves (F waves). When axonal involvement is more severe, there is an active denervation that is expressed by fibrillation and positive wave. Patients can be treated with plasmapheresis or intravenous human immunoglobulin. Respirator failure must be prevented by means of mechanical ventilation. Autonomic intercurrences are possible, especially when there is motor improvement, due to the risk of cardiac arrest and hypotension.

The onset of painful symptoms of moderate to severe intensity may occur in several parts of the body, generally in the back. Often pain begins in the lower back or lumbosacral region, and sometimes it radiates to the lower limbs, simulating sciatic pain, which is caused by the inflammatory radiculopathy. About 55% of patients present with back pain, and 72% complain of back pain during the course of the disease.[8] The presence of back pain alone, independent of the lower limbs being radiated, is not a sign of GBS onset; other symptoms must also be present, such as flaccidity, lack of strength, paresthesias, or areflexia, in order to corroborate the diagnostic hypothesis of GBS (**Tables 7.1** and **7.2**).[9]

In children younger than 10 years of age, back pain may be the initial symptom in 20% of cases.[10] However, back pain and lower limb pain may be present in 83% of children under the age of 6 at the beginning of the illness. In the acute phase, there is an association between back pain and the thickening and uptake of contrast in the nerve roots detected on magnetic resonance imaging (MRI) due to inflammation or compression of the nerve roots.[10,11]

Clinical evolution of acute or subacute back pain, with or without radiation to the lower limbs and an autonomic disorder such as bladder dysfunction for longer than 24 hours, probably is not GBS but rather a medullar lesion, such as myelitis, in which the sensory level has not yet appeared, or has been undervalued.

Myopathies

Myopathies are a heterogeneous group of diseases, in which muscle fibers, and their structures, channels, or metabolism, as well as the muscle interstice, are affected, resulting in muscle weakness.

The myopathies may present as hereditary or acquired. Hereditary myopathies generally evolve chronically; the acquired myopathies haven't muscle involvement prior the initial signals presentation. Regarding the anatomopathology, muscle fiber necrosis may be present or possibly may have been replaced by inflammatory infiltrated fatty tissue proportional to the necrosis, and by increased connective tissue; these findings indicate the presence of dystrophy. In the myopathies, the structure of the muscle fibers is affected; in inflammatory myopathy, there is a predominance of inflammatory infiltrate.

The clinical picture typical of a myopathy is symmetrical and proximal muscle weakness without any sensory involvement, in contrast to peripheral neuropathies, which are distal and symmetrical to the sensory involvement (**Tables 7.1** and **7.2**).

Myopathies can be acute, subacute, or chronic. The acute and subacute myopathies include inflammatory myopathies of the polymyositis type, dermatomyositis, and myositis due to inclusion bodies; myopathies induced by drugs such as statin; and infectious myositis. The chronic and hereditary myopathies includes muscular dystrophies, myotonias of the dystrophic type or of other types, channelopathies, and congenital and mitochondrial myopathies. This discussion focuses on lower back pain resulting from inflammatory myopathies, statin myopathy, and dystrophinopathies such as Duchenne's muscular dystrophy (DMD), Becker's muscular dystrophy (BMD), myotonic dystrophy, and facioscapulohumeral dystrophy.

Polymyositis and Dermatomyositis

Polymyositis and dermatomyositis are nonsuppurative and idiopathic inflammatory diseases of the muscles. In polymyositis only the muscles are involved, whereas in dermatomyositis both the muscles and the skin are involved.

The disease presents with proximal and symmetrical muscle weakness, often accompanied by pain that develops over weeks or months. Especially in polymyositis the "dropped head" sign can be seen, because of the weakness of the posterior cervical muscles and difficulty in swallowing. In dermatomyositis, the skin changes are characterized by edema and erythema of the eyelids (heliotrope), erythema on the extensor surfaces of the fingers (Gottron's sign), and small dark-red points on the edge of the cuticles (periungual vasculitis). The muscle enzymes of CPK are elevated, and electroneuromyography identifies the myopathic and denervation pattern.

Muscle biopsy in polymyositis shows necrosis, degeneration, and regeneration of fibers, with an inflammatory infiltrate surrounding fibers that are generally not necrotic, such as those between the muscle fibers. This inflammatory infiltrate is composed of CD8 T lymphocytes, suggesting a cytotoxic process mediated by T cells against muscle antigens that have not been well defined. In contrast, in dermatomyositis there is a vasculitis, and this inflammatory infiltration includes predominantly B cells and CD4 helper lymphocytes, hence with humoral mediation. Perifascicular atrophy is found as a result of microinfarctions that are pathognomonic, in addition to degeneration, regeneration, and necrosis of muscle fibers.

The muscle inflammation observed may cause mild or moderate pain disseminated throughout the body, including the back.

Myopathy Caused by Statins

Statins are prescribed for treating dyslipidemias; they inhibit 3-hydroxy-3-methylglutaryl coenzyme A (HMG-CoA) reductase, ultimately helping reduce myocardial and cerebral infarctions. One of the side effects is muscle alteration. Patients who use statins have a 50% greater likelihood of having musculoskeletal pain and a 50 to 60% greater likelihood of having pain in the back and legs.[12]

The clinical manifestations can vary from minor complaints of muscle fatigue that does not interfere with the patient's functioning to the very serious symptom of rhabdomyolysis. The American College of Cardiology (ACC)/ American Heart Association (AHA)/ National Heart, Lung, and Blood Institute (NHLBI) defined the following terms used for muscle symptoms of statin[13]: myalgia is muscle pain without an elevation of CPK; myopathy is any muscle disease; myositis is muscle symptoms with increased CPK; and rhabdomyolysis is muscular symptoms in association with a CPK elevation more than 10 times the normal upper limit, the elevation of creatinine, and the occasional presence of myoglobinuria.

Myalgia is expressed clinically by muscle weakness, pain in the proximal muscles, and/or back pain. The mean time to onset of myalgia after beginning statin use is still under discussion, but it usually occurs after about 1 month. The myopathic picture appears to be well correlated with the statin dose and to be independent of cholesterol reduction.[14]

Case Study

A 52-year-old man, a smoker with prior myocardial infarction, was prescribed a statin. After 3 months, he started to experience serious lower back pain, with mild radiation to the lateral and anterior portion of the right thigh, without a deficit of strength or a change in sensitivity. An extensive examination was performed of the hip and urinary system, as well as determining the possibility of radicular alterations, and the patients medications were reviewed. Nothing was found to explain his discomfort. After the statins were withdrawn, the lower back pain disappeared in 5 to 10 days.

Because statin-induced muscle abnormalities are common, physicians must seriously weigh the risk of muscle symptoms against the statin' benefit of preventing a myocardial infarction or cerebrovascular accident.

Dystrophinopathies

Dystrophin is a protein essential to the muscle structure. It is located subsarcolemmally, connecting the actin to the sarcolemma. The gene that encodes dystrophin is located on the short arm of chromosome X (locus Xp21) and it is the largest gene in humans, with 79 exons. Mutations of this gene cause a partial or total dysfunction of this protein, giving rise to two important muscular dystrophies, DMD and BMD.

Both DMD and BMD appear in boys because they are limited to chromosome X. DMD begins earlier and is more severe, and BMD is milder with a later onset. DMD can begin as early as around 18 months, but it is generally noticed around the age of 4 years. There is proximal muscle weakness, especially in the lower limbs, pseudohypertrophy of the calves, anserine gait, and Gowers's sign, with a rise from a sitting to a standing position by grasping and pulling on body parts from the knees to hips until reach an erect position (laborious escalade on itself). These findings reflect muscle involvement in general, and are not pathognomonic of the dystrophinopathies. Over time, the picture becomes more severe, with progressive difficulties until the patient stops walking between the ages of 9 and 13 years. Later there are difficulties with the upper limbs as well as scoliosis, especially in wheelchair users.

The elevation of CPK in the blood is more than 10 times the upper limit for the patient's age, and sometimes may be 50 to 100 times the upper limit. Because the transaminases rise, many children undergo liver investigation, including liver biopsies, and it must be remembered that transaminases are also part of the muscle enzymes. In more advanced cases, due to the simple fact that there is no more muscle to be degraded, the muscle enzymes may become normal. Electroneuromyography has a myopathic pattern, with normal neuroconduction, and the needle exam shows short duration and short range potentials, often polyphasic, and increased paradoxical recruitment. Muscle biopsy shows a dystrophic pattern, with immunocytochemistry evidencing almost complete absence of dystrophin in muscle fibers (**Fig. 7.2**). Molecular analysis by polymerase chain reaction (PCR) shows an abnormality in 60 to 70% of cases, and it is useful to identify the abnormality by sequencing the dystrophin gene.

A BMD presents with milder defects in dystrophin, so that although the protein is truncated, it is partially functional. The clinical picture is similar to that observed in DMD, but with a later onset of symptoms, after the age of 5 to 7 years, or sometimes in adolescence (**Fig. 7.3a**). Enzymatic alterations may be small, with a CPK that is less than 10 times the normal level or even normal. The electroneuromyographic alterations are similar to those in DMD, and the muscle biopsy may reflect the same dystrophic pattern, but in immunocytochemistry there is the partial presence of dystrophin (**Fig. 7.3b,c**). The molecular analysis by PCR may be normal.

In one study, 41% of patients with DMD/BMD experienced pain in the previous 3 months,[7] and of these patients, 76% had neck and back pain. Similar to the findings reported with SMA, nonambulating patients had more pain, especially back pain. The factors that most exacerbates the pain were sitting position in 52%, and daily activities in 44%; the factors that relieved pain were rest in 88%, change of position in 80%, and massage in 64%. The causes of the pain, both in ambulating and nonambulating patients, are the same described above for patients with SMA.

Improved patient care, especially mechanical ventilation, increases the survival of these

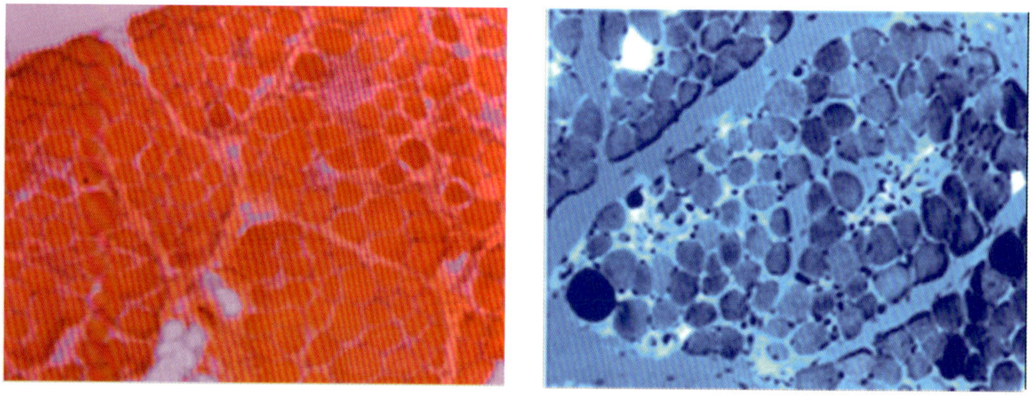

a

Fig. 7.2 Dystrophic pattern in Duchenne's muscular dystrophy. **(a)** Hematoxylin and eosin stain. **(b)** Modified Gomori trichrome stain.

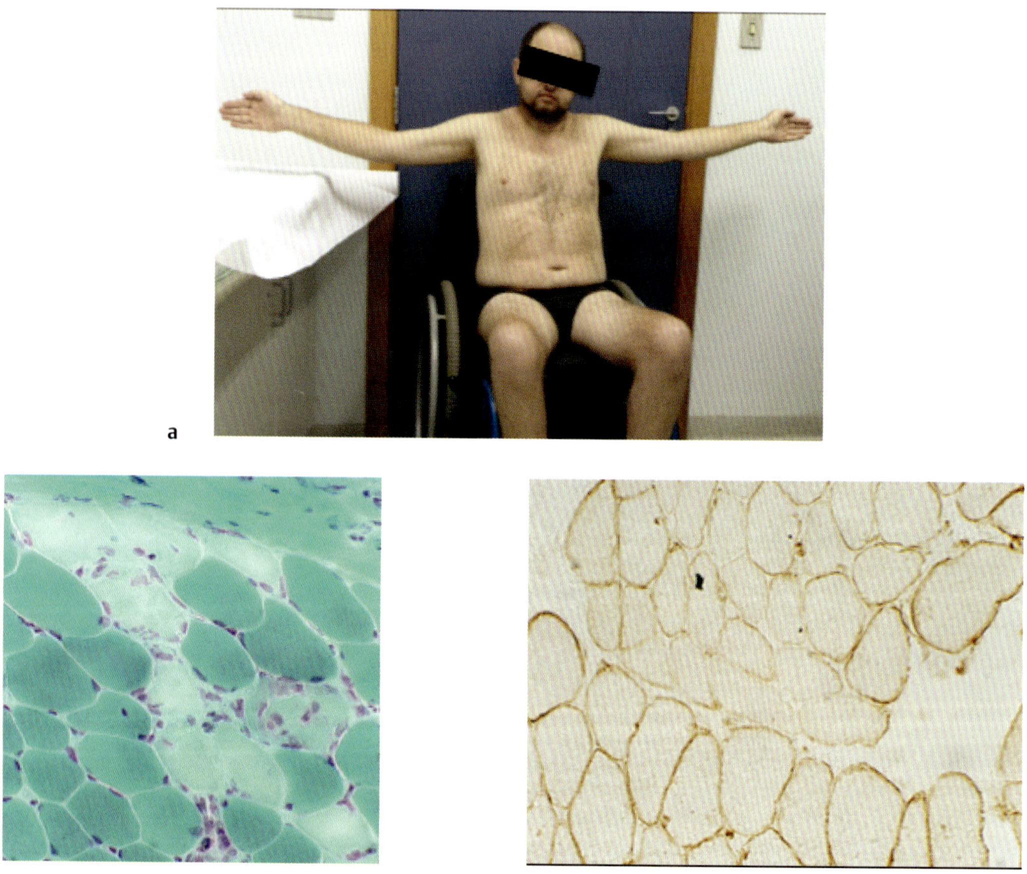

a

b

Fig. 7.3 **(a)** Becker's muscular dystrophy patient with proximal weakness in the upper limbs and atrophy of both quadríceps. **(b)** Dystrophic pattern with fiber necrosis in histological exam (modified Gomori trichrome stain). **(c)** Dystrophin with absence of immunofixation on the periphery of the fibers (immunoperoxidase stain).

patients, and in one study 85% reached the age of 30 years.[15] The incidence of pain was 73.5% in patients with DMD over the age of 20 years who were nonambulators and on mechanical ventilation; 24.1% had back pain and 11.4% neck pain.[16] Of patients with a poor quality of life, 80% reported experiencing pain and fatigue, whereas of patients with a good quality of life, the prevalence of pain was 70%.

Myotonic Muscular Dystrophy

Myotonic muscular dystrophy (MMD) is the most frequent neuromuscular disease. It is hereditary and entails a multifaceted clinical picture, as many patients do not present all the characteristics of the pathology. It is classified as type I and type II; the genetic abnormality of MMD I is located on the long arm of chromosome 19, in gene *DMPK* (myotonin protein kinase), whereas in type II the altered gene is *CBBP* (ZNF9) located on the long arm of chromosome 3. Both genes in normal people produce 3 to 37 repeats of trinucleotide CTG, but in these patients there are many more repetitions, affecting especially the chlorine channels, leading to weakness.[17] It is autosomal dominant, and has a characteristic called phenomenon of anticipation, which means that in each generation symptom onset occurs earlier than in the previous generation; for example, in one generation it may occur at 60 years of age, and in later generations, over time, it may begin immediately after birth.

Myotonia or difficulty in relaxing after muscle contraction is one of the marked symptoms of MMD I, together with muscle weakness, distal predominance, drop foot, and slapping gait. The weakness of myotonic muscular dystrophy is distal, in contrast to what is observed in myopathy, where it is proximal. There can be facial weakness (**Fig. 7.4**) with atrophy of the temporal muscles, premature and frontal baldness, endocrinologic involvement (hypogonadism, diabetes mellitus), ocular changes (cataract), cardiac symptoms (branch block), mental alterations in some patients (mental retardation), and other symptoms. Over time, the clinical picture becomes worse, both for the muscles and for other organs. MMD II has different characteristics from MMD I, such as proximal muscle weakness, pain, and stiffness.

The diagnosis may be suggested by electroneuromyography, which identifies myotonic discharges with the characteristic sound of accelerating and decelerating a motorbike, as well as a myopathic pattern. The confirmation comes with a molecular analysis showing a large number of expansion CTGs in MMD I, and in MMD II there are mutations and an expansion, with a repeated sequence of tetranucleotide.

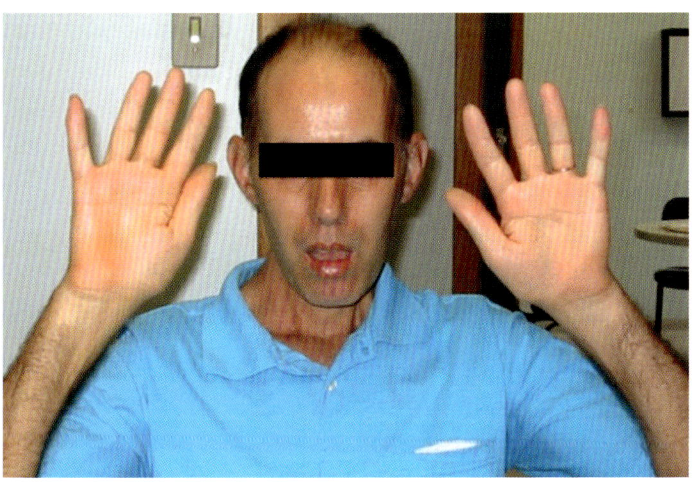

Fig. 7.4 Myotonic muscular dystrophy type I (Steinert) with facial muscle weakness, baldness, and atrophy of the hands.

Pain is one of the factors that compromise the quality of life of patients with MMD; in one study 69% of patients reported having pain within the previous week, and in 66% it was back pain.[18]

The possible causes of this back pain are discussed in the next subsection.

Facioscapulohumeral Dystrophy

This is an autosomal dominant neuromuscular disease with high penetrance and variable expression in the affected families, and the alteration is located on the long arm of chromosome 4 at locus 35 (4q35), with a contraction mutation in the DNA fragment D4Z4.

The symptoms of facioscapulohumeral dystrophy (FSHD) generally begin in adolescence or early adulthood, with weakness of the facial muscles and later of the scapular waist muscles, and with the presence of a winged scapula. Over time, weakness appears in the leg and lower region of the abdominal muscles. Generally the evolution is insidious, and patients may require a wheelchair at the most advanced stages. Some patients do not experience clinical symptoms and do not realize that they have deficits. The diagnosis is made based on the clinical characteristics of the disease and on a electroneuromyographic study that shows myopathic involvement of the more proximal muscles. The level of muscle enzymes is generally normal.

Although it is not listed among the symptoms of FSHD, pain is one of the frequent complaints.[19] In one study, 82 to 89% of patients reported pain in the previous week; in 75 to 78% it was back pain.[19] The patients whose mobility was limited and who were using wheelchairs, crutches, or canes experienced more pain, especially back pain.

Patients with MMD and FSHD more frequently present with back pain, reflecting the more marked weakness in the trunk and neck muscles.[18] In addition, the predominant weakness of the flexor muscle, compared with the extensor, favors the onset of kyphosis and scoliosis. Early degeneration of the spine also favors the occurrence of pain.[19]

Parkinson's Disease and Dystonia

Parkinson's disease (PD) is a neurodegenerative, progressive, and chronic disorder that affects mainly individuals over the age of 50 years as a result of dopamine deficiency through the nigrostriatal tract. The motor clinical manifestations are characterized by tremor, stiffness, postural alterations, and nonmotor symptoms of the autonomic, cognitive, and postural types, as well as sleep disorders; pain is reported in 68 to 85%[20] (**Table 7.1**).

Ford[17] reported five types of pain in PD:

1. Musculoskeletal pain: resulting from parkinsonian stiffness, rheumatologic disease, or skeletal deformity
2. Radicular-neuropathic pain: resulting from radicular lesion, peripheral neuropathy, or focal neuropathy
3. Dystonic pain: related to antiparkinsonian medication
4. Central neuropathic pain related to antiparkinsonian medication
5. Acathisia: induced by a drug or in an "off" period

Musculoskeletal pain is relevant because it occurs in 70% of patients, and is attributed to postural and joint involvement and cramps (**Table 7.2**).[20] The muscles of the neck, paraspinal, and calf regions are more easily affected, whereas the most affected joints are the shoulders, pelvis, knee, and ankle, with a prevalence between 45 and 74%.[21]

The prevalence of radiculoneuropathic pain ranges from 5 to 20% and appears to be associated with paresthesias and weaknesses in the areas innervated by roots or nerves.[17,22] The incidence of back and radicular pain is 74% and 38%, respectively.[22]

Both abnormal muscle tone and reduced flexibility of the spine are causes of nonradicular back pain resulting from skeletal structures, soft tissues, and muscles. The acceleration of spinal diskopathy, and, consequently, worsened pain is provoked by abnormal postural changes, dystonia, festinating gait (gait with quick start, fast short steps leaning forward), and kyphosis.[23]

If the musculoskeletal pain is the result of parkinsonian stiffness and dopaminergic therapy, physiotherapy and exercises are indicated. There is no direct relationship between the intensity of the back pain and the duration of the disease, the patient's age, the stage of the disease, the number of hours a day in the "off" phase, or subthalamic stimulation.[20]

Back pain in patients with neuromuscular disease and movement disorders is frequent and compromises their quality of life. When there are other more noticeable signs and symptoms related to the pathology, back pain may be neglected or underdiagnosed.

Chapter Summary

Patients with neuromuscular diseases, Parkinson's disease, or dystonia experience back pain because of the disease's neuromuscular consequences. Usually patients first report body pain in general, and later they report back pain. It is important to determine the patient's specific pathology so as to place the clinical findings in the disease context for treatment purposes. Parkinsonian stiffness, rheumatologic diseases, skeletal deformities, radicular lesions, and peripheral or focal neuropathy are major causes of musculoskeletal pain. Imbalance of the trunk and weakness of extensor muscles in musculoskeletal diseases contribute to pain and degeneration of the spine.

Pearls

- Evaluate and treat the patient in the context of the diagnosed neuromuscular disorders, be it Parkinson's disease or dystonia, and their various clinical findings; do not just treat the back pain symptom.
- In nonambulating patients, back pain is an important factor in a reduced quality of life. It is exacerbated by the constant sitting position. Changing position and muscle relaxation relieve the discomfort.
- Back pain, lumbosacral pain, and pain in the legs may be the initial symptom in GBS, and it is important to determine whether there has been a recent infection, generally pulmonary or gastroenterological, or symmetrical areflexia. This occurs due to inflammation or compression of the nerve roots, which can be seen on MRI.
- Back pain with urinary difficulties must be investigated for the possibility of a medullary or polyradicular lesion.
- The use of statins should be explored in patients with back pain; other muscle pains, cramps, and CPK elevation should also be evaluated.

Pitfalls

- Failing to recognize other neurologic signs and symptoms together with muscle pain
- Failing to recognize that muscle pain in these patients is generally not intense or acute, except for GBS patients
- Failing to recognize that back pain in neuromuscular diseases, PD, and dystonias is not an isolated symptom

References

Five Must-Read References

1. Almeida TF, Roizenblatt S, Tufik S. Afferent pain pathways: a neuroanatomical review. Brain Res 2004; 1000:40–56
2. Manchikanti L. Epidemiology of low back pain. Pain Physician 2000;3:167–192
3. Falavigna A, de Braga GL, Monteiro GM, et al. The epidemiological profile of a middle-aged population with low back pain in southern Brazil. Spine 2015;40: E359–E365
4. Hanisch F, Skudlarek A, Berndt J, Kornhuber ME. Characteristics of pain in amyotrophic lateral sclerosis. Brain Behav 2015;5:e00296
5. Chiò A, Canosa A, Gallo S, et al. Pain in amyotrophic lateral sclerosis: a population-based controlled study. Eur J Neurol 2012;19:551–555
6. Bürglen L, Lefebvre S, Clermont O, et al. Structure and organization of the human survival motor neurone (SMN) gene. Genomics 1996;32:479–482
7. **Lager C, Kroksmark AK. Pain in adolescents with spinal muscular atrophy and Duchenne and Becker muscular dystrophy. Eur J Paediatr Neurol 2015; 19:537–546**
8. **Ropper AH, Shahani BT. Pain in Guillain-Barré syndrome. Arch Neurol 1984;41:511–514**
9. Grant R. Backache and the Guillain-Barre syndrome. Br Med J (Clin Res Ed) 1986;293:506
10. Jones HR. Childhood Guillain-Barré syndrome: clinical presentation, diagnosis, and therapy. J Child Neurol 1996;11:4–12
11. Micó SI, Aliaga CP, Martín PP, Pérez-Gramunt MA, eds. Dolor lumbar y de miembros inferiores con rechazo de la deambulación como modo de presentación de síndrome de Guillain-Barré. An Pediatr (Barc) 2007;66:87–106
12. **Buettner C, Davis RB, Leveille SG, Mittleman MA, Mukamal KJ. Prevalence of musculoskeletal pain and statin use. J Gen Intern Med 2008;23:1182–1186**
13. Pasternak RC, Smith SC Jr, Bairey-Merz CN, Grundy SM, Cleeman JI, Lenfant C; American College of Cardiology; American Heart Association; National Heart, Lung and Blood Institute. ACC/AHA/NHLBI clinical advisory on the use and safety of statins. J Am Coll Cardiol 2002;40:567–572
14. Scandinavian Simvastatin Survival Study Group. Randomised trial of cholesterol lowering in 4444 patients with coronary heart disease: the Scandinavian Simvastatin Survival Study (4S). Lancet 1994; 344:1383–1389
15. Passamano L, Taglia A, Palladino A, et al. Improvement of survival in Duchenne muscular dystrophy: retrospective analysis of 835 patients. Acta Myologica 2012;31:121–125
16. Pangalila RF, van den Bos GA, Bartels B, Bergen M, Stam HJ, Roebroeck ME. Prevalence of fatigue, pain, and affective disorders in adults with Duchenne muscular dystrophy and their associations with quality of life. Arch Phys Med Rehabil 2015;96:1242–1247
17. Ford B. Pain in Parkinson's disease. Mov Disord 2010;25(Suppl 1):S98–103
18. **Jensen MP, Hoffman AJ, Stoelb BL, Abresch RT, Carter GT, McDonald CM. Chronic pain in persons with myotonic dystrophy and facioscapulohumeral dystrophy. Arch Phys Med Rehabil 2008;89:320–328**
19. Bushby KM, Pollitt C, Johnson MA, Rogers MT, Chinnery PF. Muscle pain as a prominent feature of facioscapulohumeral muscular dystrophy (FSHD): four illustrative case reports. Neuromuscul Disord 1998; 8:574–579
20. Beiske AG, Loge JH, Rønningen A, Svensson E. Pain in Parkinson's disease: prevalence and characteristics. Pain 2009;141:173–177
21. Fil A, Cano-de-la-Cuerda R, Muñoz-Hellín E, Vela L, Ramiro-González M, Fernández-de-Las-Peñas C. Pain in Parkinson disease: a review of the literature. Parkinsonism Relat Disord 2013;19:285–294, discussion 285
22. **Broetz D, Eichner M, Gasser T, Weller M, Steinbach JP. Radicular and nonradicular back pain in Parkinson's disease: a controlled study. Mov Disord 2007;22: 853–856**
23. Adams MA, Freeman BJC, Morrison HP, Nelson IW, Dolan P. Mechanical initiation of intervertebral disc degeneration. Spine 2000;25:1625–1636

8

Back Pain in Children and Adolescents

Katherine M. Schroeder, Erica E. Gonzalez, and John P. Dormans

Introduction

Historically, back pain in children and adolescents was considered rare and often a serious complaint. However, its prevalence has increased over recent years.[1,2] Although the cause of back pain is often associated with a condition that improves spontaneously and has a favorable natural history, providers should have a high index of suspicion for more serious pathologies. This chapter reviews the epidemiology, evaluation, differential diagnosis, and initial treatment of children and adolescents who present with complaints of back pain.

Epidemiology

Back pain in the pediatric population is more common than previously thought,[1,2] with reported rates of 7 to 58% in the literature.[3] It can be expected that 10 to 30% of the normal pediatric population will experience back pain at some point by the time they reach adolescence.[4] Reported risk factors for childhood back pain include older age, a family history of back pain, increased physical activity or participation in competitive sports, manual work, and carrying a heavy backpack.[3]

Clinical Evaluation

A detailed history and physical examination are essential when evaluating a child or adolescent with back pain. Duration, severity, frequency and inciting factors should be determined. Any history of trauma, recent illness, or infection should be documented. Potential warning signs should be further investigated, including constitutional symptoms such as night sweats or weight loss, severe pain, recurrent or worsening back pain, night pain, limp or altered gait, and back pain in a younger child, especially under the age of 5 years (**Table 8.1**).[2] A full physical exam should be performed, including inspecting the child's spine for midline lesions that may indicate intraspinal pathology. The spine should be palpated for tenderness, masses, or stepoff of the posterior elements. Range of motion of the spine, significant kyphosis or lordosis, and gait should be assessed, and the Adams forward bend test should be performed. A complete neurologic examination should be performed, including motor and sensory exams, as well as deep tendon reflexes, abdominal reflexes, and upper motor neuron signs.[1] In 2010, Fujimori et al[5] reported that the sensitivity of the abnormal superficial abdominal reflex for syringomyelia in presumed idiopathic scoliosis was 89%, with a 95% specificity.

Table 8.1 "Red Flags" in the Initial Assessment of a Pediatric Patient Presenting with Back Pain

"Red Flags" from the History	"Red Flags" on the Physical Examination
Severe, worsening, or recurring pain	Neurologic symptoms
Night pain	Limp/gait abnormality
Fever, weight loss, reduced appetite	Fever, tachycardia
Loss of bowel/bladder control	Progressive deformity
Refusal to bear weight	Abnormal bruising or bleeding
Back pain in a young child (< 5 years of age)	Lymphadenopathy or abdominal mass
Lost or delayed developmental milestones	

A cavus foot can also be a sign of intraspinal pathology. It is also often useful to do a thorough hip exam, assess pelvic obliquity, and look for a leg length discrepancy that may be associated with the patient's complaint of back pain. A wide differential diagnosis should be kept in mind during the initial evaluation (**Box 8.1**). A high index of suspicion should be maintained when evaluating a child with back pain, as pain is the most common presenting complaint for most tumors and infections in the pediatric spine and pelvis.

Box 8.1 Differential Diagnosis of Back Pain in a Child or Adolescent

- Nonspecific/mechanical low back pain
- Spondylolysis and spondylolisthesis
- Scheuermann kyphosis
- Scoliosis
- Lumbar disk herniation
- Trauma
- Infection: diskitis, vertebral osteomyelitis, sacroiliac joint infection, epidural abscess
- Benign neoplasms: Langerhans cell histiocytosis, aneurysmal bone cyst, osteoblastoma, osteoid osteoma, osteochondroma
- Malignant neoplasms: Ewing sarcoma, osteogenic sarcoma, chondrosarcoma, leukemia
- Metastatic disease: rhabdomyosarcoma, neuroblastoma, Wilms' tumor, lymphoma
- Intraspinal tumor: astrocytoma, ependymoma
- Systemic causes: osteoporosis, juvenile idiopathic arthritis
- Referred back pain: renal abnormalities, pyelonephritis, retroperitoneal lesions, pelvic inflammatory disease

Full length posteroanterior (PA) and lateral spine radiographs should be obtained in most cases. Further imaging studies should be utilized as indicated. Magnetic resonance imaging (MRI), computed tomography (CT), and bone scans all have a role in spine imaging. MRI is considered the gold standard for most spinal pathologies, particularly the more serious pathologies such as tumors or infection. It should be kept in mind that younger patients require sedation for an MRI, and this may require that the study be done at a children's hospital or at a facility with appropriate anesthesia support. Single photon emission computed tomography (SPECT) and CT scans are primarily used in the diagnosis of spondylolysis, but they can also be used in the acute trauma situation when a fracture may be suspected. The use of bone scans has decreased over recent years, but they are still used to diagnose a stress reaction in the par interarticularis. A bone scan may also be useful if the patient has multiple sites of complaints or if there is concern about a multifocal process such as leukemia, Langerhans cell histiocytosis (LCH), chronic recurrent multifocal osteomyelitis (CRMO), or metastasis. It is important to review the patient's previous imaging rather than relying on just the imaging report, as adult radiologists may be less familiar with pediatric spine conditions.

Laboratory studies are useful, particularly where there is suspicion for infection or tumor. A complete blood count with peripheral blood smear can be useful in the diagnosis of leukemia. Although nonspecific, increases in the white blood cell count and an elevated C-reactive protein and erythrocyte sedimentation rate can be seen in most patients with an infection, but may also be seen in patients with malignancies.[6] Blood cultures can be useful in identifying an organism in patients with diskitis or vertebral osteomyelitis.[6]

It is important to remember that back pain can be a referred pain, a symptom, for example, of renal, urinary, abdominal, or gynecologic problems. Lymphoma and leukemia can also present with back pain. If the picture is unclear or if one of these pathologies is suspected, it is important to involve the patient's primary care physician or other specialists.

Nonspecific Low Back Pain

Nonspecific back pain can be defined as pain when there is no identifiable etiology. Sources of nonspecific low back pain can be muscle strain, overuse, contusion, poor posture, or deconditioning. Running, lifting weight, or frequent sitting typically brings on the pain. It was originally thought that the majority of children and adolescents who present with back pain had diagnosable pathologies, but recent reports have found that mechanical or nonspecific back pain can be seen in up to 75% of adolescents presenting with back pain.[7,8] This is generally a diagnosis of exclusion after a thorough history and physical. The first line of treatment is physical therapy and activity modification, particularly if an overuse injury is suspected.

Even a patient with negative initial imaging and suspected nonspecific back pain should be followed to ensure that the pain is improving. Worsening pain or symptoms could suggest another diagnosis, and thus further workup is indicated.

Spondylolysis and Spondylolisthesis

Spondylolysis and spondylolisthesis are common causes of back pain in children over the age of 10 years and are rarely seen in children under the age of 5 years.[3,9] Spondylolysis is a defect in the pars interarticularis and most commonly affects the fifth lumbar vertebra. The isthmic type of spondylolysis is caused by a stress fracture of the pars interarticularis and is thought to result from repetitive microtrauma to the segment. Spondylolisthesis occurs in the presence of bilateral pars defects, when one vertebra translates anteriorly on the more caudal vertebra. This can cause compression of exiting nerve roots and, in some cases, subsequent neurodeficits. In children and adolescents, spondylolisthesis is most commonly seen at the L5-S1 segment.[2] The dysplastic pars defect occurs secondarily to elongation of the pars. It is thought to be a consequence of a congenital defect and is a less common source of spondylolisthesis.[1]

Spondylolysis is traditionally seen in boys who participate in sports with repetitive extension, flexion, or rotation of the lumbar spine.[1,3,8] Typical symptoms include low back pain, pain with lumbar extension, and occasionally radiating pain to the buttock or posterior thigh. In general, the patient reports a history of insidious onset of low back pain, rather than an acute injury. On exam, the patient may have tenderness over the lumbar spinous processes or paraspinal muscles and often has pain with extension of the lumbar spine.

Initial imaging should include PA and lateral radiographs of the lumbar spine. Oblique radiographs, although often used, have not been shown to increase the diagnostic accuracy beyond standard PA and lateral views, particularly for spondylolysis.[7,10] SPECT, bone scan, and MRI have all been used for the diagnosis of spondylolysis. Miller et al[7] reported that CT and plain films had higher sensitivity for diagnosis of spondylolysis compared with bone scan with lower radiation (**Fig. 8.1**). Recently, MRI has also been shown to have comparable sensitivity to CT scan in the diagnosis of spondylolysis.[11] It may also be advantageous in diagnosing an early stress reaction in the pars that may otherwise not be seen on CT scan. MRI has the additional advantages of detecting soft tissue pathology and entailing no radiation. Spondylolisthesis is best diagnosed on a standing lateral radiograph.

a 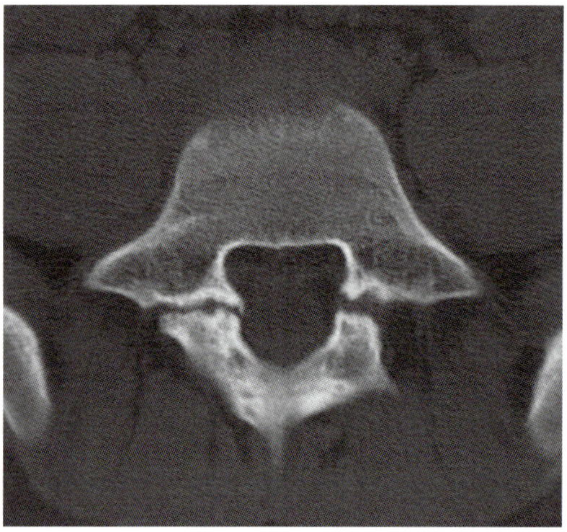

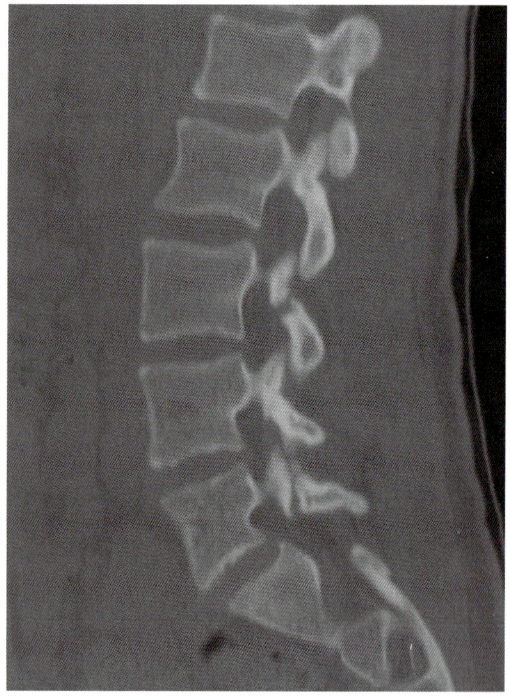

Fig. 8.1 **(a)** Axial and **(b)** sagittal computed tomography (CT) scans demonstrate spondylolysis with bilateral L5 pars defects.

Standing radiographs are essential in determining the degree of the listhesis, as it may reduce with supine positioning.

Nonsurgical management of spondylolysis includes bracing, activity modification, physical therapy, and nonsteroidal anti-inflammatory drugs (NSAIDs). A 2009 meta-analysis of spondylolysis and grade I spondylolisthesis found an 83.9% success rate of nonoperative treatment after 1 year.[12] In this study, neither bracing nor healing of the lesion correlated with successful treatment outcomes. It is generally accepted that healing of the lesion does not correlate with successful outcomes in patients with spondylolysis, and this should be discussed with the patient and family during the initial discussion of treatment goals. In patients with spondylolysis or low-grade spondylolisthesis, surgical treatment is generally reserved for patients who have continued symptoms after more than 6 months of nonoperative treatment.

Scheuermann Kyphosis

Scheuermann kyphosis can be a source of pain in older adolescents. It is a structural kyphotic deformity in the thoracic or thoracolumbar spine and can be distinguished from postural kyphosis by the inability to correct the kyphosis with extension. Patients often also present with compensatory lumbar and cervical lordosis, and sometimes complain of pain at the apex of the thoracic kyphosis or at the hyperlordotic lumbar area. A lateral radiograph of the spine demonstrates > 5 degrees of anterior wedging of at least three adjacent vertebra and > 45 degrees of regional kyphosis.[1] Schmorl nodes, end-plate irregularities, and narrowing of the disk spaces are also seen. PA and lateral radiographs should be obtained to measure the degree of kyphosis and to rule out other pathology, such as spondylolysis or spondylolisthesis.

Nonoperative treatment with bracing can be used in the growing child, and the braces should be tailored to the apex of the kyphosis. If the apex of the Scheuermann deformity is cranial to T7, a Milwaukee brace is recommended. Lower thoracic or thoracolumbar deformities can be managed with an underarm brace.[1] Physical therapy focusing on posture, trunk strengthening, and hamstring stretching can also be useful. Surgical treatment for Scheuermann kyphosis is generally reserved for those patients who have continued progression of the kyphosis despite skeletal maturity or continued pain despite nonsurgical treatment with physical therapy.

Adolescent Idiopathic Scoliosis

Patients with idiopathic scoliosis often present with shoulder asymmetry or rib prominence and may be referred by the pediatrician or school nurse. Occasionally, patients with scoliosis may present with back pain. A retrospective study of 2,442 patients with presumed idiopathic scoliosis found that 23% of the patients had back pain on presentation and another 9% developed back pain during the observation period[13]; 9% of the children with back pain and scoliosis had an underlying condition, most commonly spondylolysis or spondylolisthesis. Other diagnoses included Scheuermann kyphosis, syrinx, disk herniation, tethered cord, and intraspinal tumor.

As with all patients who present with scoliosis, a full neurologic exam should be performed and a thorough history should be taken. Standard PA and lateral radiographs of the spine should be obtained. An atypical scoliotic curve (i.e., left thoracic), rapidly progressing curve, or abnormal neurologic finding should prompt an MRI examination to further investigate another underlying condition.

Trauma

Lumbar disk herniation is less common in pediatric patients than in adults[2]; 30 to 60% of children and adolescents with symptomatic lumbar disk herniations have a history of trauma prior to the onset of pain.[1,14] Symptoms in pediatric patients tend to be similar to those seen in adults, with disk herniation, and radicular symptoms or pain with lumbar flexion. In one study, pediatric patients tended to have a greater nerve-root tension and 90% have a positive straight leg raise on exam.[14] Saddle paresthesia or bowel or bladder dysfunction should raise concern about cauda equina syndrome. Plain radiographs should be ordered, but an MRI of the lumbar spine is the imaging modality of choice for disk herniation. In a 2008 study, adolescent disk herniation was associated with separation of the apophyseal ring in 28% of patients.[15] CT scan may be used to confirm the apophyseal ring separation on axial imaging (**Fig. 8.2**).

Although the nonoperative success rate in pediatric patients is lower than that in adults,[1] most pediatric patients with lumbar disk herniation should be initially treated without surgery. Bed rest, activity restriction, anti-inflammatories, and physical therapy should be used initially. Indications for surgical management include failure of nonoperative treatment, progressive neurologic deficits, and cauda equina syndrome. Patients with apophyseal ring fragments have a higher rate of requiring surgery than those with disk herniations alone.[15] Management of apophyseal ring fractures is similar to that for disk herniation. It has been

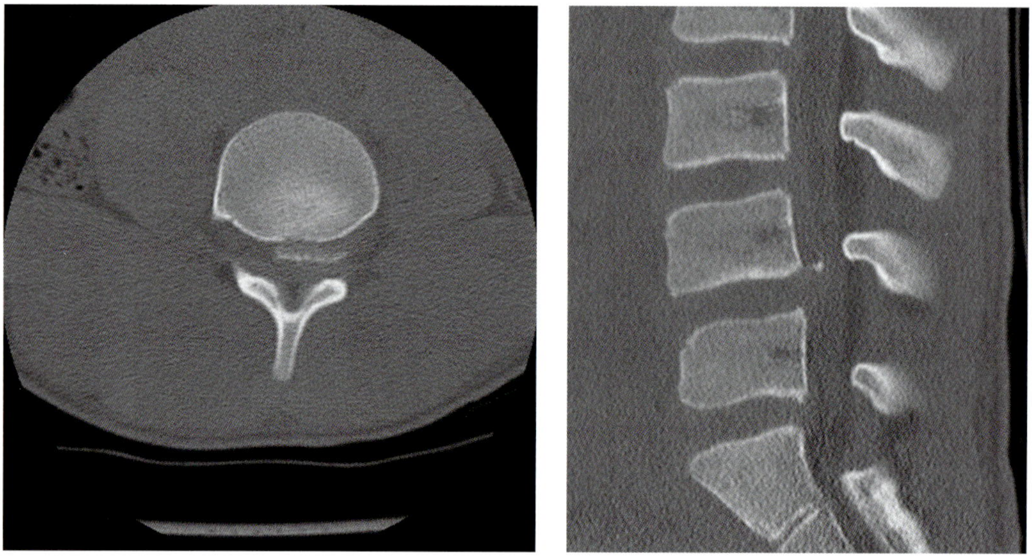

a

Fig. 8.2 **(a)** Axial and **(b)** sagittal CT scans demonstrate a posterior detached bony fragment at the border of the posterior end plate of L4, indicating a posterior end-plate fracture.

suggested that the apophyseal ring fragment should be removed along with the disk, particularly in patients with neurologic deficits.[1]

Infection

A history of fever, neurologic symptoms, gait abnormalities, night pain, or persistent back pain should raise suspicion regarding infection in a pediatric patient presenting with back pain. Infectious causes of back pain in the pediatric population include diskitis, vertebral osteomyelitis, epidural abscess, and sacroiliac joint infection.[8,16]

Diskitis refers to an infection involving the intervertebral disk space. Although it can been seen at any level, it is often localized in the lumbar or lumbosacral region of the spine.[1] Diskitis has a higher incidence in the toddler age group, where gait abnormalities, limping, and back pain represent the most common symptoms.[1,2,17] Plain radiographs are usually not diagnostic early in the disease course, but they may show disk space narrowing or loss of lumbar lordosis. MRI demonstrates a narrowing of the intervertebral disk space and is considered the most useful diagnostic tool for early detection of diskitis. MRI shows increased signal in the bone marrow or intervertebral disks on the T2-weighted images.[1] MRI is also useful in detecting a soft tissue abscess, bony destruction, or compression of neural elements.[17] Laboratory values demonstrate an elevated C-reactive protein and erythrocyte sedimentation rate, and an increased white blood cell count. Blood cultures should be obtained to diagnose concomitant bacteremia and potentially to identify a causative organism. Initial treatment involves empiric intravenous antibiotics for 1 to 2 weeks, followed by oral antibiotics for 2 to 4 weeks. Spine immobilization may be recommended for pain relief and support.[6] If there is a lack of clinical improvement, worsening symptoms, or evidence of an atypical infection, aspiration or biopsy is indicated.

In contrast to children with diskitis, patients with vertebral osteomyelitis are generally older (typically 6 to 9 years of age) and commonly present with pain, muscle spasms, and fever.[18] The preferred imaging modality is MRI, which can demonstrate the extent of vertebral involvement and the location of abscess formation.[2,6] Again, a blood culture may be useful in identifying the causative pathogen. Treatment for children with vertebral osteomyelitis includes antibiotics specific to the pathogen and spinal immobilization. The duration of antibiotic treatment for vertebral osteomyelitis is generally longer than that for diskitis, typically 4 to 6 weeks. Inflammatory markers are useful to monitor the response to treatment and should be expected to trend down with effective antibiotic treatment.

Sacroiliac joint infection in children is often associated with fever and pain in the lower back, buttock, hip, or abdomen.[5] Pain with lateral compression of the pelvis or direct palpation of the sacroiliac joint should raise suspicion for sacroiliac joint infection.[6] Also evident are elevated levels of C-reactive protein and erythrocyte sedimentation rate and increased white blood cell count. A bone scan detects an area of increased uptake and demonstrates the region of the sacroiliac joint infection. Medical therapy for sacroiliac joint infection consists of antibiotics and rest.

Surgery is rarely indicated for children with pediatric diskitis, vertebral osteomyelitis, or sacroiliac joint infections.

An epidural abscess is a rare infection of the central nervous system that often requires surgical intervention. Other indications for surgery include failure of nonsurgical management, neurologic deficits caused by cord compression or nerve root compression, major destruction of the vertebral bodies, or instability of the spine.[1] Spinal instrumentation may be needed in rare cases.

Benign Tumors

Tumors of the spine account for 2 to 8% of all musculoskeletal tumors and may arise from either the bone or the spinal cord.[8,16] In younger children, gait abnormalities may be the first sign of a spinal tumor.[1] Children who present with persistent back pain (≥ 4 weeks), night pain, neurologic symptoms, or systemic or constitutional symptoms should raise the suspicion for a tumor. MRI is the most useful modality to visualize soft tissue and demonstrate the presence of a tumor of the spine. The location of the tumor is important and can help guide the differential diagnosis, as certain tumors have a predilection for either the anterior or posterior elements of the spine. Benign tumors of the bone commonly involve the posterior elements of the spine, mainly the lamina or pedicle.[1,8] Conversely, malignant tumors have a predilection for the anterior elements[16] (**Table 8.2**).

Osteoid osteoma and osteoblastoma often have similar presentations, and diagnosis is determined by the history and imaging modalities. Osteoid osteoma is a benign bone tumor accounting for 1% of all spinal tumors and 11% of all primary benign tumors in patients between 10 and 25 years of age.[8] Children present with back pain at night, which is relieved by NSAIDs.[8] Osteoid osteomas are not locally aggressive and less than 2 cm in size. Osteoid osteomas may be difficult to diagnose on plain radiographs, but appear as a small radiolucent nidus with a sclerotic rim.[16] Advanced diagnostic techniques such as CT and bone scans are useful in identifying the location of the osteoid osteoma (**Fig. 8.3**). In general, the natural

Table 8.2 Location of Malignant Versus Benign Tumors of the Spine

	Malignant	Benign
Posterior Elements		Aneurysmal bone cyst Osteoblastoma Osteoid osteoma
Anterior Elements	Ewing sarcoma Leukemia Metastatic disease	Eosinophilic granuloma Langerhans cell histiocytosis Hemangioma Giant cell tumor

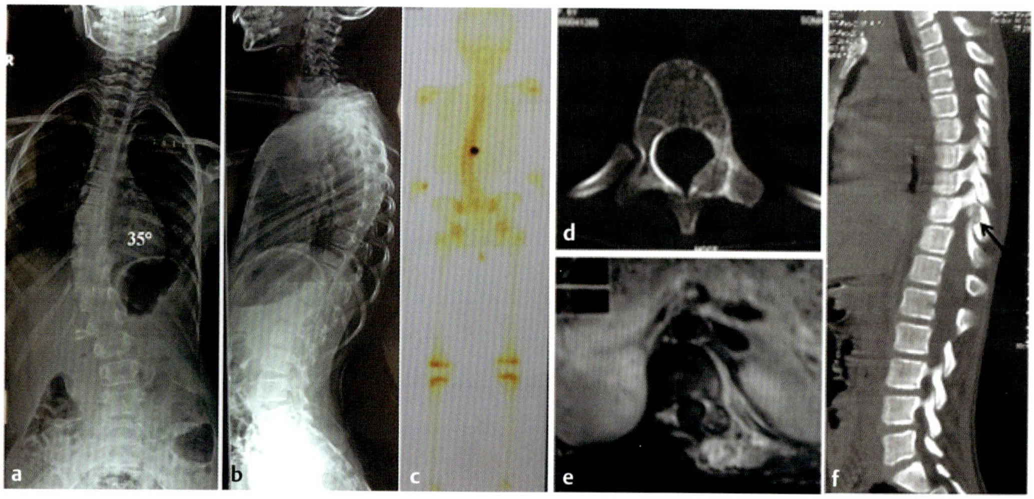

Fig. 8.3 A 12-year-old girl presented with painful scoliosis. **(a)** Anteroposterior (AP) radiograph, **(b)** lateral radiograph, **(c)** bone scan, **(d)** axial CT, **(e)** axial magnetic resonance imaging (MRI), and **(f)** sagittal CT demonstrate a nidus at the concave apex of the curve (**f,** *black arrow*), suggestive of osteoid osteoma. (From Kandwal P, Vijayaraghavan G, Goswami A, Jayaswal A. Back pain in children: how sinister? Indian J Pediatr 2015 Sep 28 [Epub ahead of print]. Reprinted by permission.)

history of an osteoid osteoma entails "burn out" over many years.

Approximately 40% of osteoblastomas occur in the spine.[1] Osteoblastomas are larger in size and may subsequently cause neurologic symptoms. Unlike with osteoid osteomas, the use of NSAIDs tends to be ineffective in osteoblastomas. Osteoblastomas tend to be more locally expansive and destructive in nature, compared with osteoid osteomas.[1,8,19] CT is helpful in determining the size and location of the lesion for surgical planning. Due to their aggressive behavior, osteoblastomas require early surgical treatment, soon after diagnosis, with intralesional curettage of the lesion and instrumentation as indicated.

Both osteoid osteomas and osteoblastomas can be associated with scoliosis, with up to 65% of patients with osteoid osteomas and 52% of patients with osteoblastomas presenting with scoliosis.[6] The tumor is located on the concave side of the apex and is thought to be induced by muscle spasm caused by the inflammatory effect of the tumor.[19] In both lesions, improvement of deformity has been documented following complete resection of the lesion, particularly in patients who have had associated scoliosis present for < 15 months.[6,19]

Aneurysmal bone cysts (ABCs) are benign but locally aggressive bone tumors; 20% are located in the spine.[5] Usually, the posterior elements of the vertebra and lumbar region of the spine are most often affected. Plain radiographs demonstrate a characteristic expansile lesion. MRI demonstrates multiloculated, expansile lesions with fluid-fluid levels that produce a low-intensity signal on T1 images and a high intensity on T2 images[1,6] (**Fig. 8.4**). Although rare, ABCs can cross the disk space and involve more than one spinal level.[16] ABCs can occasionally be associated with other bone lesions including osteosarcoma, giant cell tumor, and eosinophilic granuloma.[6,16] Although neurologic symptoms are rare in children with benign bone tumors, aneurysmal bone cysts have a > 25% incidence of neurologic involvement at presentation.[16] Due to the aggressive nature of ABCs, treatment includes surgical intralesional curettage with stabilization. Biopsy with intraoperative frozen-section analysis should be performed to confirm the diagnosis prior to resection and reconstruction[1,6]

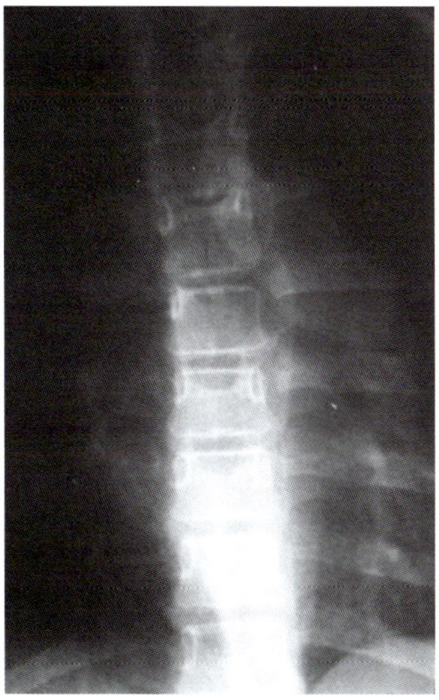

a

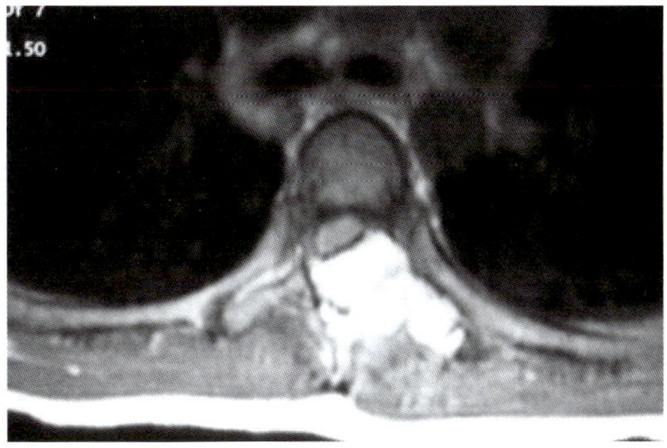

b

Fig. 8.4 **(a)** Plain posteroanterior (PA) radiograph demonstrates an "absent of pedicle" sign, indicating an infiltrative process involving the pedicle. **(b)** Axial MRI demonstrates a classic-appearing aneurysmal bone cyst in the posterior elements of the vertebra.

Although the majority of the benign lesions of the spine have a predilection for the posterior elements, eosinophilic granuloma, also known as LCH, usually occurs in the anterior column[8]; 10 to 15% are located in the spine, most commonly in the cervical spine, followed by the thoracic and lumbar spine.[1,20] Patients frequently complain of back pain over the affected region. Radiographically, eosinophilic granuloma is characterized by vertebra plana or a "coin-on-edge" appearance.[1,6,16] The collapsed vertebra usually occurs with preservation of the disk spaces above and below, and the collapse can be partial or complete.[6,16] MRI is the preferred modality to differentiate eosinophilic granuloma from malignant bone tumors or infection, as soft tissues lesions are not usually associated with the vertebral lesions of eosinophilic granuloma.[1,6] Multifocal disease is present in up to 50% of patients with eosinophilic granuloma; thus, a bone scan should be conducted to detect other areas of involvement.[1,20] A biopsy is often needed to confirm the diagnosis. Most eosinophilic granuloma lesions in children are self-resolving and typically are not associated with long-term complications. Surgical management is rarely needed and is reserved for patients who fail nonoperative treatment and patients with instability or neurologic dysfunction.[1,8]

Malignant Tumors

The most common malignant tumors of the pediatric spine include Ewing sarcoma, lymphoma, and leukemia.[2] Osteogenic sarcoma and metastatic disease can also been seen in the spine. Malignant tumors are associated with progressively worsening pain over a short period, constitutional symptoms, or gait abnormalities, and often can present like an infection. Due to the complexity of these lesions, a multidisciplinary approach is important in the management of malignant tumors of the spine.

Ewing sarcoma is the most common primary malignant bone tumor seen in children; up to 10% originate in the spine.[1,6] These tumors are most commonly seen in the sacrum, followed by the lumbar and thoracic spine, and are rarely seen in the cervical spine.[1,6] Neurologic involvement due to cord compression can be seen.[1,8] The onset of symptoms may be gradual and nonspecific, resulting in a delay in diagnosis. At the time of diagnosis, 25% of patients with Ewing sarcoma present with metastasis.[1,6] Radiographs may show vertebral collapse with an associated soft tissue mass. An MRI is needed to best evaluate soft tissue and spinal canal involvement. A biopsy is always indicated to confirm the diagnosis. Following staging, the treatment of Ewing sarcoma in the spine includes neoadjuvant chemotherapy, local control with radiation or surgical resection, and postoperative chemotherapy.[1] Stabilization with instrumentation and fusion is often necessary following resection of the lesion.

Leukemia is the most common pain-producing malignancy of the spine, and bone pain may be the presenting symptom in up to 25% of patients with leukemia.[1,6] Leukemia is the most prevalent form of cancer in children and is commonly associated with pain, lethargy, fever, pallor, and unexplained bruising or bleeding. Characteristic findings include elevated complete blood count, erythrocyte sedimentation rate, and white blood cell count, in addition to a lowered platelet count, and an increased leukocyte count.[6] Diagnosis is usually confirmed via bone marrow aspiration.[1] Radiographs are nonspecific and can show diffuse osteopenia, vertebral body compression, sclerosis, osteolysis, or periosteal new bone formation.[1,6] Treatment of leukemia primarily involves chemotherapy and radiation. Bracing may be useful to provide pain relief while collapsed vertebrae are allowed time to heal.[4]

Metastatic lesions to the spine in children can occur as a consequence of rhabdomyosarcoma, neuroblastoma, or Wilms' tumor.[1,6] Most children present with pathological fractures, and some may have compression of the spinal cord. MRI is the imaging modality of choice, and a biopsy is mandatory for a definitive diagnosis.[6]

Although rare, spinal cord tumors can also present as pain in the pediatric population. The most common spinal cord tumors are astrocytomas and ependymomas, and they are primarily located in the cervical spinal cord.[2,8] Back pain is the most common presenting symptom followed by weakness, gait disturbance, torticollis, and neurologic dysfunction.[2] Physical examination demonstrates tenderness to palpitation of the spine in patients with spinal cord tumors.[6] Radiographs of the spine may detect tumors, but further evaluation with MRI is usually needed.

Chapter Summary

The number of pediatric patients presenting with back pain has increased over recent years, and many of these patients, particularly in the adolescent population, have nonspecific back pain. However, a high index of suspicion should be maintained for more severe pathology in any child presenting with back pain. The initial assessment should focus on a detailed history and physical exam. It is important to note any "red flags" on the initial exam or history to rule out a more serious pathology. Most causes of back pain are benign, particularly in the adolescent age group. However, a broad differential diagnosis should be kept in mind. Constitutional symptoms such as fever or weight loss are more consistent with tumor or infection. Mechanical symptoms or pain with activity may be more indicative of spondylolysis or a lumbar disk herniation. Plain radiographs should be ordered on the majority of pediatric patients who present with back pain. CT scan, bone scan, and MRI may also be useful as additional imaging as indicated, and laboratory studies can be helpful when infection or malignancy is suspected.

Knowing the clinical and radiographic features of the most common etiologies of back pain in the pediatric population is imperative for a timely diagnosis and effective treatment of this population.

Pearls

- There is no test that can substitute for a thorough history and physical exam in the initial assessment of a pediatric patient who presents with back pain.
- Be mindful of "red flags" on the initial evaluation of the child with back pain.
- Back pain in a child may be referred pain rather than based in the spine or paraspinal muscles. Involve the patient's primary care doctor if the exam is unclear or if there is suspicion regarding visceral, pelvic, or retroperitoneal causes.

Pitfalls

- Do not rely on prior imaging reports alone; try to obtain the actual imaging scans. Be sure to review the current imaging when focusing on the differential diagnosis after obtaining a history and performing a physical exam.
- Patients who present with spinal tumors may have nonspecific pain or symptoms, which may contribute to a delay in diagnosis.
- Not all scoliosis is idiopathic, even in an adolescent girl. Be sure to rule out an underlying pathology before deeming a scoliosis idiopathic.

References

Five Must-Read References

1. Shah SA, Saller J. Evaluation and diagnosis of back pain in children and adolescents. J Am Acad Orthop Surg 2016;24:37–45
2. Davis PJ, Williams HJ. The investigation and management of back pain in children. Arch Dis Child Educ Pract Ed 2008;93:73–83
3. Altaf F, Heran MK, Wilson LF. Back pain in children and adolescents. Bone Joint J 2014;96-B:717–723
4. Burton AK, Clarke RD, McClune TD, Tillotson KM. The natural history of low back pain in adolescents. Spine 1996;21:2323–2328
5. Fujimori T, Iwasaki M, Nagamoto Y, Sakaura H, Oshima K, Yoshikawa H. The utility of superficial abdominal reflex in the initial diagnosis of scoliosis: a retrospective review of clinical characteristics of scoliosis with syringomyelia. Scoliosis 2010;5:17
6. Dormans JP, Moroz L. Infection and tumors of the spine in children. J Bone Joint Surg Am 2007;89(Suppl 1):79–97
7. Miller R, Beck NA, Sampson NR, Zhu X, Flynn JM, Drummond D. Imaging modalities for low back pain in children: a review of spondylolysis and undiagnosed mechanical back pain. J Pediatr Orthop 2013; 33:282–288
8. Kandwal P, Vijayaraghavan G, Goswami A, Jayaswal A. Back pain in children: how sinister? Indian J Pediatr 2015 Sep 28 [Epub ahead of print]
9. Turner PG, Green JH, Galasko CS. Back pain in childhood. Spine 1989;14:812–814
10. Beck NA, Miller R, Baldwin K, et al. Do oblique views add value in the diagnosis of spondylolysis in adolescents? J Bone Joint Surg Am 2013;95:e65
11. Rush JK, Astur N, Scott S, Kelly DM, Sawyer JR, Warner WC Jr. Use of magnetic resonance imaging in the evaluation of spondylolysis. J Pediatr Orthop 2015; 35:271–275
12. Klein G, Mehlman CT, McCarty M. Nonoperative treatment of spondylolysis and grade I spondylolisthesis in children and young adults: a meta-analysis of observational studies. J Pediatr Orthop 2009;29: 146–156
13. Ramirez N, Johnston CE, Browne RH. The prevalence of back pain in children who have idiopathic scoliosis. J Bone Joint Surg Am 1997;79:364–368
14. Dang L, Liu Z. A review of current treatment for lumbar disc herniation in children and adolescents. Eur Spine J 2010;19:205–214
15. Chang CH, Lee ZL, Chen WJ, Tan CF, Chen LH. Clinical significance of ring apophysis fracture in adolescent lumbar disc herniation. Spine 2008;33:1750–1754
16. Garg S, Dormans JP. Tumors and tumor-like conditions of the spine in children. J Am Acad Orthop Surg 2005;13:372–381
17. Early SD, Kay RM, Tolo VT. Childhood diskitis. J Am Acad Orthop Surg 2003;11:413–420
18. Fernandez M, Carrol CL, Baker CJ. Discitis and vertebral osteomyelitis in children: an 18-year review. Pediatrics 2000;105:1299–1304
19. Kan P, Schmidt MH. Osteoid osteoma and osteoblastoma of the spine. Neurosurg Clin N Am 2008;19: 65–70
20. Garg S, Mehta S, Dormans JP. Langerhans cell histiocytosis of the spine in children. Long-term follow-up. J Bone Joint Surg Am 2004;86-A:1740–1750

9

Back Pain in Adults

Max Aebi

Introduction

The aging of the population in industrialized countries appears to be a nonreversible phenomenon. Increasing life expectancy, due in a great part to advances in health care, combined with a drastic decrease in the birth rate, has led to this situation.[1] World demographics have shifted from a pattern of high birth rates and high mortality rates to one of low birth rates and delayed mortality.[1,2] In Europe, the proportion of the population over the age of 65 was 10.8% in 1950, 14% in 1970, and 19.1% in 1995, and is projected to be 30.1% in 2025 and 42.2% in 2050.[3] The proportion of the population over the age of 75 has grown from 2.7% in 1950 to 5.2% in 1995, and is projected to be 9.1% in 2025 and 14.6% in 2050.[3] And this trend is not limited to industrialized countries; the developing countries' share of the world's population over the age of 65 is projected to increase from 59% to 71%. The global consequences of this distortion of the age pyramid on health care development, access, and costs are huge.[4] For example, 59% of United States residents over the age of 65 have osteoarthritis, which is the main cause of disability and the most frequent cause of back and neck pain. Osteoarthritis is the most frequently encountered complaint of people of all ages, and the nature of the spine renders this problem difficult to investigate and to treat.

The aging of the spine is characterized by two major parallel and independent processes, which lead to different clinical situations:

1. The reduction of bone mineral density, hence bone mass
2. The development of degenerative changes of the diskoligamentous complex (disks, ligaments, facet joint capsules, and facet joints), resulting in instability, deformity, and narrowing of the spinal canal and the exit of the nerve roots (spinal and foraminal stenosis), with secondary neurologic problems such as myelopathy, cauda equina, radicular syndromes, and disability

Hence, degeneration alone, or in combination with bone mass reduction by osteoporosis or metastatic tumor involvement, contributes to a different degree to the development of a variety of lesions and often to several painful and invalidating disorders.

Osteoporotic Compression Fractures

Osteoporotic compression fractures of vertebral bodies as an expression of age-related diminution of the bone mass is an increasing problem due to aging of the Western population as well as the Japanese and Chinese population, resulting in increasing numbers of severely osteoporotic patients, mostly women. Recent studies have shown that osteoporotic vertebral fractures are associated with an increased risk of mortality and a decreased quality of life.[5,6] The prevalence of these fractures is 39% in patients over the age of 65 years.[4,7]

Degeneration of the Spinal Structures

Degeneration of the spinal structures induces interactive alterations at many levels: bones, disks, facet joints, and ligaments. Some of these degenerative lesions can be responsible for compressive damage to the neural elements, as in the case of disk herniation or spinal stenosis.

Disk degeneration begins when the balance between synthesis and degradation of the matrix is disrupted; at the microscopic level, disk degeneration includes a net loss of water as a consequence of a breakdown of proteoglycans in so-called short chains, which are unable to bind water.[8,9] Furthermore, there is disruption of collagen fiber organization, specifically in the annulus, and increased levels of proteolytic enzymes. Disk degeneration can be seen in 16% of 20-year-olds and 98% of 70+-year-olds[10,11] (**Fig. 9.1**).

Women reach the same level of degeneration about 10 years later than men (**Fig. 9.1**). In the aging of the spine there is a predetermined cell viability (endogenous = genetic) and decreasing cellular activity in the disk over the years due to exposure of the disk to repetitive mechanical loads.[9,12,13] This leads to a loss of extracellular matrix, with proteoglycans degrading, and decreased capability to bind water. The collagen organization is dissociated, which leads to a loss of height of the disk. This is always combined with a secondary deterioration of the facet joints, ligaments, and muscles. Through this process, the boundaries between the annulus and nucleus are less distinct, and the collagen is increasing in the nucleus and replacing the proteoglycans. With that we see concentric fissuring at radial tears, which weakens the disk, starting in the third and fourth decade of life. There is substantial variation in this cascade of events. But these changes clearly have biomechanical consequences for the motion segment.[12]

The role of vascularization in the aging disk is most crucial. The nutritional supply of the cells in the disk diminishes because the adjacent vertebral end-plate permeability is decreasing, leading to a blood supply decrease with a secondary tissue breakdown, which starts in the nucleus, and mechanical impact on the cells (sensitive to mechanical sickness), which leads to a qualitative and quantitative modulation of the matrix proteins.[13–15] The variation of the proteoglycan content as well as the water content is age-dependent and operating

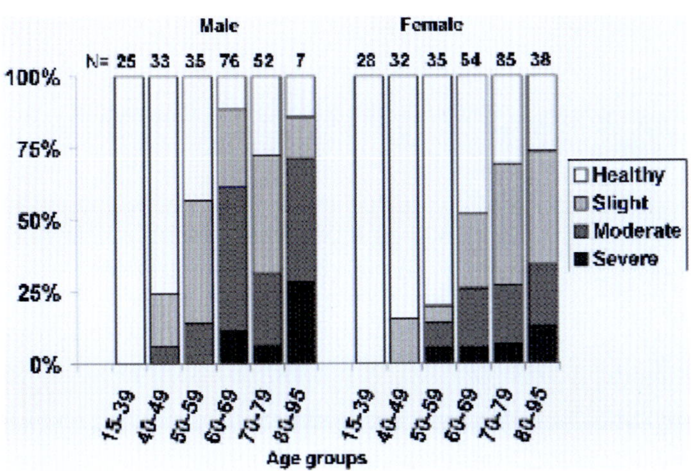

Fig. 9.1 The prevalence of macroscopic disk degeneration based on autopsies by age for men and women. The women reach the same level of degeneration about a decade later than men. (Data from Ref. 10.)

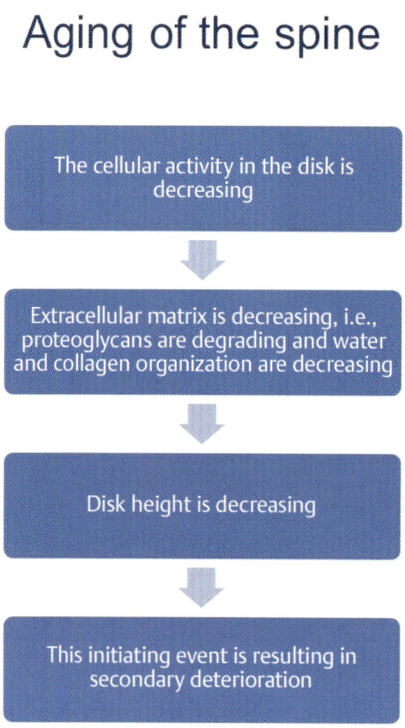

Fig. 9.2 The cascade of events in the degenerative process of the intervertebral disk.

in parallel: more degradation of the proteoglycans, less water content, and higher probability of disintegration of the disk (**Fig. 9.2**).

Thus, we can see that orthopedic surgeons, musculoskeletal specialists, and dedicated spine specialists are going to be treating huge numbers of patients affected by diseases that result from the aging of the musculoskeletal system.

Typical Disorders of the Aging Spine

Typical disorders of the aging spine that express themselves as back or neck pain with or without neurologic symptoms or signs include the following:

- Degenerative disease of the disks, osteochondrosis, and disk prolapse/herniation
- Degenerative disease of the facet joints resulting from joint incongruences due to disk height loss and arthritis, secondary instability, and deformity
- Degenerative spondylolisthesis with or without spinal stenosis and instability
- Spinal stenosis: central, recess, and foraminal stenosis due to narrowing of the elements of the spinal canal, following hypertrophy of the ligamentum flavum and the joint capsules and the facet joint by itself—pathomorphology that may lead to compression of the neural structures of the spinal canal
- Spinal deformities: scoliosis, kyphosis, and concomitant secondary instability and neurologic deficit
- Osteoporosis with vertebral compression fractures (VCFs) alone or in combination with degenerative defects, which may be followed by a secondary deformity
- Pathological fractures of the vertebrae due to metastatic disease
- Infection of the spine, spondylodiskitis, and spondylitis

Disk Degeneration, Osteochondrosis, and Disk Herniation

Symptomatic, isolated, or multilevel disk degeneration can be seen in the lumbar and cervical spine.[16] The clinically most relevant disk degeneration with subchondral edema, possible secondary spondylolisthesis or translational and rotatory dislocation, and consecutive spinal deformity is most frequently seen in the lumbar spine at the following levels, in decreasing order: L3-L4, L2-L3, L4-L5, and L1-L2. The asymmetrical degeneration may lead to a disk herniation with major or mass dislocation of whole disk fragments (annulus and nucleus parts), leading usually to at least a major neurologic complication, such as root compression or cauda compression with significant radicular pain or sensorimotor deficit.

This pathology can occur in the context of previous surgery in the lower lumbar spine that led to a fusion or at least a poorly mobile spinal segment, with overload and stress rising to the adjacent superior or inferior segment, with rapid degeneration of the disk and with

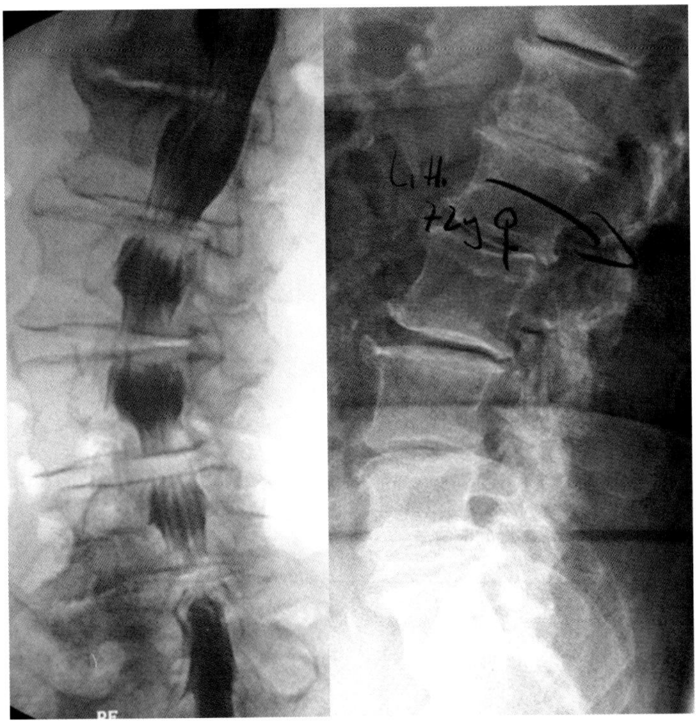

Fig. 9.3 Multilevel disk degeneration with instability in LH, a 72-year-old female. *Arrow:* maximum reklination demonstrates air inclusion L2-L3 and then L12 as an expression of a pathological movement.

potential instability, spinal stenosis, and possible extrusion of major disk fragments as an acute event. In almost all these situations, decompression of the segment and a stabilization may become necessary[17–19] (**Fig. 9.3**).

Asymmetric degeneration of the disk may lead to further deterioration of the adjacent motion segments and may end with a progressive degenerative scoliosis[5] that may need surgical treatment (see below). This may also occur as a long-term process in patients who suffer from an asymmetric transitional anomaly of the lumbosacral junction or early disk pathology at the lower lumbar spine (**Fig. 9.3**).

It is sometimes difficult to differentiate the active subchondral bony damage from osteoporotic compression fractures. Obtaining a thorough history, performing a physical examination, and requesting imaging scans such as magnetic resonance imaging (MRI) with short tau inversion recovery (STIR) sequences, computed tomography (CT), and bone scintigraphy will facilitate arriving at a diagnosis.

Symptomatic isolated or multilevel disk degeneration can be seen in the lumbar spine as well as in the cervical spine. This disk degeneration with osteochondrosis and sometimes significant subchondral edema, as an expression of inflammation, and occasionally combined with significant disk protrusion, can occur in elderly patients primarily without relevant deformity or instability. This degeneration can start at a younger age and can be asymptomatic or can be combined with off-and-on back pain over the course of years and even decades.[16]

For mostly mechanical reasons, disk degeneration can aggravate and become highly symptomatic, specifically when it is combined with segmental instability and osteochondritis (**Fig. 9.4**). Because these disks are severely degenerated and dehydrated over many years, a herniation consists almost always of a large, combined annulus and fibrotic nucleus sequester. The consequence of this disk degeneration may be a secondary deformity, with typical translatory dislocation of vertebrae in a segment or several segments, rotation and scoliosis, and kyphoscoliosis.[5,16] It is also possible that disk degeneration and facet joint arthritis can

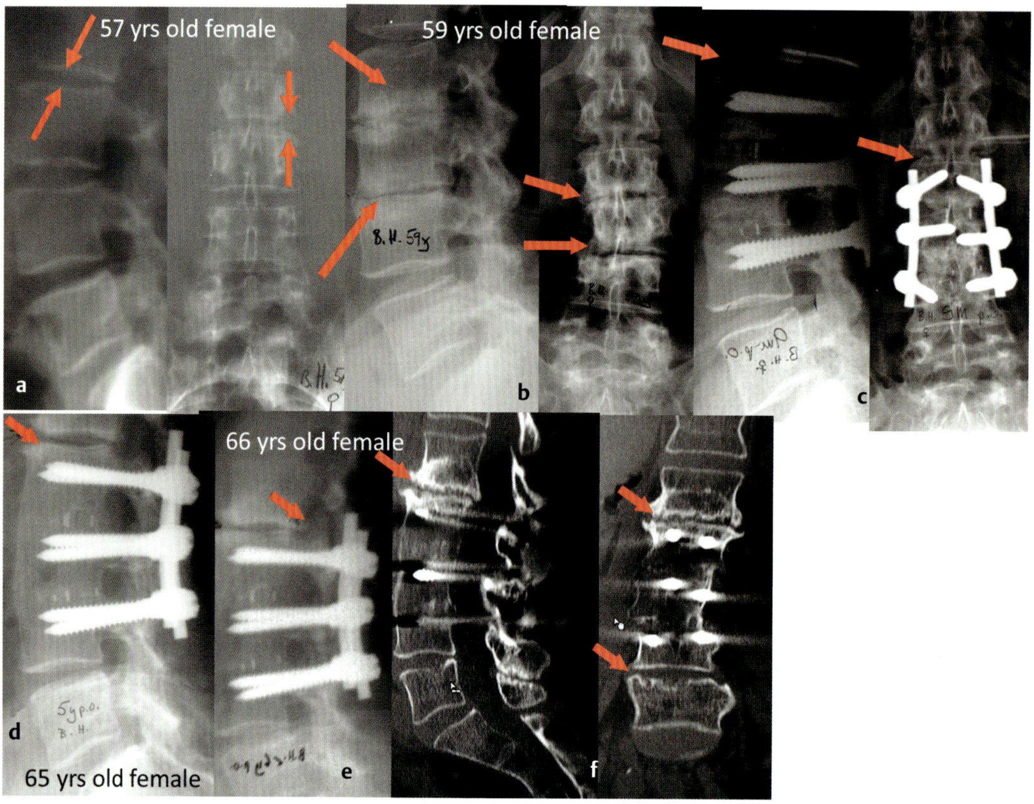

Fig. 9.4 Adjacent segment disease. **(a)** A 57-year-old woman with severe back pain but no leg pain. Segment L2-L3 osteochondrosis with beginning degenerative lumbar scoliosis. Nonsurgical treatment. **(b)** A 59-year-old woman with severe back pain and new leg pain and claudication symptomatology. Clear progression of the degenerative scoliosis. **(c)** Decompression, correction, and stabilization of the degenerative deformity of the same patient, with pedicular screw system and transforaminal lumbar interbody fusion (TLIF) in L2-L3 and L3-L4. **(d)** The now 65-year-old woman, who was almost pain-free for 5 years, experiences back pain in the upper lumbar spine. **(e)** Now 66 years old and more than 6 years postoperative, the woman experiences severe back pain and irradiation into the groin on the right more than on the left. **(f)** Severe adjacent segment degeneration noted at L1-L2 and beginning at L4-L5.

lead to a degenerative spondylolisthesis.[20–22] As long as the disk degeneration is isolated on one to three levels without a major deformity, a typical axial "instability" pain may occur, mostly during rotational movement, lifting when upright, or turning in bed during sleep. If conservative treatment with isometric reinforcement exercises of the abdominal and paravertebral muscles is not successful, surgery may be necessary.[21,23–26]

If surgery is necessary, many minimally invasive surgical techniques have been suggested, using a retroperitoneal anterior approach, a posterior approach, a far lateral approach (extreme lateral interbody fusion [XLIF]) (**Fig. 9.5**), or a combination of these approaches. Anterior surgery with stand-alone cages (anterior lateral interbody fusion [ALIF]) that are fixed with screws is straightforward in non-obese patients, and is quite feasible from L3-L4, L4-L5, and L5-S1, that is, in the lower lumbar spine. In obese or osteoporotic patients, or in those with previous abdominal surgery, it is advisable not to do an anterior surgery (ALIF or

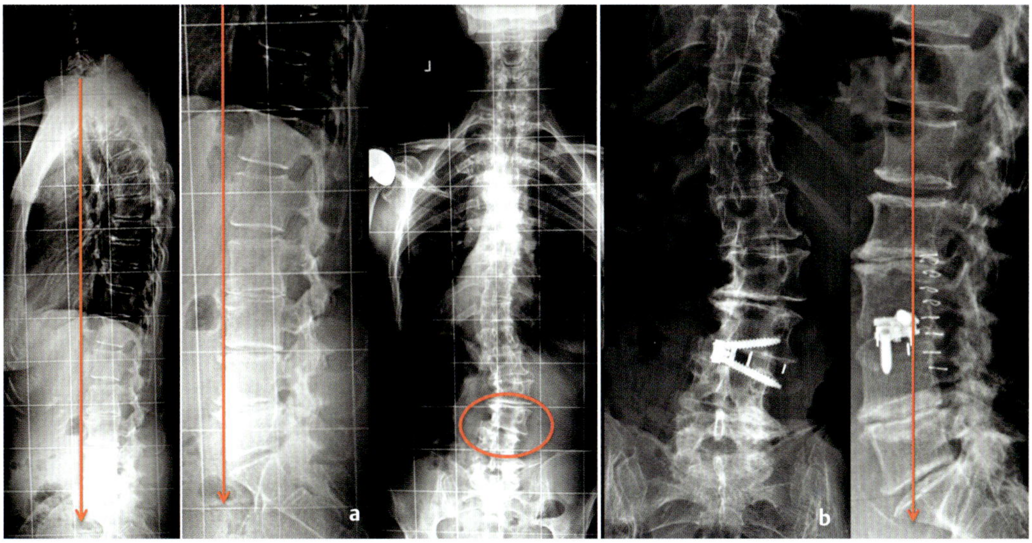

Fig. 9.5 A 68-year-old woman with severe movement- and activity-dependent left leg pain. **(a)** Degenerative left convex lumbar scoliosis with significant osteophyte formation in several segments, except at L3-L4 *(circle)*. Here a translational rotatory instability can be demonstrated *(circle)*, which is most probably the cause of motion-dependent pain. Therefore, only this "strategic" segment has been immobilized and fixed by a stand-alone extreme lateral interbody fusion (XLIF) cage with plate fixation, leaving the deformity otherwise alone. **(b)** Instant pain relief and improved sagittal alignment are noted postoperatively.

XLIF) alone, but rather combined with a posterior surgery with pedicle fixation and posterior lateral interbody fusion (PLIF) or transforaminal lumbar interbody fusion (TLIF) procedure, or just as an isolated posterior surgery. This is particularly true when decompression of the neurostructures in the spinal canal is the main purpose of the surgery.

Specifically in the frail elderly, where surgery is the only remaining option after all other treatments have failed, minimally invasive surgery, such as a far lateral approach (XLIF),[27–30] is most appropriate, as it entails little blood loss, little surgical trauma, and brief anesthesia duration. However, to avoid posterior surgery, stand-alone cages should be used that can be fixed either by an additional plate or with the plate incorporated with the cage (**Fig. 9.5**). This technique facilitates achieving indirect decompression of a foraminal and sometimes a recess stenosis. However, it is limited in osteoporotic bone (the cage may migrate in the vertebral body) and in central stenosis, which is fixed, but nevertheless it may be appropriate in dynamic (mechanical unstable segment) central stenosis.[29,31] In these cases it is sometimes necessary to do a posterior pedicle screw fixation with cement reinforcement and even to fill the intervertebral space after removing the disk with cement, that is, a so-called diskoplasty. In some cases where the disk height is significantly reduced and there is significant concomitant facet joint arthritis, which contributes to the pain generation, a microsurgical interlaminar decompression with resection of the flavum, capsule, and partial arthrectomy, combined with a translaminar facet screw fixation, may be sufficient (**Fig. 9.6**). This is an atraumatic surgery suitable for very elderly patients who have considerable morbidity, a reduced life expectancy, and little demand for physical activity; this surgery entails little blood loss, and one of its major purposes is to control pain, which is fulfilled by immobilizing each facet joints with a screw and with sufficient decompression.

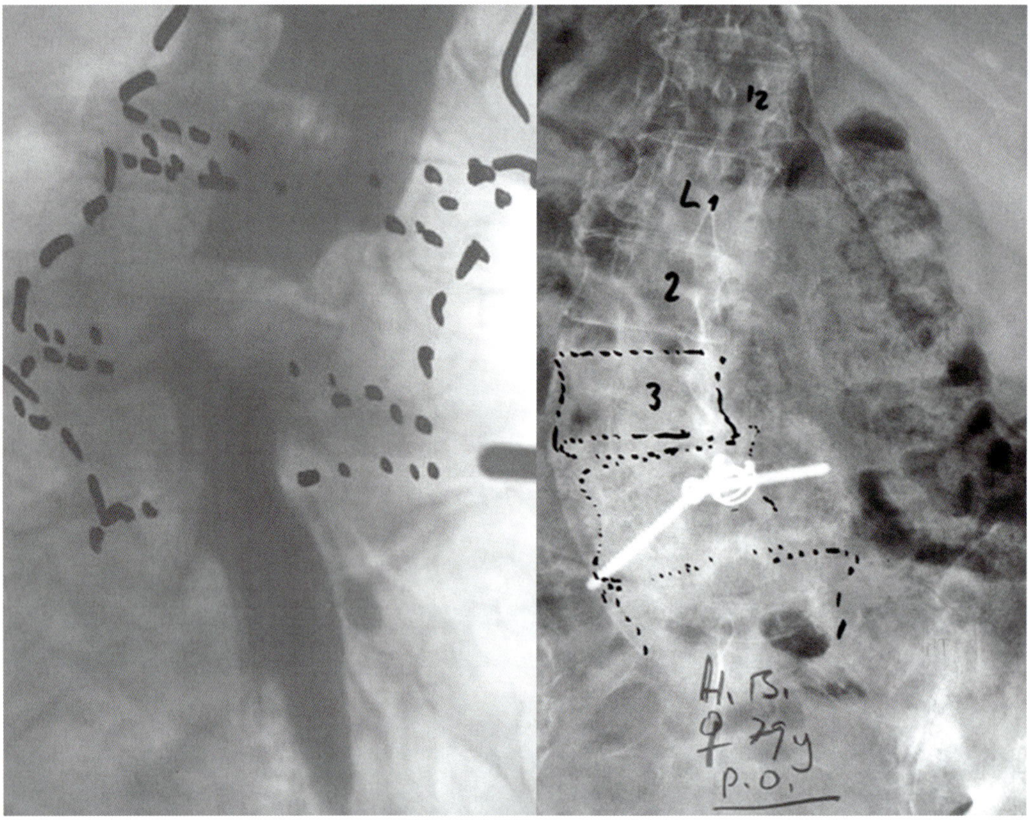

Fig. 9.6 Translaminar screw fixation as a minimal intervention for decompression and immobilization of arthritic facet joints in a 79-year-old polymorbid patient. The markings outline the poorly identifiable contours of the vertebral bodies.

Spinal Stenosis in the Elderly

Spinal stenosis is a very common condition in the elderly, and it is important to differentiate among central stenosis, lateral stenosis, and root canal stenosis. In some cases there can be combination of two of these types, or one type can be combined with degenerative spondylolisthesis. Other conditions include Paget's disease, a degenerative disease that may cause spinal stenosis with or without neurologic complications, and secondary spinal stenosis due to fracture, mostly osteoporotic fracture, or due to tumor compression of the spinal canal, mostly from metastatic disease. Finally, there is iatrogenic stenosis, which can occur as a late result after any spine surgery at any age. In these cases, spinal stenosis may occur as a so-called adjacent segment problem after fusion surgery, or it may be a part of a degenerative deformity (scoliosis and kyphosis).[32]

In most cases, spinal stenosis is due to degenerative changes or a preexisting narrow canal. These changes can lead to symptoms, but so-called stenotic images sometimes are present on imaging studies in several symptom-free individuals. The relationship among degenerative lesions, abnormal imaging, and patient complaints is still unclear. Lumbar stenosis with a claudication symptomatology, however, is a common reason for decompressive surgery or fusion. The investigation of stenotic symptoms should be extremely careful and thorough, and should include the appropriate auxiliary examinations, such as infiltration techniques (extraforaminal root blocks, epidural blocks, facet joint infiltrations, diskography, sacral blocks) as well as functional X-rays (flexion/extension lateral view with the patient in the supine position, and traction films), including vascular investigation. This is of the utmost importance, especially if surgery is deemed necessary for good results.[33]

Surgical management of spinal stenosis can consist of purely decompressive surgery. Different techniques are available, such as classic laminectomy, laminotomy, partial laminectomy, resection of ligamentum flavum and scar tissue, simple foraminal decompression, and others. In recent years it has been suggested in some cases to use a so-called interspinous process distraction, in which the foramina are opened and the canal is widened and indirectly decompressed.[23,33] The interspinous process distraction also unloads the disks as well as the facet joints. The most appropriate patients for this procedure are those with increasing symptoms when doing lumbar extension movements. There is still a quite significant debate about whether a decompression needs to be accompanied by instrumentation.[23,33] Depending on the osteophyte formations in the anterior column as well as the osteoarthritis of the facet joints, and in the absence of any instability, such as degenerative spondylolisthesis, a simple decompression without instrumentation may be sufficient. If there is a need for significant resection of hypertrophic facet joint parts to decompress the dural sac as well as the exiting roots, it may be necessary to stabilize the segment either by simple translaminar/transarticular screw fixation or by pedicle fixation. The first method provides a less rigid fixation than the alternative with pedicle fixation. The risk of pedicle fixation in spinal stenosis patients without a deformity or obvious instability is that is generates a rigid spine section, which affects the adjacent segment, including the disks as well as the vertebral bodies.[17,18,34–36] This increases the risk of fatigue fractures in these vertebral bodies and a disruption of the posterior ligament complex as an expression of the aging of ligaments and muscles (**Fig. 9.7**).

In a patient with a severely degenerated cervical spine with spinal stenosis, compression of the cord may be treated with consecutive myelopathy or root compression. The spinal stenosis of the cervical spine often goes together with a deformity usually in kyphosis and sometimes in a minor scoliotic deformity in the frontal plane. If there is a relevant deformity of the cervical spine combined with a narrow spinal canal, diagnostic traction may be applied to explore how far the deformity can be reduced and the cervical spine can be realigned. In case this is possible, surgery may be done under traction in the reduced position. In this case there is no manipulation for reduction necessary during the surgery, but only the decompressive, and if necessary, the stabilization part.

In the cervical spine, there are different ways in which the spinal stenosis can be addressed. It can be done with an anterior surgery, either by a uni- or multilevel diskectomy, and resection of the posterior, inferior, and superior corner of the adjacent vertebra. In cases in which the compression of the spinal cord is mainly due to disks on several levels, this technique can be applied on each individual level by maintaining the main part of the vertebral body. This method facilitates placing intervertebral spacers and restoring the cervical lordosis. In cases in which there is more compression due to relevant osteophytes, extension of the compression beyond the disk space, or concomitant ossification of the posterior longitudinal ligament (OPLL), one or even two level vertebrectomies may be necessary, with an anterior reconstruction with (expandable or rigid) cages or bony struts (fibula or iliac crest) and plate fixation. If this stabilization seems to be insufficient and does not restore the lordosis, a combined posterior fixation with tension banding and realigning of the cervical spine in lordosis may be necessary. There is also the option of posterior surgery through laminectomy, laminotomy on several levels, or laminoplasty. In cases in which there is insufficient physiological lordosis (in fact kyphosis), a simultaneous fixation of the decompressed cervical spine along with the decompression may be necessary. Most often, the technique of choice is lateral mass screws combined with rod systems. This surgery is combined with a posterolateral fusion, either by bone substitutes or with cancellous bone from the iliac crest. Because cervical spine surgery is not as invasive as lumbar spine surgery, elderly people with significant

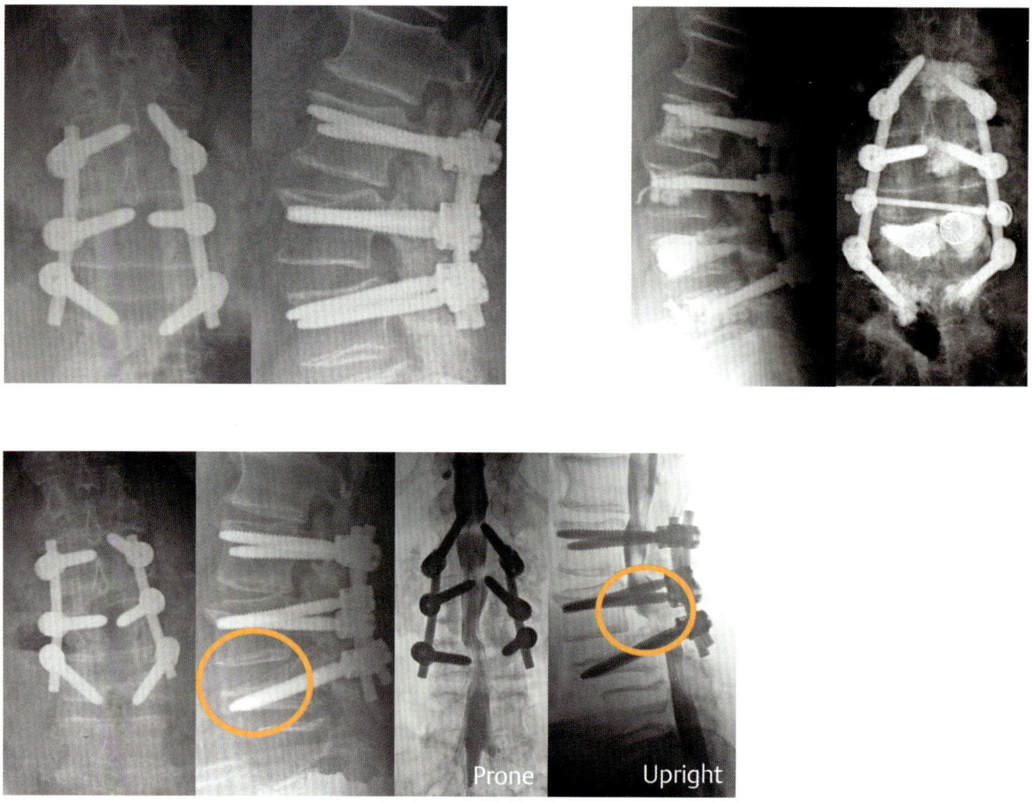

a

b

Fig. 9.7 A 75-year-old woman with a body weight of 120 kg experienced severe claudication symptomatology as well as position- and movement-dependent low back pain. She was almost completely immobilized at home. Spinal stenosis and position-dependent spondylolisthesis was demonstrated at L3-L4 and partially at L2-L3. Osteopenia was diagnosed. She was decompressed at two levels, and fixed with a pedicle screw system from L2 to L4. In order not to create too rigid a spine, intervertebral cages were not used. **(a)** Three weeks postoperative. The patient was mobilized, and she experienced considerable reduction in her pain. **(b)** Five weeks postoperative. During rehabilitation, massive pain and incapacity of walking suddenly returned. A vertebral compression fracture of the instrumented L4 vertebral body was performed, with a secondary instability and dynamic massive compression of the dural sac. **(c)** After revision. The patient was instrumented further down to L5, with cement augmentation of the screws in each vertebra and stent kyphoplasty of L4.

comorbidities can be treated specifically by anterior surgery under neuromonitoring, as it entails relatively little blood loss, and the surgical trauma is mostly "local," not involving the homeostasis of the body, as in a surgery of the lumbar spine performed with the patient in the prone position which takes longer.

Degenerative Spondylolisthesis

Degenerative spondylolisthesis occurs usually at the level of L4-L5, and less frequently at the level of L3-L4 and L5-S1. Very often, degenerative spondylolisthesis is combined with spinal stenosis. The spondylolisthesis is a consequence of a disk degeneration and insufficiency of the facet joints to maintain the stability of the segment. In these cases very often the facet joint effusion can be demonstrated, as well as air inclusion in the disk and in the facet joints. The spondylolisthesis can also be combined with a facet joint synovial cyst, which may add to the compressive effect of the spondylolisthesis, with a secondary narrowing of the spinal canal.

Whether this pathology needs to be decompressed and stabilized or whether simple decompression is sufficient is debated.[20,21,37] If instability can be demonstrated in functional X-rays with maximal bending and maximal extension over a hypomochlion of the lumbar spine in supine position and accompanying low back pain in combination with irradiation into the legs, stabilization may well be indicated (**Fig. 9.7**). Here again, whether this should be a pedicle fixation alone or in combination with an interbody fusion, such as PLIF or TLIF, with all the potential risks of failure, is debated (**Fig. 9.4**).[11,20,21,24,26]

According to the guidelines of the North American Spine Society (NASS),[29] there is very little evidence for determining whether a spondylolisthesis is to be surgically treated with decompression alone, or in combination with fusion with or without implants (screws and cages), or whether a reduction is necessary.

Degenerative Deformity (Scoliosis and Kyphosis)

The degenerative deformity mainly of the lumbar spine and the thoracolumbar spine is a typical disease of the elderly, particularly women. This is basically a disk disease with the whole cascade as described earlier: disk degeneration as the initial starting point, usually unilateral or asymmetrical, and incongruence of the facet joints with subluxation and rotatory deformity, which appears in the anteroposterior (AP) view as a translational dislocation, mostly at the level of L2-L3 or L3-L4.[5] The deformity in the frontal plane (scoliosis) is practically always combined with a lumbar kyphosis, and this deformity very frequently is combined with recess or foraminal stenosis, occasionally appearing as a so-called dynamic stenosis, and being clinically relevant only when the patient is in upright position or in a certain position while lying or sitting (de novo scoliosis)[5] (**Fig. 9.4**). The clinical appearance of the degenerative deformity is pain, mostly back pain, with frequent irradiation into the legs, be it a so-called pseudoradicular irradiation or as a real radicular irradiation and claudication symptomatology. Therefore, the clinical problem to be addressed is the progressing deformity, the instability of one or several segments, the neurocompression in the spinal canal, be it centrally or laterally, and very frequently the combination with osteoporosis. These patients are usually unbalanced, not only in the frontal plane but more importantly in the sagittal plane. There is very little substantial nonsurgical treatment for these patients.[38] Occasionally, a brace can be tried, and a walker or canes may be used to maintain balance.

These patients are generally experience improvement while walking in water, because of the water's buoyancy. But the only efficient treatment is surgery, which entails risks and complications.

Surgical treatment is almost always indicated when progression of the curve can be demonstrated over time, and in cases of relevant central, recess, or foraminal stenosis with significant radicular pain or neurologic deficit. There is not only a segmental instability, visible in many of these deformities, but also a global instability of the spine, which means that the spine is collapsing along the sagittal axis, which increases the deformity in the upright position and decreases the deformity in the prone position,[5] and even more so when the patient is under axial traction.

In general, this surgery is demanding for both the patient and the surgeon. Because many of these patients are older than 65 and usually have several risk factors due to polymorbidity, such a surgery needs to be well planned and thoroughly discussed with the patient and family, pointing out the risks and postoperative consequences. The patient and family must understand that the surgery could be fatal. Considerable effort has focused in recent years on facilitating the surgery and reducing the inherent risks for elderly patients. One of the key problems is blood loss during surgery, so different techniques have been tried, such as returning the blood with a cell saver and lowering the patient's blood pressure as much as possible. Also, approaching the surgical procedure from the back and using a staged incision can help to diminish the blood loss[24]; that is, the spine is opened portion by portion, then instrumented, and finally corrected and stabilized. This reduces the exposure field of the wound and therefore the potential blood loss. In most degenerative scoliosis or deformity patients who need surgery, a pedicle fixation is indicated to correct the deformity to a certain degree, specifically in the sagittal plane. In recent years it has become an increasing challenge to determine the extent of the fixation, because experience has shown that many patients develop secondary problems, such as adjacent segment disease (**Fig. 9.4**), proximal and distal junctional kyphosis/failure, and osteoporotic compression fractures above the fixation, sometimes skipping the immediately adjacent segments.

Whether cages need to be placed intervertebrally in elderly patients with concomitant osteoporosis has been debated.[5] By correct restoration of the lordosis and establishing the plumb line out of C7 through the end plate of S1, or at least less than 6 cm in front of the promontorium and behind the hip joints, the force transmission goes through the posterior elements, and therefore anterior support with a cage placed in the disk space may not be necessary. Avoiding cage surgery in elderly patients is a major step in reducing blood loss and surgical risk, especially the risk of a too rigidly stabilized spine. Depending on the presenting problem, the physical demands on the patients, and the patient's comorbidities, different surgical options with various levels of invasiveness are available (**Fig. 9.6**). In recent years, the use of a far lateral trans-psoas approach with selected correction of the most severely involved segments ("strategic" segments) has helped diminish the surgical trauma in frail patients[27,36,39,40] (**Fig. 9.5**).

Vertebral Compression Fractures

In recent years different options have been proposed to treat vertebral compression fractures in elderly patients, but these different methodologies have engendered controversy. Several techniques have been developed to augment compressed vertebrae as a consequence of osteoporotic fractures (**Fig. 9.8**). The simplest is the so-called vertebroplasty, in which transpedicular injection of cement into a fractured vertebral body can stabilize it. However, this technique cannot reduce a fracture, except by positioning of the patient. This treatment entails several risks involved, and there has been considerable debate in randomized clinical trials about whether surgical augmentation is preferable to conservative treatment of these fractures.[41,42]

The major risk of this treatment is cement leak, most relevantly into the spinal canal through the posterior wall. Cement leak can also occur to the side or to the front, which is less problematic if it is only a small amount of cement. The second relevant risk is that cement can enter the venous sinuses of the vertebral body, and from there enter the venous system, causing cement thrombosis or embolism in the lung.[43] Significant progress in cement technology has reduced these risks.

Vertebroplasty entails placing the working tubes through the pedicle into the vertebral body. There is a risk that the tubes inadvertently might be placed into the spinal canal or outside the pedicle and into the lateral paravertebral area, causing vascular damage. However, just as in pedicle screw placement, today's X-ray technology has made the percutaneous placement of a cannula into a pedicle a standard procedure, and so performing this procedure should not be a problem if the technique guidelines are followed.

The pedicle projection must be visualized carefully in the AP view, and the guiding Kirschner wire (K-wire) must be placed so that it projects completely within the oval contour of the pedicle in the frontal plane. The K-wire is slightly convergent toward the midline, and it can cross the inner wall of the pedicle projection contour when the K-wire tip is already in the vertebral body in the lateral view. Therefore, it is important to observe the forward drilling K-wire in the pedicle projection in the AP view by quickly checking the lateral view for each step, to follow the progress of the tip in the depths of the vertebral body. A Jamshidi needle can be used instead of the K-wire, which saves a step in the procedure.

Once the K-wire is placed, the Jamshidi needle or an analogue instrument like the working tube can be introduced over the K-wire and

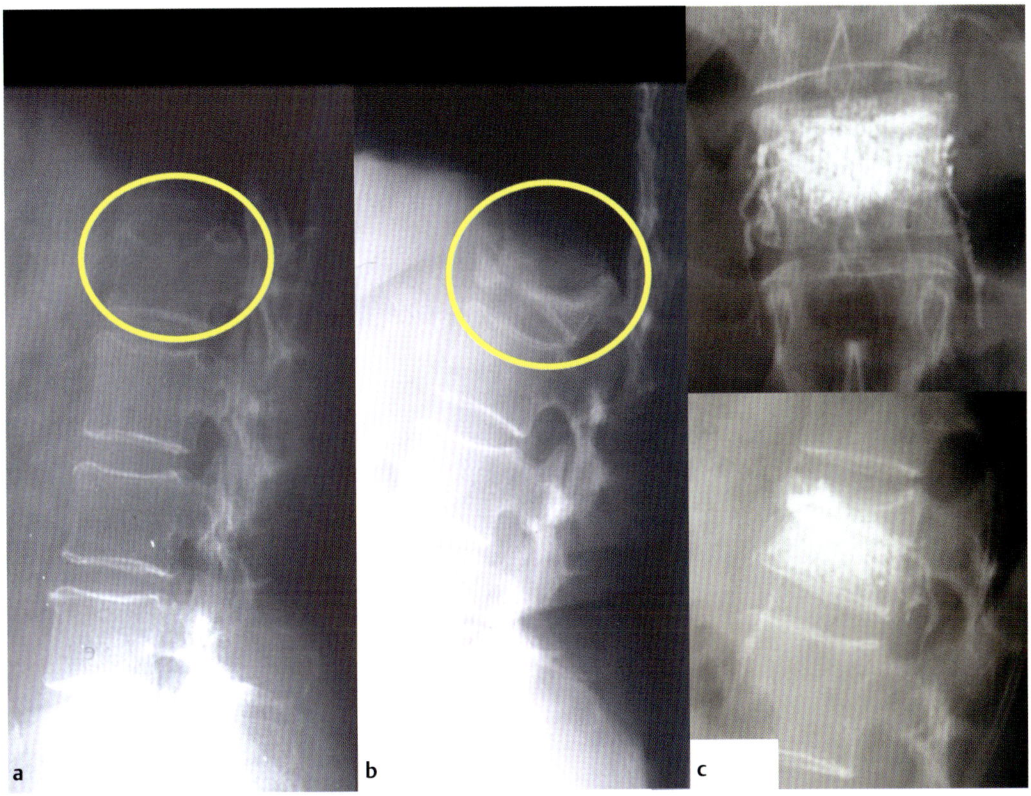

Fig. 9.8 A 76-year-old woman with vertebral compression fracture (VCF) and osteoporosis. **(a)** Fracture *(circle)* 2 weeks after back pain spontaneously began. **(b)** Four weeks later: vertebra plana *(circle)*. **(c)** Balloon kyphoplasty restored the vertebral height and integrity.

progressed into the vertebral body. When the working cannula is positioned properly in the posterior third of the vertebral body, the vertebral body can be drilled to prepare a seat for the balloon catheter or the cement applicator (in a simple vertebroplasty). Through this working channel, biopsies can also be taken. In cases of an additional kyphoplasty, the balloon catheter can be driven into the working cannula and placed in the prepared seat in the vertebral body. The same is true for the balloon catheter, which is armed with a stent, which then is inflated by the balloon and expanded as a vertebral body supporter and partial corrector of the compression fracture. With a simple vertebroplasty, no correction can be performed directly with cement. In an early stage of fractures, a kyphoplasty balloon, with or without a stent, can facilitate a reduction of the impressed end plate. The introduction of the balloon kyphoplasty and stent kyphoplasty technology has made this procedure of cement augmentation safer. According to some meta-analyses, the kyphoplasty procedure entails lower morbidity and mortality and fewer cement complications compared with a simple vertebroplasty procedure.[44] But augmentation technology has failed to prove its superiority over conservative treatment in randomized clinical trials.[28,41] However, there are several flaws in these prospective trials; basically, the trials do not replicate the real-life clinical experience.[6]

Prospective case series have demonstrated that augmentation surgery is highly beneficial and successful in patients with vertebral body compression fractures who are in severe pain.[44] The indication for such augmentation surgery should be primarily pain in still active fractures,

a

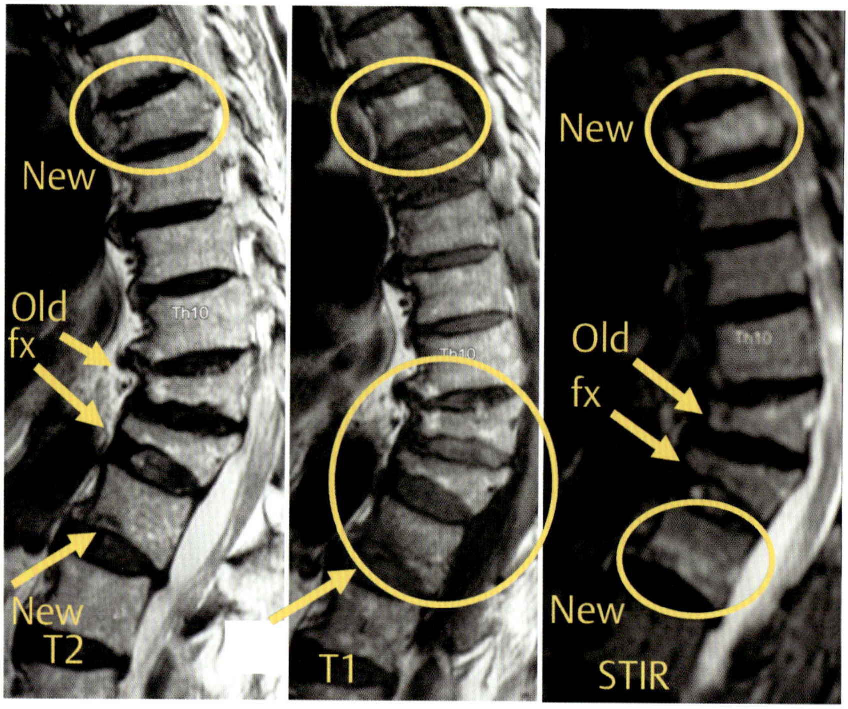

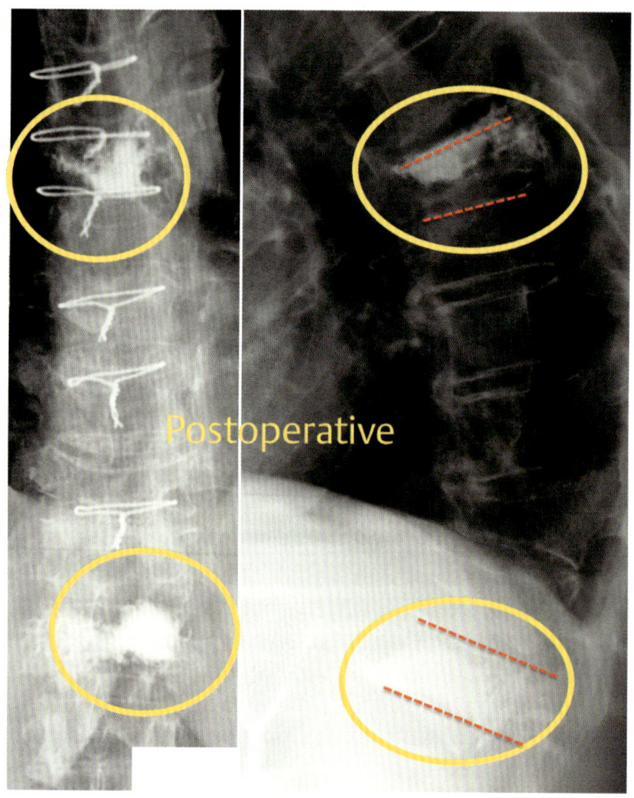

Fig. 9.9 Multilevel vertebral compression fractures in osteoporosis with secondary kyphosis. Old fractures with wedge-type vertebral bodies. No white uptake on magnetic resonance imaging (MRI) T2 and short tau inversion recovery (STIR) sequences, whereas new fractures show white uptake in T2 and STIR sequences (on T1 there is black uptake).

that is, fractures that are not healed and that are demonstrated as white vertebrae on MRI with STIR sequences. The usual practice is try conservative treatment first; if it fails, then augmentation surgery can be performed, but only after 6 weeks postfracture (**Fig. 9.9**).

Another benefit of augmentation surgery, namely the correction of the vertebral body wedge shape and indirect correction of a secondary kyphosis, is less well supported in the literature. However, if there are several fractures with wedge deformity of vertebral bodies, a significant kyphosis can develop, with a significant disturbance of the sagittal balance, which is detrimental in the long term for the elderly patient. In such cases, the surgical treatment with augmentation of the vertebral body to avoid further progression of kyphosis may be extremely beneficial (**Fig. 9.8**).

Other Typical Disorders of the Spine in Elderly Patients

As the treatment options for cancer are becoming more sophisticated, yielding increased survival time, there is a concomitant higher probability that elderly patients will develop metastases in the spine. Many metastases can be managed without surgical treatment, using chemotherapy and local irradiation. However, some patients experience significant pain due to metastatic fractures of the spine or compression of the spinal canal due to tumor expansion. The most frequent tumors are metastases of breast cancer in women and of prostate cancer in men, as well as the multiple myeloma disease of the spine.[45]

With today's available minimally invasive technology, augmentation can be combined with less invasive stabilization as a palliative procedure in elderly patients who experience spinal metastases.

Spinal infections in elderly patients are also becoming more frequent. Spondylodiskitis and spondylitis can be quite destructive, interrupting the anterior column and causing secondary kyphosis. The early stage of spondylodiskitis can be treated with antibiotics and partial immobilization. The indications for surgical treatment are pain that is unrelieved by pain medication, persistent high infection parameters in the blood (C-reactive protein, blood sedimentation rate, leukocytes), increasing secondary deformity, and neurologic deficit. The procedures are very similar to those in tumor surgery. Surgery in frail elderly patients with an infection of the spine, which is generally secondary to an infection elsewhere (bladder, lungs, lower limbs, skin), entails a high risk of septic complications, and thus surgery should be considered only for the above-mentioned criteria.

Chapter Summary

Spinal disorders in frail elderly patients with polymorbidity have become a major challenge in spinal surgery. It is a major challenge not only in terms of technical and surgical demands, but also in terms of the consequences of the treatment. These patients are best treated with an interdisciplinary approach. The surgeon's role is that of a highly specialized consultant for the specific spinal problem that needs to be treated in the context of the patient's overall medical care. Therefore, complex spinal problems in elderly patients should be treated in major medical centers in which interdisciplinary teams have experience in treating these cases.

The golden years are not so golden for elderly patients with severe forms of back pain. Whereas many elderly patients with moderate back pain can benefit from medications, lifestyle modifications, and other procedures, most of which are covered by Medicare and other health insurance plans, some elderly patients who suffer from severe back pain have too many comorbidities to undergo the necessary procedures. These frail patients present a challenge to the field of back pain management.

Pearls

- The world's demographics have shifted from a pattern of high birth rates and high mortality rates to one of low birth rates and delayed mortality. The consequence is a steady increase in the number of elderly people.
- A significant part of health care costs for the elderly is related to the restoration of quality of life and the maintenance of an independent lifestyle.
- Back pain due to degenerative disease and loss of bone mass of the spine are typical disorders of the elderly.
- Typical nosological entities in the elderly spine are osteochondritis, disk prolapse/herniation, facet joint arthritis, degenerative spondylolisthesis, spinal stenosis, degenerative spinal deformities, osteoporotic compression fractures, and pathological fractures due to metastatic disease.
- Apart from the typical spinal pathology of the elderly, such as spinal stenosis, degenerative spondylolisthesis, and cervical myelopathy, degenerative deformity represents one of the biggest challenges in spinal surgery. There are few alternatives to surgical treatment.
- New surgical techniques have been developed to minimize surgical risk and exposure in frail elderly patients with comorbidities.

Pitfalls

- The inability of the elderly spine to compensate for imbalance and deformities makes surgical treatment, specifically rigid fixation, a major challenge.
- Adjacent-segment disease is a specific problem of rigid fixation in the elderly and is due to imbalance and low-quality bone and connective tissue.
- The loss of bone mass is responsible for spine failure in the elderly.
- Major spine surgery in the elderly entails risks and complications due the polymorbidity of the elderly and to bad tissue quality. Therefore, surgery needs to be well thought out and well planned to reduce the inherent risks.

References

Five Must-Read References

1. Szpalski M, Gunzburg R, Mélot C, Aebi M. The aging of the population: a growing concern for spine care in the twenty-first century. Eur Spine J 2003;12(Suppl 2):S81–S83
2. Kinsella K, Velkoff V. An Aging World. U.S. Census Bureau. Washington, DC: U.S. Government Printing Office, series p95/01–1; 2001
3. International Institute for Applied Systems/Environmental Resources and Development. Analysis database, 2002. Laxenburg, Austria: International Institute for Applied Systems Analysis; 2003
4. National Center for Chronic Disease Prevention and Health Promotion. Chronic Disease Notes and Reports, Special Focus Healthy Aging. Atlanta: Centers for Disease Control and Prevention; 1999
5. Aebi M. The adult scoliosis. Eur Spine J 2005;14:925–948
6. Aebi M. Vertebroplasty: about sense and nonsense of uncontrolled "controlled randomized prospective trials". Eur Spine J 2009;18:1247–1248
7. Pluijm SM, Tromp AM, Smit JH, Deeg DJ, Lips P. Consequences of vertebral deformities in older men and women. J Bone Miner Res 2000;15:1564–1572
8. Ohshima H, Urban JP. The effect of lactate and pH on proteoglycan and protein synthesis rates in the intervertebral disc. Spine 1992;17:1079–1082
9. Roughley PJ. Biology of intervertebral disc aging and degeneration: involvement of the extracellular matrix. Spine 2004;29:2691–2699
10. Battié MC, Videman T, Parent E. Lumbar disc degeneration: epidemiology and genetic influences. Spine 2004;29:2679–2690
11. Battié MC, Videman T, Levälahti E, Gill K, Kaprio J. Genetic and environmental effects on disc degeneration by phenotype and spinal level: a multivariate twin study. Spine 2008;33:2801–2808
12. Adams MA, Roughley PJ. What is intervertebral disc degeneration, and what causes it? Spine 2006;31:2151–2161
13. Horner HA, Urban JP. 2001 Volvo Award Winner in Basic Science Studies: effect of nutrient supply on the viability of cells from the nucleus pulposus of the intervertebral disc. Spine 2001;26:2543–2549
14. Bibby SR, Jones DA, Ripley RM, Urban JP. Metabolism of the intervertebral disc: effects of low levels of oxygen, glucose, and pH on rates of energy metabolism of bovine nucleus pulposus cells. Spine 2005;30:487–496
15. Urban JP, Smith S, Fairbank JC. Nutrition of the intervertebral disc. Spine 2004;29:2700–2709
16. Cheung KM, Samartzis D, Karppinen J, Luk KD. Are "patterns" of lumbar disc degeneration associated with

low back pain?: new insights based on skipped level disc pathology. Spine 2012;37:E430–E438
17. Anandjiwala J, Seo JY, Ha KY, Oh IS, Shin DC. Adjacent segment degeneration after instrumented posterolateral lumbar fusion: a prospective cohort study with a minimum five-year follow-up. Eur Spine J 2011;20: 1951–1960
18. Ekman P, Möller H, Shalabi A, Yu YX, Hedlund R. A prospective randomised study on the long-term effect of lumbar fusion on adjacent disc degeneration. Eur Spine J 2009;18:1175–1186
19. Lee CS, Hwang CJ, Lee SW, et al. Risk factors for adjacent segment disease after lumbar fusion. Eur Spine J 2009;18:1637–1643
20. North American Spine Society. Evidence-based clinical guidelines on diagnosis and treatment of degenerative lumbar spondylolisthesis, 2008. https://www.spine.org/Documents/ResearchClinicalCare/Guidelines/Spondylolisthesis.pdf
21. Resnick DK, Choudhri TF, Dailey AT, et al; American Association of Neurological Surgeons/Congress of Neurological Surgeons. Guidelines for the performance of fusion procedures for degenerative disease of the lumbar spine. Part 9: fusion in patients with stenosis and spondylolisthesis. J Neurosurg Spine 2005;2:679–685
22. Sengupta DK, Herkowitz HN. Degenerative spondylolisthesis: review of current trends and controversies. Spine 2005;30(6, Suppl):S71–S81
23. Resnick DK, Choudhri TF, Dailey AT, et al; American Association of Neurological Surgeons/Congress of Neurological Surgeons. Guidelines for the performance of fusion procedures for degenerative disease of the lumbar spine. Part 10: fusion following decompression in patients with stenosis without spondylolisthesis. J Neurosurg Spine 2005;2:686–691
24. Schwarzenbach O, Rohrbach N, Berlemann U. Segment-by-segment stabilization for degenerative disc disease: a hybrid technique. Eur Spine J 2010;19: 1010–1020
25. Suratwala SJ, Pinto MR, Gilbert TJ, Winter RB, Wroblewski JM. Functional and radiological outcomes of 360 degrees fusion of three or more motion levels in the lumbar spine for degenerative disc disease. Spine 2009;34:E351–E358
26. Tsahtsarlis A, Wood M. Minimally invasive transforaminal lumber interbody fusion and degenerative lumbar spine disease. Eur Spine J 2012;21: 2300–2305
27. Anand N, Baron EM. Minimally invasive approaches for the correction of adult spinal deformity. Eur Spine J 2012
28. Isaacs RE, Hyde J, Goodrich JA, Rodgers WB, Phillips FM. A prospective, nonrandomized, multicenter evaluation of extreme lateral interbody fusion for the treatment of adult degenerative scoliosis: perioperative outcomes and complications. Spine 2010;35(26, Suppl):S322–S330
29. Le TV, Baaj AA, Dakwar E, et al. Subsidence of polyetheretherketone intervertebral cages in minimally invasive lateral retroperitoneal transpsoas lumbar interbody fusion. Spine 2012;37:1268–1273
30. Rodgers WB, Gerber EJ, Patterson J. Intraoperative and early postoperative complications in extreme lateral interbody fusion: an analysis of 600 cases. Spine 2011;36:26–32
31. Labrom RD, Tan JS, Reilly CW, Tredwell SJ, Fisher CG, Oxland TR. The effect of interbody cage positioning on lumbosacral vertebral endplate failure in compression. Spine 2005;30:E556–E561
32. Szpalski M, Gunzburg R. Lumbar spinal stenosis in the elderly: an overview. Eur Spine J 2003;12(Suppl 2):S170–S175
33. North American Spine Society. Evidence-based clinical guidelines on diagnosis and treatment of spinal stenosis, 2009. https://www.spine.org/Documents/ResearchClinicalCare/Guidelines/SpinalStenosis.pdf
34. Chen BL, Wei FX, Ueyama K, Xie DH, Sannohe A, Liu SY. Adjacent segment degeneration after single-segment PLIF: the risk factor for degeneration and its impact on clinical outcomes. Eur Spine J 2011;20: 1946–1950
35. Everett CR, Patel RK. A systematic literature review of nonsurgical treatment in adult scoliosis. Spine 2007;32(19, Suppl):S130–S134
36. Schulte TL, Leistra F, Bullmann V, et al. Disc height reduction in adjacent segments and clinical outcome 10 years after lumbar 360° fusion. Eur Spine J 2007; 16:2152–2158
37. Abdu WA, Lurie JD, Spratt KF, et al. Degenerative spondylolisthesis: does fusion method influence outcome? Four-year results of the spine patient outcomes research trial. Spine 2009;34:2351–2360
38. Harding IJ, Charosky S, Vialle R, Chopin DH. Lumbar disc degeneration below a long arthrodesis (performed for scoliosis in adults) to L4 or L5. Eur Spine J 2008;17:250–254
39. Cho KJ, Suk SI, Park SR, et al. Arthrodesis to L5 versus S1 in long instrumentation and fusion for degenerative lumbar scoliosis. Eur Spine J 2009;18:531–537
40. Crawford CH III, Carreon LY, Bridwell KH, Glassman SD. Long fusions to the sacrum in elderly patients with spinal deformity. Eur Spine J 2012;21:2165–2169
41. Buchbinder R, Osborne RH, Ebeling PR, et al. A randomized trial of vertebroplasty for painful osteoporotic vertebral fractures. N Engl J Med 2009;361: 557–568
42. Kallmes DF, Comstock BA, Heagerty PJ, et al. A randomized trial of vertebroplasty for osteoporotic spinal fractures. N Engl J Med 2009;361:569–579

43. Hulme PA, Krebs J, Ferguson SJ, Berlemann U. Vertebroplasty and kyphoplasty: a systematic review of 69 clinical studies. Spine 2006;31:1983–2001
44. Hübschle L, Borgström F, Olafsson G, et al; SWISSspine Registry Group. Real-life results of balloon kyphoplasty for vertebral compression fractures from the SWISSspine registry. Spine J 2014;14:2063–2077
45. Aebi M. Spinal metastasis in the elderly. Eur Spine J 2003;12(Suppl 2):S202–S213

10

Back Pain in Spinal Infections

Rishi Mugesh Kanna, Ajoy Prasad Shetty, Emiliano Vialle, and Shanmuganathan Rajasekaran

Introduction: Pyogenic Spondylodiskitis

The spine is a common site of infection in pyogenic spondylodiskitis. Within the spine, the anterior structures (i.e., the vertebral body and the discs) are affected in more than 95% of patients.[1] The incidence of pyogenic vertebral infection is reported to be 3 to 16% of all bone and joint infections, with a small increase in its incidence each year.[2,3] The incidence is higher in less developed and developing nations due to malnutrition, immune deficiency states such as human immunodeficiency virus (HIV), delayed diagnosis, and lack of access to medical facilities. In developed nations, the increase is probably due to increased awareness, increased numbers of spinal surgeries, better diagnostic modalities, and the expanding at-risk group. Diabetes mellitus, malnutrition, intravenous substance abuse, HIV infection, malignancy, long-term steroid use, chronic renal failure, liver cirrhosis, septicemia, and previous spine surgery are the common predisposing factors identified. Protein malnutrition, defective cellular and antibody-mediated immunity, and steroid-mediated immunosuppression are also important. With the increase in the number of spinal surgeries, postoperative iatrogenic diskitis accounts for up to 30% of all cases of pyogenic spondylodiskitis.[4]

A bimodal age distribution has been observed, with the first peak occurring in young children and a second peak at approximately the fifth to sixth decades of life. Males are twice as commonly affected as females, for reasons that are not clear.[5] Because of its rarity and vague presentation, diagnosis is often delayed, which can result in abscess formation and severe compression of the neural structures, leading to neurologic deficit and rarely septicemia and mortality in 2 to 4% of cases.[6]

Etiology

Most infections occur due to bacterial spread from a distant site to the spinal column through the bloodstream. The skin, the respiratory tract, and the genitourinary tract are the common primary foci. But in 30 to 70% of patients, a primary focus of infection cannot be detected.[7] Earlier, tubercular bacilli accounted for most infections of the spine, and recent studies have found that pyogenic organisms are the common isolates. Among these, *Staphylococcus aureus* and *Streptococcus* species account for more than 50% of cases. Gram-negative organisms such as *Escherichia coli* and *Proteus* are causative in patients with urinary tract infections and intravenous drug abusers. *Klebsiella pneumoniae* and *Pseudomonas* are common isolates in patients with hospital-acquired infections. Anaerobic organisms and organisms of low virulence are common in patients with diabetes mellitus and those with penetrating spine trauma. Despite the best investigative efforts, including blood, urine, and tissue cultures to isolate the organism, in one third of cases, the infective organisms are never identified.[8]

Pathophysiology

The arterial route is the common route of bacterial spread to a vertebra following bacteremia. About 90 to 95% of pyogenic spinal infections affect the vertebral body or disk, and the posterior elements of the spine are infrequently involved. This is due to the increased blood supply of the cancellous bone of the vertebral body and its rich, cellular marrow. The circulating bacteria readily colonize in the subchondral end plates when the blood flow stagnates in the metaphyseal arterial loops just beneath the vertebral end plates. Due to the avascularity of the disk and the peculiar arterial anatomy of the vertebral subchondral region on either side of the disk, the subchondral region of the disk is infected first and the disk is secondarily invaded by bacteria from the end-plate region. Communicating vascular plexus of the paravertebral and epidural region enable the spread of infection from one metaphysis to the other. Vertebral body infections commonly occur in the lumbar spine because of the high blood flow to this region of the spine. In children, the intervertebral disk has penetrating arteries, and hence direct invasion of the disk can occur, resulting in primary diskitis, followed by vertebral body involvement.

Retrograde seeding of venous blood via the Batson's venous plexus can also play a role. Whenever intra-abdominal or intrathoracic pressure increases, venous blood is shunted from the abdominal and pelvic organs toward the valveless paravertebral venous plexus. Thus, infections from pelvic and abdominal organs can reach the spine through retrograde veins. Rarely, contiguous spread of infection from a nearby infected focus such as a renal abscess, aortic vascular implants, or paravertebral nodes can infect the vertebra and disk, producing infective spondylitis.

In pyogenic spondylitis, the involvement is usually focal, but multiple-site involvement can infrequently occur in immune-deficient patients. As destruction proceeds, the vertebral canal can be invaded by pus and granulation tissue, which can cause cord compression, neurologic deficit, and systemic dissemination of bacilli, resulting in sepsis. Continued destruction of the vertebral body results in pathological collapse, kyphosis, and spinal instability. Unlike tubercular infection, where the spread of abscess is slow, in pyogenic spondylitis the abscess formation is rapid, associated with intense inflammation, resulting in early neurological deficit.

Clinical Presentation

A precipitous onset with signs of acute pyogenic infection is rare, and the usual presentation is one of insidious onset, with back pain being the most common symptom, developing in 1 or 2 weeks. The pain is initially localized to the level of infection, but vague distribution to the paraspinal areas is common. With progression, the pain is quite severe even at rest, being aggravated by the least spinal movement. Onset of severe pain can indicate severe instability, due to either gross destruction of the vertebral bodies or involvement of posterior structures, especially the facet joints. Radicular pain along the distribution of a nerve root can occur when the abscess and granulation tissue presses the corresponding nerve root.

Because low back pain is a common and nonspecific symptom, a high degree of suspicion is needed to make an early diagnosis of pyogenic spondylitis. The presence of clinical "red flags," such as pediatric age or age > 65 years, chronic steroid intake, cancer chemotherapy, renal disease, diabetes mellitus, HIV infection, and high fever, must prompt a laboratory investigation and radiological workup.

Although fever is present in less than one third of adult patients, children with vertebral osteomyelitis can present with an abrupt onset of malaise and fever. Young children may not directly complain of back pain but rather present with refusal to eat, stiffness of the back with restricted spinal movements, and guarded walking.

Neurologic involvement occurs due to vertebral body collapse with kyphosis or with the development of large epidural abscess. It is manifested as numbness and weakness in one or both lower limbs and bladder or bowel disturbances. Where neurologic involvement is suspected, a meticulous neurologic examination must be performed, including a rectal examination to detect early cauda equina compression. This is important, as early surgical intervention in such cases would be beneficial.

Investigations

Laboratory Studies

The total and differential white cell counts, erythrocyte sedimentation rate (ESR), and C-reactive protein (CRP) are the common blood tests performed to aid in the diagnosis of diskitis. Other tests including a complete hemogram and renal and liver function tests are mainly indicated for initiating antimicrobial chemotherapy and anesthetic purposes if surgical treatment is considered.

Leukocytosis (> 10,000 cells/mm^3) is common in patients with pyogenic spondylitis but nonspecific. Elevation of the ESR, although nonspecific, is the most common laboratory abnormality. Elevated ESR is positive in more than 90% of patients with spinal infections.[9] The average ESR in patients with pyogenic spondylitis ranges from 43 to 87 mm per hour in different studies.[10,11] Unexplained back pain associated with spinal stiffness and an increased ESR should lead the clinician to suspect infective spondylitis.

The CRP is also an excellent indicator of acute inflammation. It is elevated in more than 90% of patients with spinal infection and is more specific than ESR.[12] Because both ESR and CRP are sensitive markers but not specific for spinal infection, they assume more significance in combination with clinical features and imaging findings. Also, rather than single values, serial ESR and CRP values help in predicting infection in postoperative spondylodiskitis[13,14] and in assessing the response to treatment.

In evaluating the treatment response to spinal infections, both ESR and CRP have significant roles. Carragee et al[15] found that a 25% reduction of the initial value of the ESR after 1 month of treatment was a good prognosis marker in the treatment for spondylodiskitis. However, 50% of those with no change in the ESR values during the treatment period also had good outcome. Thus, in patients clinically responding to therapy, a raised ESR should not be a cause for concern and should not lead to unnecessary interventions or prolonged therapy.

Urine cultures are advised in situations where the genitourinary tract is considered the primary focus. Blood cultures should always be obtained in all patients, preferably during a febrile episode and prior to administration of antibiotics. But they are not sensitive and are positive in only 60% of patients.

Histopathology

A computed tomography (CT)-guided or image intensifier–guided percutaneous biopsy of the infected vertebra or disk is advised to acquire tissue for microbiological studies. This is especially useful in patients without significant neural compression, where tissue biopsy is required to initiate appropriate therapy. Trocar biopsies are better than fine needle aspiration because a larger amount of material from the infected area is available for examination. The acquired tissue is sent for aerobic cultures, Gram's stain, tubercular polymerase chain reaction gene assay, culture for tubercular bacilli, and histopathological assessment. Although tissue aerobic cultures are positive in only 50 to 60% of patients, histological findings are helpful to identify the infective process and to differentiate diskitis from tuberculosis, tumors, and pathological fractures. The presence of infiltration of neutrophils, necrosis, and inflammatory changes are diagnostic of acute infective diskitis. In tubercular infections, epithelioid granulomas, lymphocytic infiltrates, and multinucleated giant cells are the typical findings. If blood cultures and percutaneous biopsy techniques fail to identify the infecting organism and the patient does not respond to empirical therapy, then open surgical biopsy during spinal debridement and stabilization is indicated.

Radiological Studies

Plain radiographs are not helpful initially, as they are normal in the early stages of the disease. The earliest findings are observed by 2 to 3 weeks and include loss of delineation of the trabeculae of the subchondral bone and destruction of the end plates with narrowing of the disk space (**Fig. 10.1**). In advanced disease, complete collapse of the disk space, destruction of vertebral bodies, asymmetrical kyphosis, and spinal instability due to subluxation may be evident (**Fig. 10.2**). CT is useful in assessing the degree of bone destruction, detecting cavities within the bone, and examining the surrounding soft tissues (**Fig. 10.3**). Hence, it is mainly useful if surgical treatment is planned. It is also used as a guide for accurate placement of the biopsy needle while performing a percutaneous biopsy.

Magnetic resonance imaging (MRI) is now the investigation of choice due to its ability to depict changes even in the early stages of the disease. MRI has been shown to have a sensitivity of 96%, a specificity of 92%, and an accuracy of 94% in patients with spinal infections.[16] In fact, MRI has such high sensitivity that the marrow changes observed on MRI look more extensive than the actual extent of vertebral destruction. The standard sequences performed are T1- and T2-weighted images, short tau inversion recovery (STIR) sequences, and contrast studies (**Fig. 10.4**). T1-weighted images show decreased signal intensity changes in the vertebral bodies and disk spaces due to the presence of edema. In T2-weighted images, the signal intensity is increased in the vertebral disk and the body. The extension of infection in the adjoining tissue is better delineated by fat-suppression STIR sequences and contrast studies. MRI also clearly documents the location and size of the epidural abscess, the presence of sequestrum, the extent of compromise of the spinal canal, the degree of compression of the spinal cord, and any signal intensity changes in the cord (**Fig. 10.5**). Asymptomatic

a

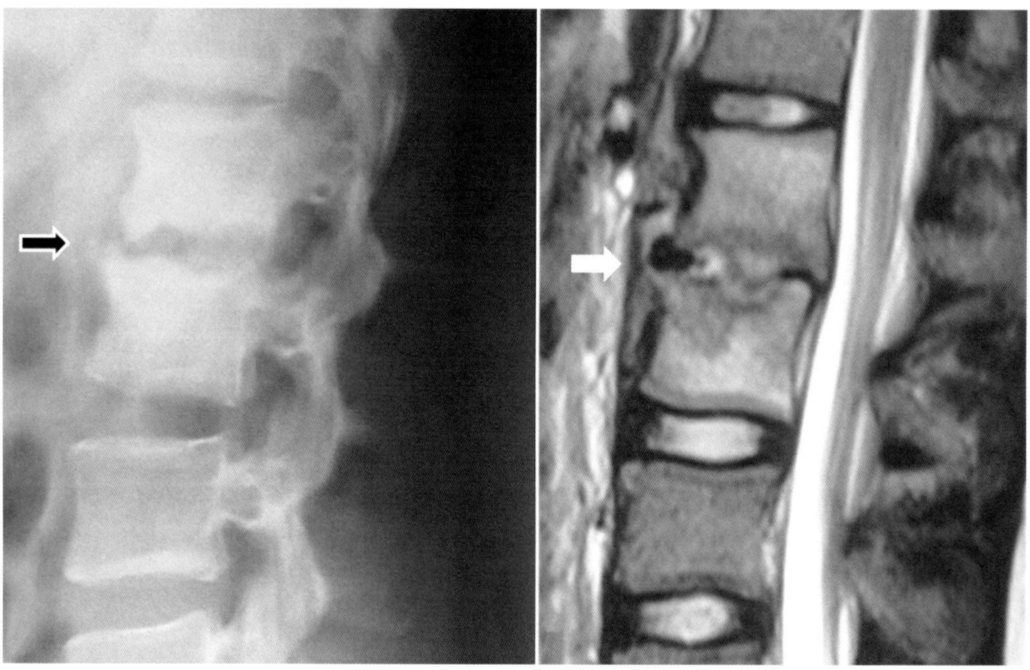

Fig. 10.1 **(a)** Lateral radiograph of the thoracolumbar spine in a patient with diskitis. The disk margins are irregular with subchondral haziness *(black arrow)*. **(b)** Sagittal T2-weighted magnetic resonance imaging (MRI) of the same patient shows loss of disk, hyperintense signal changes within the disk, and paradiskal regions *(white arrow)* indicative of diskitis.

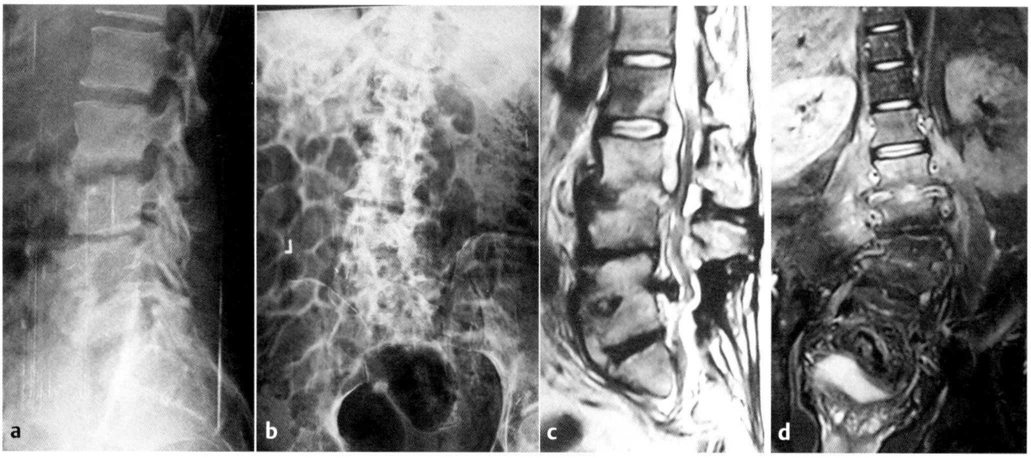

Fig. 10.2 Anteroposterior **(a)** and lateral **(b)** radiographs of the lumbar spine showing extensive vertebral destruction with loss of disk space, scoliosis, bony irregularities, and vertebral erosions. Sagittal **(c)** and coronal **(d)** MRI of the same patient showing multilevel diskitis and spondylitis with epidural and paravertebral abscess formation.

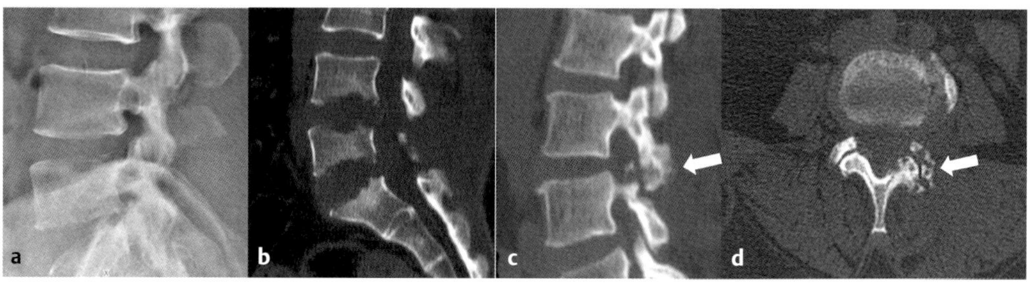

Fig. 10.3 Lateral radiograph **(a)** and sagittal computed tomography (CT) **(b)** of a patient with L4–L5, L5-S1 diskitis. The widespread erosion of the subchondral region and cavitation are better shown on CT. This is essential for surgical planning. Sagittal **(c)** and axial **(d)** CT images of another patient with facet joint pyogenic arthritis *(arrow)* on the left side. CT is ideal to evaluate infections of the posterior elements, which are not clearly seen in radiographs.

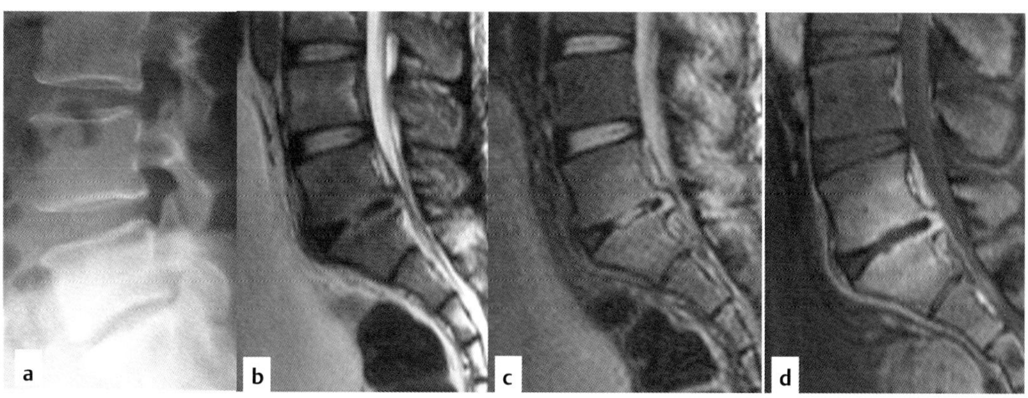

Fig. 10.4 **(a)** Lateral radiograph of a patient who presented with axial back pain and systemic features of infection. The radiograph shows a reduction in the L5-S1 disk space. Sagittal T2 **(b)**, short tau inversion recovery (STIR) **(c)**, and contrast T1 **(d)** sections show diskitis at the L5-S1 level, a thin epidural abscess, and edema within the vertebral bodies.

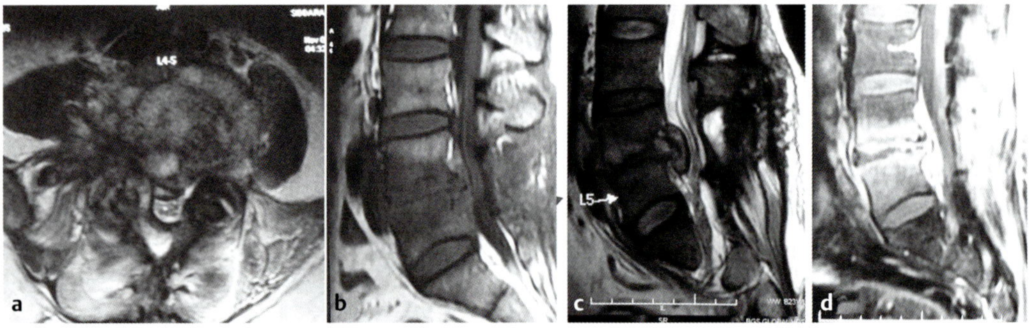

Fig. 10.5 MRI features of advanced diskitis. **(a)** Axial T2 image shows extensive perivertebral and epidural abscess formation with spinal canal obliteration. Sagittal T1 **(b)**, T2 **(c)**, and STIR **(d)** sequences show extensive diskitis at L4–L5 with disk erosion, subchondral damage, and epidural and paravertebral abscess formation.

multilevel skip lesions can be present in other vertebral segments, and hence MRI must evaluate the whole spine.

Also, MRI aids in differentiating pyogenic spondylitis from Modic changes, tubercular infections, benign osteoporotic fractures, and tumorous conditions (**Table 10.1** and **Fig. 10.6**). The presence of disk space involvement favors infection as compared with neoplasm. Usually type 2 Modic changes are painful and can mimic infections but show hyperintense signals on both T1 and T2 sequences. Type 1 Modic changes may mimic pyogenic diskitis but do not enhance with contrast, and typically the disk is not affected. Tuberculous spondylitis has an extensive bone destruction pattern with relative sparing of the intervertebral disk in the early stages, heterogeneous enhancement of the vertebral body, subligamentous spread of abscess, and large paravertebral abscesses with thin smooth walls.

Furthermore, MRI is also useful in assessing the healing response to treatment. The healing of the vertebral lesion is diagnosed on follow-up MRI based on typical features of resolution of marrow edema, replacement of marrow by fat seen as a bright signal on T1- and T2-weighted images, and complete resolution of paravertebral collections (**Fig. 10.7**). However, Kowalski et al[17] suggested that despite the clinical improvement, MRI findings of healing may lag clinical resolution and should not lead the surgeon to unnecessary invasive treatments.

A radionuclear scan with technetium (Tc) 99m is very sensitive (> 90%) for an early diagnosis of pyogenic vertebral osteomyelitis, but it has lower specificity (< 80%).[18] Any inflammation or degenerative changes in the spine can also result in increased tracer uptake, and hence the radionuclear changes are nonspecific. Radioactive gallium scan and indium 111–labeled leukocyte scintigraphy are more

Table 10.1 Typical MRI Features of Pyogenic Spondylitis and Its Mimics

Diagnosis	MRI features
Pyogenic spondylitis	Early disk space involvement with hypointensity on T1 and hyperintense signals on T2 sequences
Tubercular spondylitis	Extensive involvement of subchondral region and adjacent vertebral body; huge, multiple, thin-walled abscesses
Modic changes	Signal changes are confined to the subchondral region; disk is spared; nonenhancing; no abscess
Pathological fractures (metastasis)	Multilevel noncontiguous affliction; disk is spared; no abscess formation

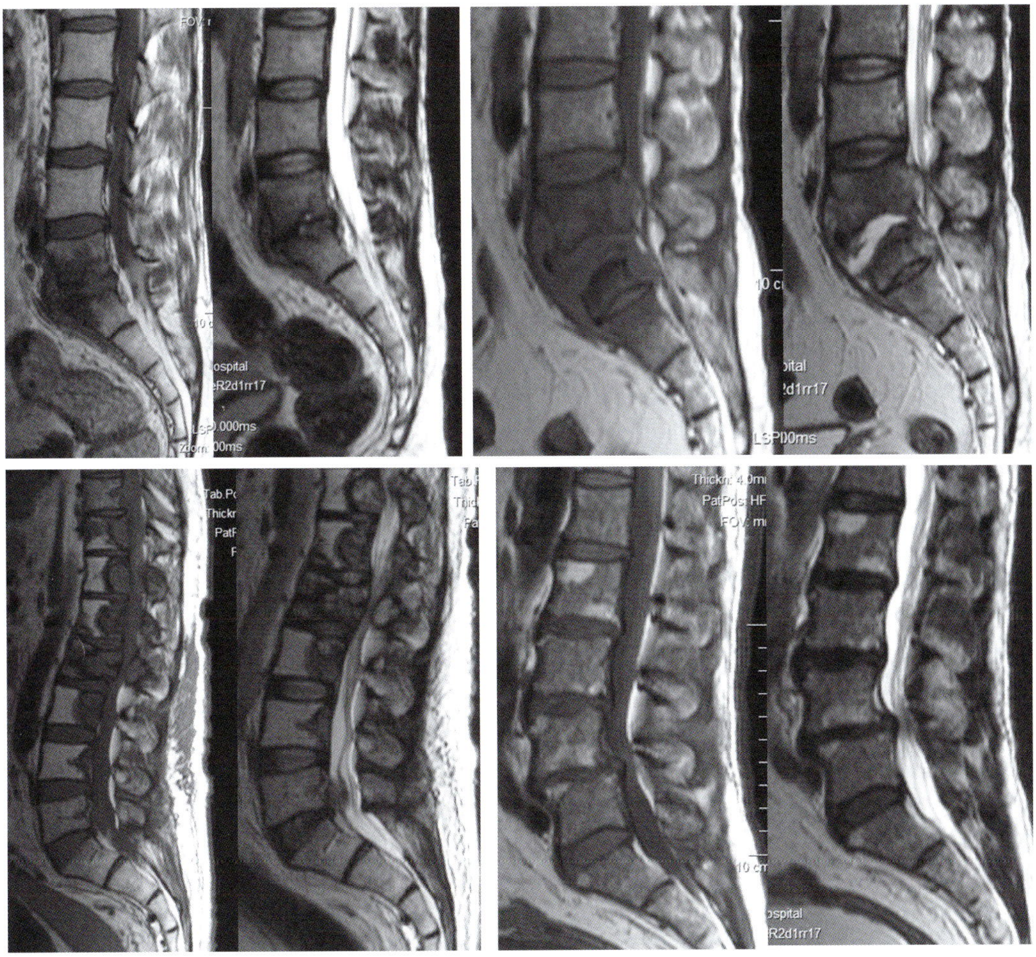

Fig. 10.6 Diskitis and its common differential diagnosis. **(a)** Diskitis. Sagittal MRI sequences show typical hypointense signals in T1 sections at L5-S1 and hyperintense changes in T2 sequences. **(b)** Tubercular spondylitis. Note the extensive abscess formation in the prevertebral and epidural regions, and the abscess wall is thin. **(c)** Metastasis involves multiple vertebral segments, heterogeneous signal changes, and no abscess formation. **(d)** Modic end-plate changes mirroring signal changes on either side of the disk. The disk signal is intact and no abscess formation is seen.

specific, with 80 to 85% specificity rates, but they have very low sensitivity. Owing to the high rate of false-negative results, they are not used routinely in diagnosing spinal infections.

Differential Diagnosis

A high degree of suspicion is required for an early diagnosis of spinal infection, especially in patients with risk factors, as the presenting symptoms may be vague. Often initial investigations are normal, and imaging may need to be treated within short intervals if clinical suspicion is very high (**Fig. 10.8**). The important differential diagnoses are metastasis, osteoporotic fractures, and degenerative vertebral changes. In postoperative diskitis, the clinical picture and blood investigations are more important than radiological investigations, as normal signal intensity changes seen in the immediate postoperative period may mimic infection.

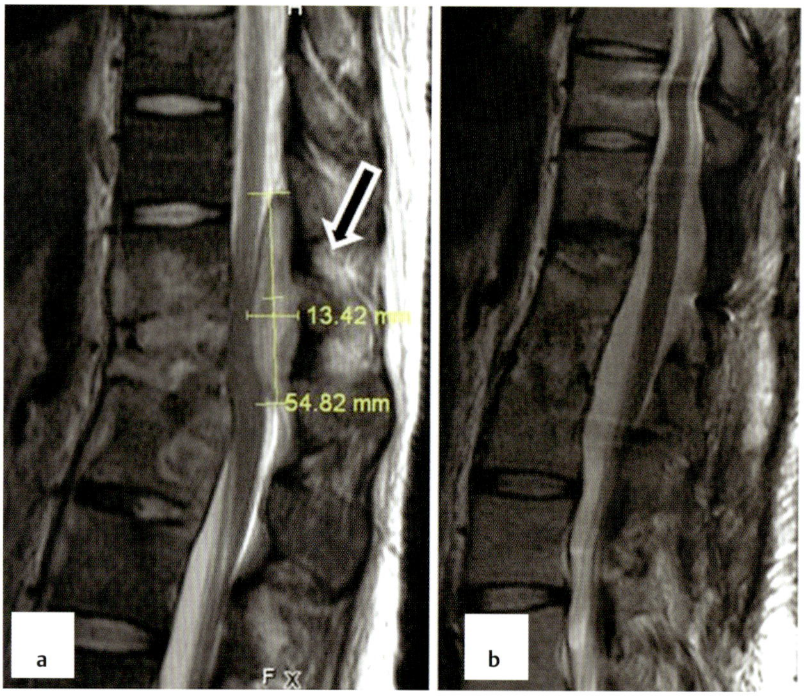

Fig. 10.7 Successful resolution of spinal infection at completion of treatment. **(a)** Sagittal MRI in the pretreatment phase shows abscess *(arrow)* in the epidural space with hyperintense signals within the disk and bone suggestive of infection. **(b)** Sagittal MRI after the completion of treatment shows resolution of the abscess and healing of the bone infection characterized by fatty replacement of the marrow.

a 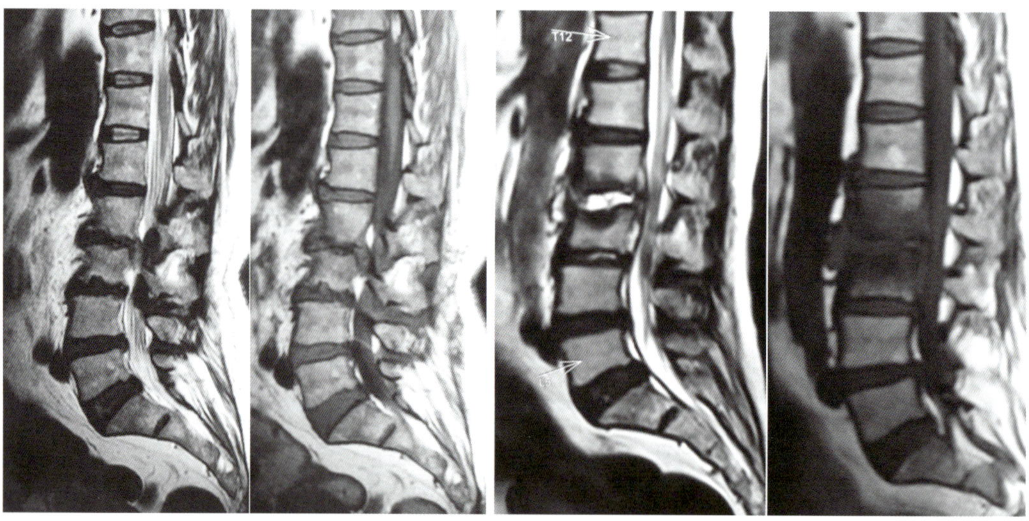 b

Fig. 10.8 **(a)** Sagittal T1 and T2 MRI of a patient who presented with back pain radiating to the leg. The images show a disk prolapse at the L2–L3 level. Because the patient's symptoms were not classic for disk prolapse, she was treated conservatively. Her back pain worsened significantly and manifested even at rest. **(b)** MRI scans 4 weeks later show L2–L3 diskitis with abscess formation. In patients for whom the physician has a high clinical suspicion about infective spondylitis, MRI should be performed.

Conservative Treatment

Conservative treatment is usually successful in the early stages of the disease, when the diagnosis is certain, the infective organism is identified, and appropriate antibiotics can be instituted before the development of severe destruction or neurologic complications. Even in situations where the organism could not be isolated, conservative treatment with empirical antibiotics provides good results (**Fig. 10.9**). Bed rest, bracing, and antibiotics are the key features of conservative therapy. Management of comorbid factors such as diabetes mellitus, anemia, malnutrition, and associated diseases is also important. Immobilization of the affected region of the spine with a rigid thoracolumbar brace and bed rest is essential for conservative treatment.

Isolation of the organism either from blood/urine culture or through a trocar biopsy of the lesion is important before the start of antibiotics. After the harvest of the material, it is prudent to start a first-generation cephalosporin empirically, as *S. aureus* is the most common organism. In patients with methicillin-resistant *S. aureus* (MRSA), vancomycin is the drug of choice. For immunocompromised patients and intravenous drug abusers, a third-generation cephalosporin along with coverage for gram-negative bacteria is advised. Recent studies show that rifampicin provides good results in pyogenic spondylitis because it is active against biofilm-embedded bacteria and has synergistic effects with other β-lactam antibiotics.[19] It is an excellent oral antibiotic to prescribe after initial intravenous therapy in infections with gram-positive organisms.

There is no clear consensus on the exact duration of antibiotic therapy, but generally intravenous antibiotics are given for a period of 3 to 4 weeks followed by 6 weeks of oral antibiotic therapy. Although several studies have recommended 6 to 8 weeks of intravenous therapy, others recommend only 4 weeks.[20–22] Antibiotic therapy for less than 4 weeks may result in an unacceptably high recurrence rate. Roblot et al[23] found no difference in the risk of relapse among patients treated for 6 weeks or longer in a retrospective analysis of 120 patients. Serial monitoring with ESR and CRP levels and clinical improvement are important parameters to judge control of infection, and it is advisable to continue antibiotics for at least a month after the ESR and clinical symptoms have returned to normal. Failure of resolution of clinical symptoms, persistently high inflammatory parameters like ESR and CRP, progressive destruction in radiographs, and epidural abscess formation on the MRI indicate failure of conservative therapy. Nonoperative treatment has a success rate of 75%, and at the end

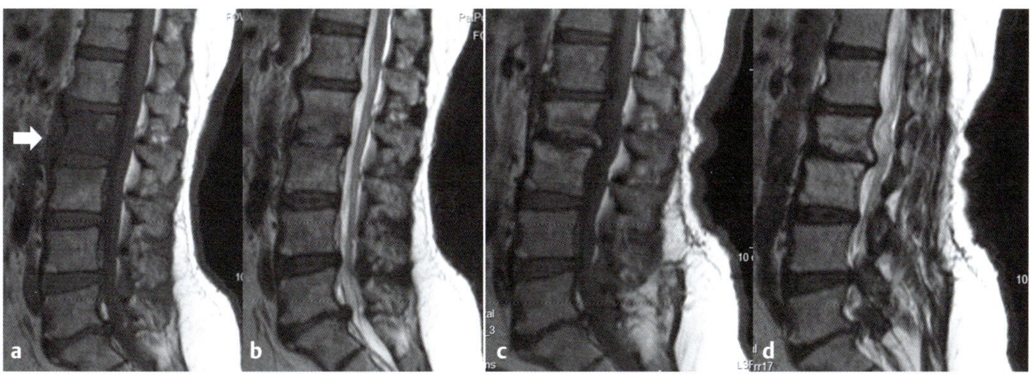

Fig. 10.9 Sagittal T1 **(a)** and T2 **(b)** images of a 72-year-old man with L1–L2 spondylodiskitis. Note the hypointense L1 vertebral body *(arrow)* on the T1 sequence and hyperintense signals on the T2 sequence. The patient was treated with antibiotics for 12 weeks. **(c,d)** Posttreatment MRIs. T1 **(c)** and T2 **(d)** sequences show complete resolution of lesion, characterized by hyperintense fatty marrow replacement of the subchondral region.

of 1 to 2 years spontaneous interbody fusion can be observed as radiological evidence of complete healing.

Surgical Treatment

Surgical treatment is required in only 10 to 15% of patients, and the indications include severe persistent symptoms, extensive vertebral destruction with or without radiological instability, increasing kyphosis, significant neurologic deficit, epidural abscess, sepsis, an ambiguous diagnosis, and inability to isolate the organism. The goals of surgical treatment are to obtain adequate tissue for both bacteriologic and histological diagnosis, to adequately decompress neural structures, and to provide spinal stability. The extent of surgery and the type of surgical approach must be planned individually based on the severity of the vertebral involvement and the general condition of the patient. Yoshimoto et al,[24] in a review of 45 cases of pyogenic spondylitis in the elderly, observed that 42% of patients with neurologic deficits were treated conservatively due to poor general condition. But the neurologic status still showed improvement in 74% of these patients with conservative treatment.

The surgical options include percutaneous abscess drainage, posterior debridement with or without pedicle screw fixation, anterior debridement and fixation, and combined anterior and posterior debridement and fixation. The choice of treatment depends on the location of the lesion, the extent of vertebral destruction, and the experience of the surgeon. One should remember that there are no randomized trials to prove the superiority of one approach over another, and studies have shown good outcomes with all techniques. Regardless of the technique, the goals of treatment—decompression, debridement, stabilization, and reconstruction—should be safely achieved.

Percutaneous Drainage

Percutaneous drainage of abscess from the disk space has been described in the literature. Hadjipavlou et al[25] studied 28 patients with primary hematogenous pyogenic spondylodiskitis treated with bilateral percutaneous transpedicular drainage and debridement of abscess. They found that immediate relief of pain was experienced by 75% of patients, and in long-term follow-up the success rate was 68%. However, they do not recommend this technique in postlaminectomy infection or in the presence of instability, kyphosis from bone destruction, or neurologic deficit. This technique appears useful in early uncomplicated diskitis and in moribund patients who may not tolerate invasive procedures.

Anterior Approach

Because spinal infections commonly afflict the vertebral body, an anterior surgical approach is recommended. It provides direct access to the diseased area, and it enables wide debridement of the infection and placement of a structural bone graft or cage to reconstruct the vertebral column (**Fig. 10.10**). Bone grafting with tricortical iliac autograft is commonly used, but to avoid donor-site morbidity, structural bone allograft can be used alternatively. In the lumbar spine, a retroperitoneal approach is used to access from L1–L2 to L4–L5, and a transperitoneal approach is used for L5-S1. Fang et al[26] reported a series of 39 patients who underwent an anterior decompression and debridement with fusion for pyogenic spondylitis, and concluded that anterior debridement and fusion give good early and long-term results, with rapid recovery of the patient and low morbidity and mortality. If anterior reconstruction is not biomechanically strong, then additional posterior instrumentation for stabilization can be used.

Liljenqvist et al[27] reported a 100% fusion rate and good results in 20 patients treated with anterior column reconstruction using an expandable titanium cage and posterior stabilization. With the recent increase in minimally invasive spine surgeries, some surgeons have successfully used percutaneous pedicle fixation in the treatment of spinal infection. Lin et al[28] retrospectively reviewed 45 patients treated for pyogenic spondylodiskitis with anterior debridement and interbody fusion followed by a second-stage procedure involving either

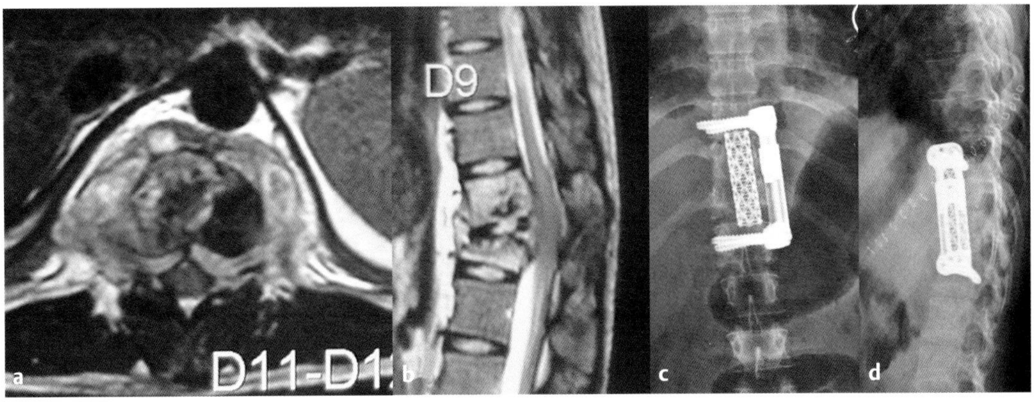

Fig. 10.10 Anterior surgery for infective spondylitis. **(a,b)** The patient presented with destruction at the T11–T12 vertebral levels with abscess formation, cord compression, and vertebral collapse. **(c,d)** He was treated with anterior decompression, corpectomy, and fusion with a cage and plate.

traditional open posterior pedicle screw fixation or percutaneous posterior pedicle screw fixation. Patients who underwent the minimally invasive surgery had lower visual analogue scale scores for pain, significantly less blood loss, and at 2 years there was no significant difference in functional outcomes.

Posterior Approach

Recently, posterior approaches have gained popularity and are becoming the standard treatment for pyogenic diskitis of the lumbar spine. In a standard posterior approach, anterior debridement of the disk and body are performed through a transforaminal/transpedicular route supplemented with posterior pedicle screw fixation. The aims of this approach are to stabilize the spine with multilevel pedicle screws, perform a wide decompression circumferentially around the spinal cord, and reconstruct the anterior vertebral void. The wide lumbar canal and the ability to retract the thecal sac without risking neural deficits and the safe transforaminal route enable anterior reconstruction of vertebral defects even up to 20 to 25 mm, comfortably through the posterior approach (**Figs. 10.11** and **10.12**). The safety of the titanium pedicle screw system even in the presence of abscess has been proved in several studies, and it is extensively used now. Gonzalvo et al[29] studied nine patients with

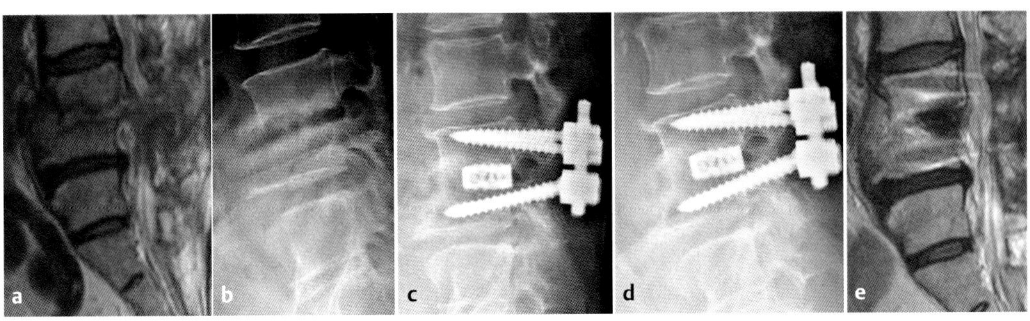

Fig. 10.11 Sagittal MRI **(a)** and lateral radiograph **(b)** of a patient with spondylodiskitis at the L3–L4 level. **(c,d)** Lateral radiographs show healing of the lesion at L3–L4 treated with transforaminal debridement and reconstruction and pedicle screw stabilization. **(e)** Follow-up MRI shows healing of the lesion with complete resolution of the abscess and bone healing.

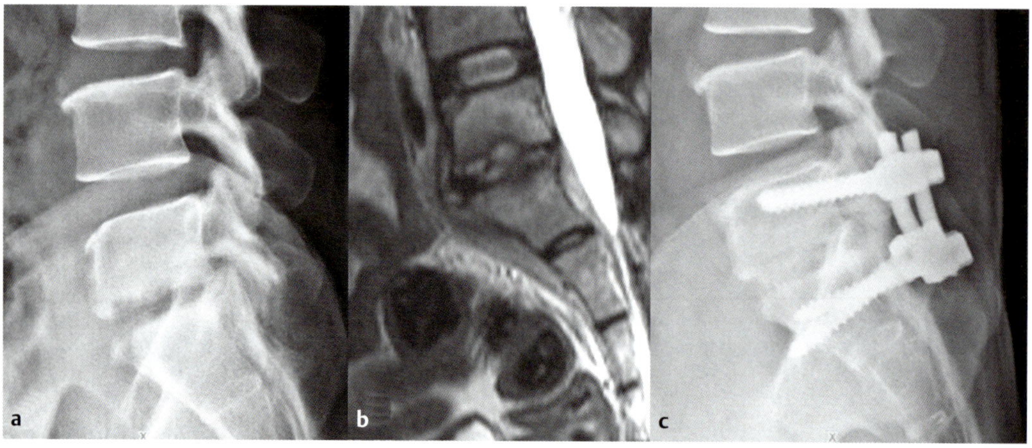

Fig. 10.12 Lateral radiograph **(a)** and sagittal MRI **(b)** of a patient with L5-S1 diskitis with disk space destruction. The patient was treated with posterior decompression, stabilization, and debridement alone, which yielded good healing of the lesion with bony fusion across the disk space. **(c)** Postoperative lateral radiograph.

pyogenic diskitis who underwent a single-level/single-stage debridement and posterior instrumented fusion with pedicle screws and an interbody and posterolateral autogenous bone graft. Preoperative neurologic deficits improved in all nine patients, and solid bone fusion was achieved in all nine, with complete healing of infection at 12 months.

The advantages of the posterior approach are its familiarity, a 360-degree exposure for spinal cord decompression, ease of multilevel instrumentation, and better deformity correction, and it enables performing a simultaneous anterior reconstruction without violating body cavities. In patients with early disease and less deformity, a posterior transpedicular decompression with pedicle screw stabilization alone provides immediate pain relief and prevents severe deformity and neurologic sequelae (**Fig. 10.13**). The transpedicular approach serves as an excellent portal for debridement of the vertebral body and decompression of the spinal cord.

Conclusion

The incidence of pyogenic spondylitis is on the rise due to an increased at-risk population, an increased number of spinal surgeries, and increased awareness leading to better diagnosis. A high index of clinical suspicion, supplemented with appropriate laboratory investigations and radiological studies, help in early diagnosis. With the advent of antibiotics, improved techniques of management, and early recognition, most patients can be treated with rest, bracing, and antibiotics. Several risk factors such as elderly age, delayed diagnosis, diabetes, renal disease, cancer chemotherapy, presence of neurologic deficit, and sepsis are associated with poor outcomes. Surgical debridement with or without stabilization is indicated in patients with neurologic deficit, sepsis, abscess formation, or increasing vertebral destruction. Currently, posterior debridement with transforaminal interbody fusion is the preferred approach.

Postoperative Pyogenic Spondylitis

Postoperative diskitis can potentially occur after any invasive procedure in the disk space, such as diskogram, diskectomy, and fusion surgeries. The incidence of postoperative diskitis varies from 1 to 7% depending on the type of surgery and the use of instrumentation.[30] Because the intervertebral disk is avascular, it is particularly

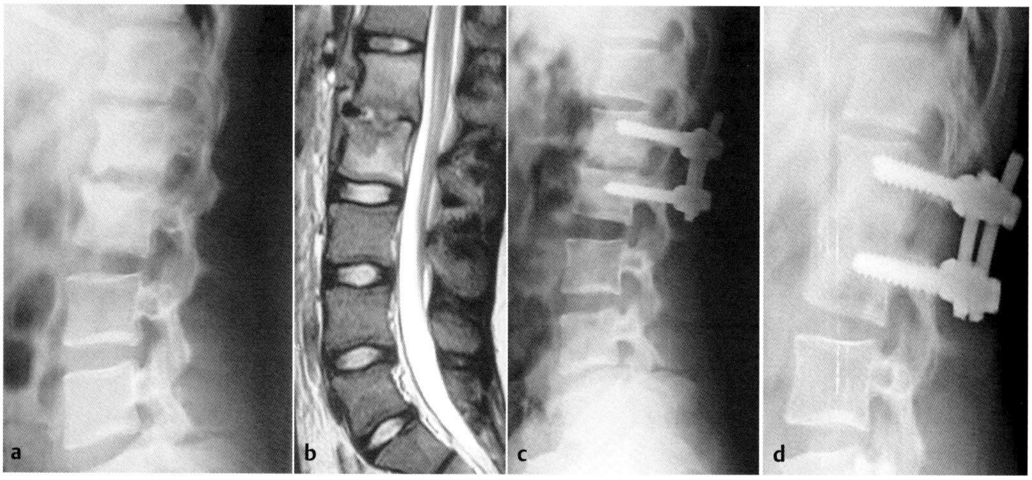

Fig. 10.13 **(a)** Lateral radiograph of thoracolumbar spine and sagittal T2 MRI **(b)** of a patient with diskitis at the L1–L2 level. **(c)** The patient has been treated with transpedicular decompression, debridement, and spinal stabilization. **(d)** Follow-up radiograph performed at 6 months shows good healing of the lesion.

prone to infection, even with a small inoculum. Normally in an uncomplicated healing after a disk surgery, the postoperative back pain improves in 2 to 3 days. Any abnormal back pain 2 to 3 days after surgery, present even at rest, or increasing with the movements of the spine, should raise the suspicion of diskitis. Obvious external signs of infection over the operative site such as local warmth and tenderness may not be present. The patient usually has significant difficulty in sitting, turning in the bed, and mobilizing. The neurologic examination may be normal.

The white cell counts, ESR, and CRP levels are considerably elevated. A deviation from the normal postoperative pattern of changes of these inflammatory markers helps in diagnosis. In the postoperative period, severe back pain associated with prolonged peak serum levels and persistent high levels of ESR and CRP at 2 to 3 weeks is considered 80% specific for infection.[13] In a study by Rosahl et al,[14] it was observed that although ESR remained markedly elevated 10 days after anterior cervical diskectomy and fusion, with a peak on postoperative day 3, the CRP levels returned to less than 50% of its peak level by postoperative day 5.

The radiographs are normal and do not show any obvious vertebral erosions until the third week. Hence, MRI is performed if there is a strong clinical suspicion. The caveat here is that sometimes it is difficult to differentiate normal postoperative changes and diskitis on the MRI. However, the presence of hyperintense signal changes in the disk space and the vertebral body on T2 sequences, which enhances with contrast, and the occurrence of a perivertebral abscess confirms the diagnosis (**Fig. 10.14**). Blood cultures and image-guided biopsy help in isolating the infective organism. But an organism is isolated in only 50% of the patients.

Early cases with fewer symptoms, minimal vertebral destruction, and a thin abscess do well with rest and appropriate parenteral antibiotic therapy. Usually parenteral antibiotic therapy is given for a period of 3 to 4 weeks followed by oral antibiotics for up to 8 weeks. The duration of therapy depends on various factors, such as the severity of infection, the type and virulence of the organism, the immune status of the patient, the presence of comorbid factors, and the magnitude of the surgery performed. Some authors believe that postlaminectomy diskitis is less amenable to conservative care, and patients do have persistent instability back pain on continued nonoperative care.[25] Surgical treatment is indicated in patients with significant pain, sepsis, abscess formation,

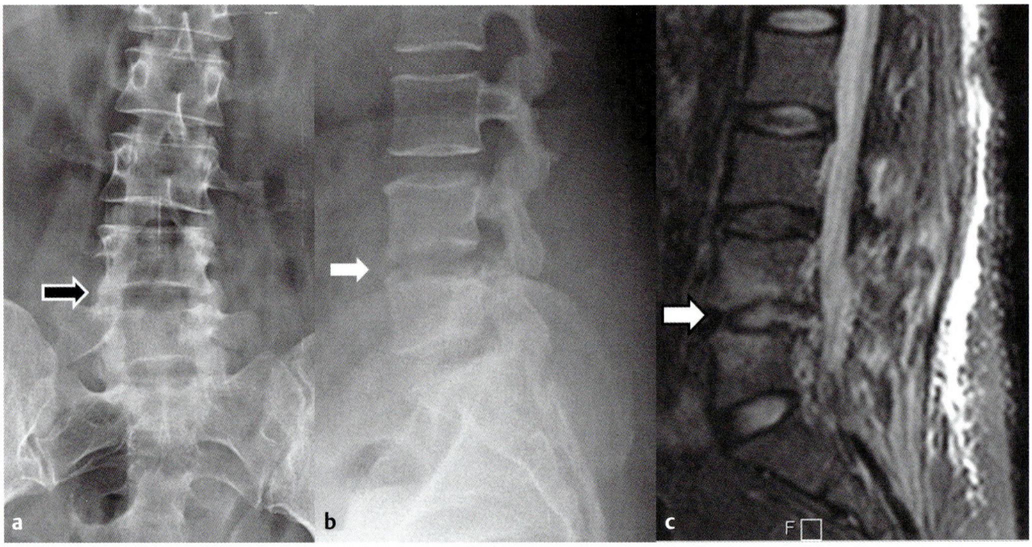

Fig. 10.14 A 45-year-old patient who underwent L4-L5 diskectomy and laminectomy one month ago presented with significant back pain and elevated inflammatory parameters at 4 weeks. **(a)** The wide laminectomy defect is seen in the anteroposterior (AP) view of the lumbar spine *(black arrow)*. **(b)** The lateral radiograph shows hazy end plates of the L4-L5 disk space *(white arrow)*. **(c)** Sagittal MR with contrast shows hyperintense signals within the disk space extending into the vertebral body and thin epidural abscess formation.

severe vertebral destruction, and neurologic deficit. In early stages, a thorough debridement is performed, and in patients who present late with a large anterior column defect, a cage or a bone graft should be used to reconstruct the anterior column and provide stability along with posterior spinal instrumentation.

Spinal Tuberculosis

Spinal tuberculosis is more common than pyogenic diskitis in underdeveloped and developing countries. It is caused by *Mycobacterium tuberculosis*. Infection results from hematogenous dissemination from a primary focus, usually the lungs, kidneys, lymph nodes, or intestinal viscera. The lumbar vertebrae can be involved with infection through the Batson's perivertebral venous plexus. The most common infection is the paradiskal type with secondary involvement of the disk. Posterior structures are involved in only 10%, and skip lesions can be identified in 15 to 20% of patients.

Chronic insidious-onset back pain associated with restriction of movements of the spine is the usual presenting feature. Constitutional symptoms of malaise, loss of appetite and weight, rise of temperature in the evening, and night sweats can be present in 40% of patients. Exuberant abscess formation is a typical feature of tuberculosis. This abscess is not warm to the touch and does not have features of inflammation; hence, it is described as a cold abscess. As the disease progresses, vertebral destruction occurs, resulting in kyphosis and neurologic deficit. Neurologic involvement results from direct compression of the cord due to an abscess, inflammatory granulation tissue, or canal compromise due to kyphosis and instability. In the late stages, neurologic deficit can result from stretching of the cord at the apex of the kyphotic deformity. Kyphosis is an important sequela of spinal tuberculosis. As the disease progresses, collapse of the vertebral body occurs, resulting in a localized kyphotic deformity. The degree of kyphosis varies depending on the number of vertebrae affected and the extent of vertebral body damage. Apart from causing deformity, the vertebral bodies at the apex of kyphosis can retropulse into the canal, causing neurologic deficit.

In adults, the kyphosis increases only during the active stages of the disease, and the final deformity depends on the severity of vertebral body damage. But in children, the kyphosis can worsen during growth, even after complete healing of the disease. Hence, children with healed tuberculosis need periodic follow-up until they achieve skeletal maturity. Rajasekaran[31,32] described four "spine at risk" radiological signs to identify children with spinal tuberculosis who are at risk for progressive deformity. These signs appear early in the course of the disease, and prophylactic surgical fusion and column reconstruction is advised for children with two "spine at risk" signs (**Fig. 10.15**).

Investigations

The ESR may be markedly elevated (> 70 mm/h), and lymphocytosis is present. The Mantoux skin test is not useful in endemic regions, as a positive test just indicates a previous tuberculous infection. In nonendemic regions, a positive Mantoux test indicates the possibility of tuberculosis.

Imaging forms a major role in the diagnosis of tuberculosis. Earliest features observed on plain radiographs are vertebral osteoporosis, narrowing of the joint space, and an indistinct paradiskal margin of vertebral bodies. In the thoracic spine, the cold abscess is visible on plain radiographs as a fusiform or globular radiodense shadow (bird's nest appearance). Wedging of one or two vertebral bodies leads to a kyphotic deformity (**Fig. 10.16**).

A CT scan is useful in assessing the extent of bony destruction; it provides early identification of posterior element involvement. It is also helpful in identifying tuberculosis in "hidden" sites, such as the craniovertebral and cervicodorsal junction, the sacroiliac joints, and the sacrum, and when a percutaneous biopsy is planned. But MRI is the gold standard for demonstrating the extension of disease into soft tissues and the spread of tuberculous abscess. MRI is the most effective method for

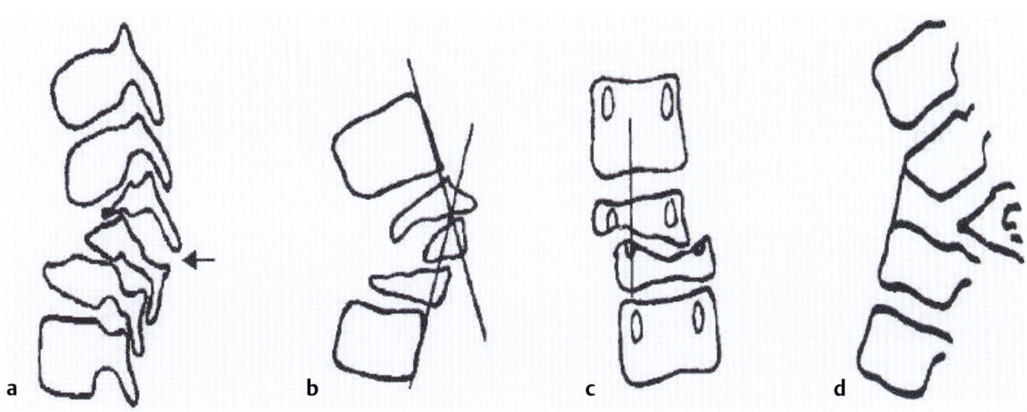

Fig. 10.15 Spine-at-risk radiological signs. **(a)** Separation of the facet joint. The facet joint dislocates at the level of the apex of the curve, causing instability and loss of alignment. **(b)** Posterior retropulsion. This is identified by drawing two lines along the posterior surface of the first upper and lower normal vertebrae. The diseased segments are found to be posterior to the intersection of the lines. **(c)** Lateral translation. This is confirmed when a vertical line drawn through the middle of the pedicle of the first lower normal vertebra does not touch the pedicle of the first upper normal vertebra. **(d)** Toppling sign. In the initial stages of collapse, a line drawn along the anterior surface of the first lower normal vertebra intersects the inferior surface of the first upper normal vertebra. Tilt or toppling occurs when the line intersects higher than the middle of the anterior surface of the first normal upper vertebra.

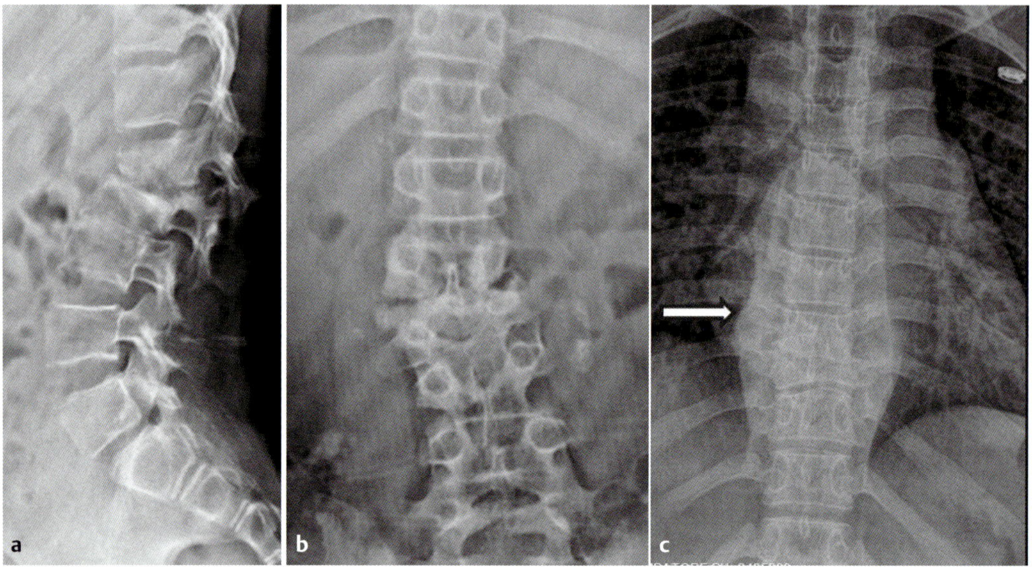

Fig. 10.16 Typical radiographic features in tuberculosis. **(a)** Multiple adjacent vertebral collapse and kyphosis. **(b)** Lateral translation and asymmetrical wedging. **(c)** A paravertebral abscess collection on either side of the vertebra is observed in the anteroposterior (AP) radiograph of the spine as widened soft tissue shadow *(arrow)* around the paravertebral region (bird's nest appearance).

demonstrating neural compression (**Fig. 10.17**). MRI with contrast is also helpful in differentiating tuberculosis from vertebral lesions of other noninfectious causes.

Tissue studies are essential to confirm the diagnosis of tuberculosis. Bone tissue or abscess samples are obtained to stain for acid-fast bacilli (AFB), and isolate organisms for culture and sensitivity. The tissue is analyzed for a tubercular polymerase chain reaction (PCR) test, which has sensitivity and specificity > 85% and also identifies drug resistance.[33] Histopathological examination is the gold standard to diagnose tuberculosis, and typical histopathological findings include large caseating necrotizing granulomatous lesions with epithelioid and multinucleated giant cells with lymphocytic infiltration.

Treatment

General supportive measures include bed rest, external bracing, nutritious diet, vitamins as required, care of bladder and bowels, and good nursing care. Modern antitubercular drugs are able to achieve therapeutic levels in caseous tissues and abscesses, and are the mainstay of treatment for spinal tuberculosis. In uncomplicated tuberculosis, ambulant multidrug chemotherapy is administered for all patients along with external bracing in the initial period. The patient is followed carefully until complete healing. Surgical treatment is recommended for certain specific indications in these patients. The World Health Organization (WHO) guidelines for the type and duration of antitubercular chemotherapy consider spinal tuberculosis to be severe extrapulmonary (category 1), and treatment is advised for 6 months. In cases of relapse or treatment failure, treatment is prescribed according to category 2, that is, for 9 months. The currently recommended first-line drug regime is four-drug therapy. This includes isoniazid 5 mg/kg, rifampicin 10 mg/kg, pyrazinamide 20 to 25 mg/kg, and ethambutol 15 mg/kg for 2 to 3 months followed by isoniazid and rifampicin for 4 to 6 months. In children, ethambutol is replaced by streptomycin, as it may cause optic neuritis. Recently, drug resistance to standard antitubercular drugs has become an increasing problem. Tuberculosis caused by organisms resistant to isoniazid and

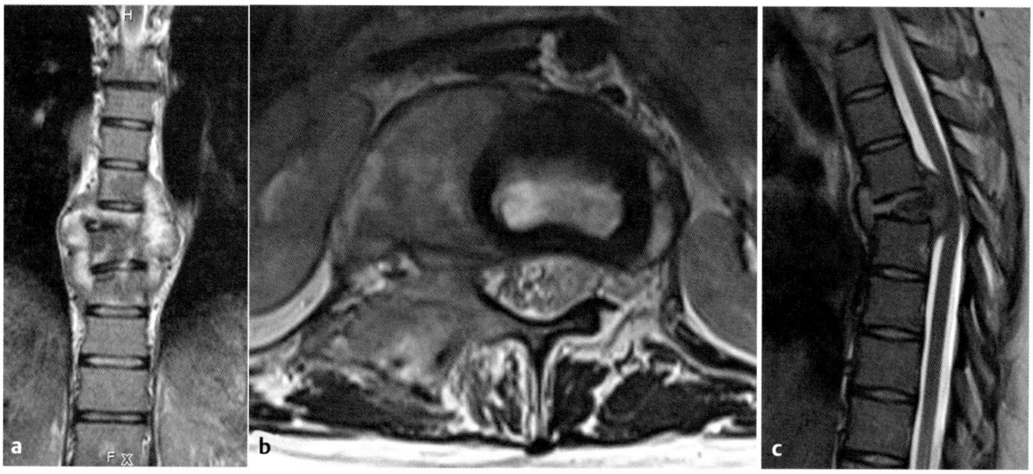

Fig. 10.17 MRI demonstrates the extent of abscess formation, spinal canal occlusion, and cord signal changes in tuberculosis. **(a)** A paravertebral abscess collection on either side of the vertebra is well seen on this coronal MRI. **(b)** Axial MRI showing a well-defined paraspinal, epidural, and intraosseous abscess with thin and smooth abscess walls, and subligamentous spread of the abscess. **(c)** Sagittal MRI showing complete destruction of T3 vertebra with prevertebral and epidural abscess formation causing cord compression.

rifampicin is defined as multidrug resistant (MDR) tuberculosis. The reported median prevalence of MDR pulmonary tuberculosis is 3 to 25%. The management of MDR tuberculosis is complex and should involve infectious disease specialists.

Before the advent of antituberculosis medications and surgery, nonoperative treatment resulted in deformity, contractures, and death. Surgical excision of the disease foci was ventured, but surgical treatment in the absence of chemotherapy resulted in poor results, including sinus formation, neurologic deficit, and high mortality. The introduction of antitubercular chemotherapy in the 1960s achieved spectacular success in the control of disease. Although a significant number of patients could be treated with chemotherapy, those who presented late had significant morbidity due to kyphosis and neurologic deficit. Over half a century ago, Hodgson and Stock[34] attempted surgical excision of an infected lesion along with chemotherapy, and achieved good results. Hodgson popularized the concept of anterior surgery for spinal tuberculosis with radical debridement and placement of rib strut grafts (known as the Hong Kong surgery). The approach enabled complete clearance of the abscess and cord decompression, acquired tissue for diagnosis, and enabled reconstitution of the anterior column. Soon it was realized that such a radical surgery is unnecessary in spinal tuberculosis, and most patients can be treated with an ambulant short course of chemotherapy with surgery being performed in select cases (known as the middle-path regimen).[35]

Currently, surgery in spinal tuberculosis is performed to achieve debridement and drainage of large cold abscesses, decompression of spinal cord and neural structures, spinal deformity correction, and stabilization and reconstruction of the anterior column. These goals can be achieved through different surgical approaches selected on an individual basis. The different surgical techniques include a direct anterior approach, a combined anterior and posterior approach, and an all-posterior approach. The addition of instrumentation in spinal tuberculosis is well accepted and advised, especially where instability is present or expected after decompression. Previously, anterior surgery was frequently performed, but of late, many surgeons prefer the all-posterior approach, in which the anterior debridement

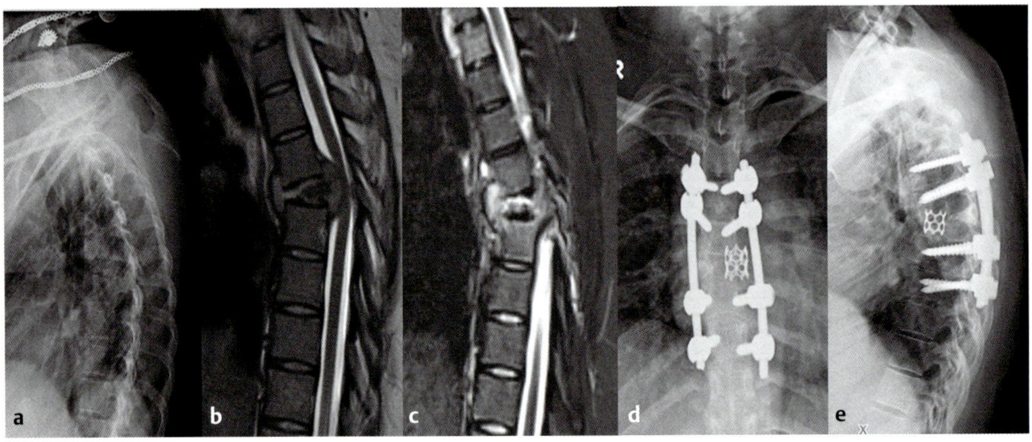

Fig. 10.18 Lateral radiograph **(a)** and sagittal MR images **(b,c)** of a patient with T7 tuberculosis and cord compression. **(d,e)** The patient has been treated by all-posterior costotransversectomy approach, anterior reconstruction, and posterior stabilization.

and reconstruction and posterior stabilization are performed through a single-stage posterior approach. Anterior reconstruction of vertebral defects up to one or two vertebral levels can be performed comfortably through the posterior approach (**Fig. 10.18**). The availability of the pedicle screw system, which provides excellent reconstruction possibilities, along with the development of surgical techniques that enable anterior reconstruction through a posterior approach, have recently tilted the balance in favor of all-posterior surgeries in spinal tuberculosis.

The aims of surgery in spinal tuberculosis are to obtain tissue sample for biopsy, to drain an abscess cavity, to achieve debridement of the disease focus, and to stabilize the spine. These aims can be achieved by anterior, posterior, or combined procedures, either staged or in a single stage.

Inflammatory Back Pain

Inflammatory back pain (IBP) can be defined as back pain arising from inflammation of the facet joints, the ligament attachments, or the sacroiliac joints. The first clinical description of IBP was provided in 1949 by Harland and colleagues: "A frequent feature of this pain and stiffness was the aggravation caused by immobility. Waking in the morning stiff and in pain, the patient gradually became more supple during the day, feeling at his best from the afternoon until bedtime." Patients tend to be young at disease onset, and the typical features of IBP are morning stiffness, chronic back pain present for at least 3 months or more, and pain relieved by movement and physical therapy.

Recently the Assessment of SpondyloArthritis International Society (ASAS) has developed criteria to diagnose IBP[36]:

1. Age at onset < 40 years
2. Insidious onset
3. Improvement with exercise
4. No improvement with rest
5. Pain at night (with improvement upon getting up)

The presence of four criteria has a sensitivity of 77.0% and a specificity of 91.7% for diagnosing IBP.[37]

The common causes of IBP include ankylosing spondylitis and undifferentiated spondyloarthropathies (including undifferentiated spondyloarthropathies, reactive arthritis, inflammatory bowel diseases, and psoriasis). IBP in these conditions is the most common symptom and the first manifestation in 75% of patients.

The pain is typically dull and poorly localized to the gluteal and sacroiliac joints. Patients commonly experience morning stiffness for at least 30 minutes, which improves with moderate physical activity. The pain often begins unilaterally and intermittently, and as the disease progresses, it becomes more persistent and bilateral. In severe cases, it extends proximally, associated with ossification of the annulus fibrosus, resulting in fusion of the spine.

The diagnosis of ankylosing spondylitis and other spondyloarthropathies is based on clinical features, laboratory results, and imaging studies. Inflammatory parameters such as ESR and CRP are elevated. More than 80% of patients with ankylosing spondylitis are human leukocyte antigen (HLA)-B27 positive. In patients suspected of having a spondyloarthropathy, determining HLA-B27 status helps in diagnosis. It is a class I surface antigen encoded by the B locus in the major histocompatibility complex, and it is strongly associated with diseases such as psoriasis, ankylosing spondylitis, inflammatory bowel disease, and Reiter syndrome.

Radiographic studies are most helpful in establishing a diagnosis. MRI shows early findings of bone marrow edema, and bone erosions around the sacroiliac joints, which helps in confirming the diagnosis (**Fig. 10.19**). Involvement of the sacroiliac joint is a requirement for the diagnosis of ankylosing spondylitis. In advanced cases, new bone formation, sclerosis and fat

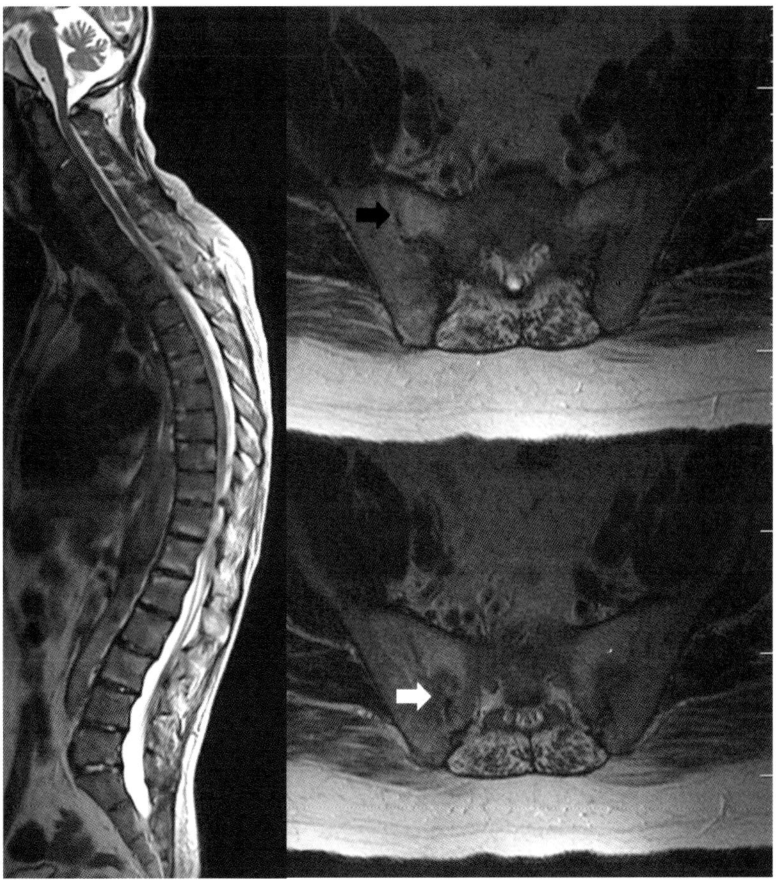

a b c

Fig. 10.19 (a) Sagittal MRI of a patient with ankylosing spondylitis shows typical vertebral corner hyperintense signals, squaring of the vertebral bodies, global kyphosis, and loss of disk space. **(b,c)** Axial sections through the sacroiliac joints shows bilateral hyperintense signals on either side *(black arrow)* of the joint with bony erosions *(white arrow)* typical of ankylosing spondylitis.

infiltration, squaring of the vertebral bodies caused by vertebral corner erosions, ossification of the annulus, and bridging syndesmophytes can be observed.

Management of these conditions involves a combination of physical therapy, analgesics, and biological treatment such as tumor necrosis factor-α (TNF-α) inhibitors. These illnesses are best managed by rheumatologists; a full description of treatment is beyond the scope of this chapter.

Chapter Summary

Infections are a frequent and ominous cause of back pain, and should be differentiated from the more common mechanical back pain. Infective spondylitis can be caused by pyogenic, granulomatous, or fungal organisms. Pyogenic vertebral osteomyelitis is the most common vertebral infection, whereas tuberculosis is still the most common in developing countries. Infection usually develops from hematogenous spread of the organism from a distant primary focus, and uncommonly by direct inoculation, through contiguous spread from adjacent structures and iatrogenic causes. With the increase in the number of spinal surgeries and instrumentation, the incidence of postoperative infective spondylitis is on the rise.

Early diagnosis and appropriate treatment can lead to near-normal function without surgery. In contrast, delay in diagnosis can lead to permanent neurologic deficits, significant spinal deformity, sepsis, or even death. The eventual outcomes depend on the extent of the disease, the type of pathogen, the severity of neurologic and vertebral damage, and the patient factors including age and comorbidities. A high clinical suspicion, appropriate laboratory investigations, and judicious use of MRI can facilitate an early diagnosis. Management principles include identification of the organism, appropriate antimicrobial chemotherapy, and supportive treatment. Surgical treatment in the form of debridement, spinal stabilization, and deformity correction is indicated in patients with extensive vertebral destruction, epidural abscess, neurologic deficits, kyphosis, or severe pain due to instability.

Pearls

- The presentation of pyogenic bacterial infections can be innocuous, and hence a high index of clinical suspicion is required in managing patients with clinical red flags, such as extremes of age, renal and liver failure, diabetes, patients on steroids, and immunosuppressive therapy.
- All attempts should be made to isolate the potential organism through blood culture, urine culture, and tissue studies, including culture, smear, and PCR studies, as this has a significant bearing on the management.
- An adequate dose of appropriate antibiotics for a period of at least 6 to 8 weeks based on the isolated organism is the mainstay of treatment.
- Stabilization of affected vertebral segments with pedicle screws is an important aspect of surgical treatment, as it enables wide decompression, thorough debridement, and early healing of the lesion.
- Children with spinal tuberculosis may develop worsening of kyphotic deformity despite bony healing. Hence, they should be carefully followed periodically until skeletal maturity.

Pitfalls

- Radiographs can be normal in the early stages of spondylodiskitis, and hence MRI should be performed with a low threshold to diagnose early spondylodiskitis.
- Prolonged delay in surgical treatment in order to try bed rest and antibiotic therapy should be avoided because early surgical debridement and stabilization enable early healing and return to normal activities.
- Avoiding internal fixation in the presence of abscess and active infection for fear of a worsening infection is incorrect because instability at the site of infection deters healing and recovery.
- In tuberculous spondylodiskitis, compliance with chemotherapy is the key and should be ensured for drug dosage and duration of therapy.
- The general condition of patients with spinal infections should be improved by optimizing their immunity, increasing their serum albumin levels, and correcting their anemia.

References

Five Must-Read References

1. Mylona E, Samarkos M, Kakalou E, Fanourgiakis P, Skoutelis A. Pyogenic vertebral osteomyelitis: a systematic review of clinical characteristics. Semin Arthritis Rheum 2009;39:10–17
2. Stäbler A, Reiser MF. Imaging of spinal infection. Radiol Clin North Am 2001;39:115–135
3. Danner RL, Hartman BJ. Update on spinal epidural abscess: 35 cases and review of the literature. Rev Infect Dis 1987;9:265–274
4. Silber JS, Anderson DG, Vaccaro AR, Anderson PA, McCormick P; NASS. Management of postprocedural discitis. Spine J 2002;2:279–287
5. Tali ET. Spinal infections. Eur J Radiol 2004;50:120–133
6. Fantoni M, Trecarichi EM, Rossi B, et al. Epidemiological and clinical features of pyogenic spondylodiscitis. Eur Rev Med Pharmacol Sci 2012;16(Suppl 2):2–7
7. Govender S. Spinal infections. J Bone Joint Surg Br 2005;87:1454–1458
8. Leong JC, Fraser RD. Spinal infection. In: Diesel SW, ed. The Lumbar Spine, 2nd ed. Philadelphia: WB Saunders; 1996
9. Carragee EJ. Pyogenic vertebral osteomyelitis. J Bone Joint Surg Am 1997;79:874–880
10. Guo LX, Ma YZ, Li HW, Xue HB, Peng W, Luo XB. [Variety of ESR and C-reactive protein levels during perioperative period in spinal tuberculosis]. Zhongguo Gu Shang 2010;23:200–202
11. Jain AK, Jena SK, Singh MP, Dhammi IK, Ramachadran VG, Dev G. Evaluation of clinico-radiological, bacteriological, serological, molecular and histological diagnosis of osteoarticular tuberculosis. Indian J Orthop 2008;42:173–177
12. Basu S, Ghosh JD, Malik FH, Tikoo A. Postoperative discitis following single-level lumbar discectomy: Our experience of 17 cases. Indian J Orthop 2012;46:427–433
13. Dall BE, Rowe DE, Odette WG, Batts DH. Postoperative discitis. Diagnosis and management. Clin Orthop Relat Res 1987;224:138–146
14. Rosahl SK, Gharabaghi A, Zink PM, Samii M. Monitoring of blood parameters following anterior cervical fusion. J Neurosurg 2000;92(2, Suppl):169–174
15. Carragee EJ, Kim D, van der Vlugt T, Vittum D. The clinical use of erythrocyte sedimentation rate in pyogenic vertebral osteomyelitis. Spine 1997;22:2089–2093
16. An HS, Seldomridge JA. Spinal infections: diagnostic tests and imaging studies. Clin Orthop Relat Res 2006;444:27–33
17. Kowalski TJ, Layton KF, Berbari EF, et al. Follow-up MR imaging in patients with pyogenic spine infections: lack of correlation with clinical features. AJNR Am J Neuroradiol 2007;28:693–699
18. Rodiek SO. [Diagnostic methods in spinal infections]. Radiologe 2001;41:976–986
19. Norden CW. Lessons learned from animal models of osteomyelitis. Rev Infect Dis 1988;10:103–110
20. Friedman JA, Maher CO, Quast LM, McClelland RL, Ebersold MJ. Spontaneous disc space infections in adults. Surg Neurol 2002;57:81–86
21. Jaramillo-de la Torre JJ, Bohinski RJ, Kuntz C IV. Vertebral osteomyelitis. Neurosurg Clin N Am 2006;17:339–351, vii
22. Viale P, Furlanut M, Scudeller L, et al. Treatment of pyogenic (non-tuberculous) spondylodiscitis with tailored high-dose levofloxacin plus rifampicin. Int J Antimicrob Agents 2009;33:379–382
23. Roblot F, Besnier JM, Juhel L, et al. Optimal duration of antibiotic therapy in vertebral osteomyelitis. Semin Arthritis Rheum 2007;36:269–277
24. Yoshimoto M, Takebayashi T, Kawaguchi S, et al. Pyogenic spondylitis in the elderly: a report from Japan with the most aging society. Eur Spine J 2011;20:649–654
25. Hadjipavlou AG, Katonis PK, Gaitanis IN, Muffoletto AJ, Tzermiadianos MN, Crow W. Percutaneous transpedicular discectomy and drainage in pyogenic spondylodiscitis. Eur Spine J 2004;13:707–713
26. Fang D, Cheung KM, Dos Remedios ID, Lee YK, Leong JC. Pyogenic vertebral osteomyelitis: treatment by anterior spinal debridement and fusion. J Spinal Disord 1994;7:173–180
27. Liljenqvist U, Lerner T, Bullmann V, Hackenberg L, Halm H, Winkelmann W. Titanium cages in the surgical treatment of severe vertebral osteomyelitis. Eur Spine J 2003;12:606–612
28. Lin TY, Tsai TT, Lu ML, et al. Comparison of two-stage open versus percutaneous pedicle screw fixation in treating pyogenic spondylodiscitis. BMC Musculoskelet Disord 2014;15:443
29. Gonzalvo A, Abdulla I, Riazi A, De La Harpe D. Single-level/single-stage debridement and posterior instrumented fusion in the treatment of spontaneous pyogenic osteomyelitis/discitis: long-term functional outcome and health-related quality of life. J Spinal Disord Tech 2011;24:110–115
30. Jiménez-Mejías ME, de Dios Colmenero J, Sánchez-Lora FJ, et al. Postoperative spondylodiskitis: etiology, clinical findings, prognosis, and comparison with nonoperative pyogenic spondylodiskitis. Clin Infect Dis 1999;29:339–345
31. Rajasekaran S. The problem of deformity in spinal tuberculosis. Clin Orthop Relat Res 2002;398:85–92

32. Rajasekaran S. Buckling collapse of the spine in childhood spinal tuberculosis. Clin Orthop Relat Res 2007; 460:86–92
33. Steingart KR, Sohn H, Schiller I, et al. Xpert® MTB/RIF assay for pulmonary tuberculosis and rifampicin resistance in adults. Cochrane Database Syst Rev 2013;1:CD009593
34. Hodgson AR, Stock FE. Anterior spinal fusion a preliminary communication on the radical treatment of Pott's disease and Pott's paraplegia. Br J Surg 1956;44:266–275
35. Tuli SM. Results of treatment of spinal tuberculosis by "middle-path" regime. J Bone Joint Surg Br 1975; 57:13–23
36. Sieper J, van der Heijde D, Landewé R, et al. New criteria for inflammatory back pain in patients with chronic back pain: a real patient exercise by experts from the Assessment of SpondyloArthritis international Society (ASAS) Ann Rheum Dis 2009;68:784–788
37. Weisman MH. Inflammatory back pain: the United States perspective. Rheum Dis Clin North Am 2012; 38:501–512

11

Conservative Treatment: Drugs, Physiotherapy, and Alternative Medicine

Christopher C. Ornelas and Mona Zall

Introduction

Low back pain (LBP) has a high prevalence in the adult and geriatric population. Up to 70% of adults are affected at some point in their lives with LBP.[1] It is the second most common cause of disability in the developing world and has major social welfare and economic implications.[2,3] When evaluating a patient with LBP, the physician should elicit a thorough history and perform a detailed musculoskeletal and neurologic examination. If the diagnosis remains unclear or if the patient does not respond to initial treatments, imaging may be necessary. LBP is usually classified as acute, subacute, or chronic, and can be described as either axial or radicular. The differential diagnosis for axial LBP is broad, and the etiology can involve intervertebral disk syndromes, facet joint–mediated pain syndromes, sacroiliac joint arthritis or strain, and muscle strain involving the paraspinal musculature.[4] Lumbar radiculopathy, or pain associated with irritation or injury to lumbosacral nerve roots, is also associated with a broad differential and can present as pain, numbness, or weakness in the affected extremity. Most episodes of acute LBP resolve, but some patients develop chronic or recurrent pain. Typically, those who have persistent LBP are older and have greater baseline pain and dysfunction, depression, an ongoing compensation claim, or fear of pain persistence. This chapter discusses nonsurgical treatment options for patients with LBP, including physical therapy, exercise, pharmacotherapy, topical modalities, therapeutic steroid injections, and neuromodulation.

Etiology and Epidemiology of Axial and Radicular Low Back Pain

Facet or zygapophyseal joints in the lumbar spine are responsible for 15 to 45% of axial LBP.[5,6] Facet pain may also cause a local referred pain pattern, and is innervated by lumbar medial branch nerves of the lumbar dorsal rami nerves. Each facet joint is innervated by the medial branch nerves cephalad and caudal to the joint. The onset of facet pain is generally insidious, and it occurs more commonly in patients of ages 65 years and older. Typically, pain is worse with prolonged standing and extension of the lumbar spine, and is alleviated by sitting, forward flexion, or recumbency. No test is considered sensitive for the identification of facet pain, and it is not always associated with obvious X-ray evidence of facet arthritis. However, small studies have shown that pain with extension and rotation may be indicative of facet pain.[4] Facet pain may be due to the intrinsic abnormalities of the joint or because of extrinsic compression of the descending root in the lateral recess or exiting nerve root in the intervertebral foramen. Facet pain can be managed in several ways, including physical therapy, intra-articular facet injections, medial branch nerve blocks, and medial branch nerve radiofrequency ablation (RFA).[4]

Radiculopathy is a type of neuropathic pain that results from a lesion or disease affecting the somatosensory system and is caused by nerve root irritation and lumbar stenosis. Radicular pain is generated by discharges from an irritated spinal nerves and presents as pain in a dermatomal distribution. Although radicular pain is most commonly associated with herniated disks, it can also be caused by ligamentum flavum thickening, facet arthropathy, body spurs, or trauma.[4] Lumbar radicular pain is managed with physical therapy, medications, and epidural steroid injections.

Lumbar stenosis occurs when there is narrowing of the vertebral canal by surrounding bone and soft tissues, which in turn leads to compression of neural structures.[4] The cause of lumbar stenosis is multifactorial, and usually involves the combination of intervertebral disk protrusion or herniation, facet joint hypertrophy, congenital narrowing of the central spinal canal, hypertrophy of the ligamentum flavum, and spondylolisthesis.[4] Lumbar stenosis can be associated with both axial and radicular pain. The hallmark symptom of lumbar stenosis is neurogenic claudication. Patients with claudication have pain that increases with standing and walking and decreases with sitting. The pain is typically located in one or more dermatomes and often affects the lower extremities symmetrically. It is distinguished from vascular claudication due to peripheral vascular disease in that it may present with prolonged standing alone, whereas vascular claudication is usually associated with ambulation.

Sacroiliac (SI) joint pain is responsible for 15 to 30% of axial LBP in individuals; 40 to 50% of patients with SI joint pain develop the pain after an acute trauma. The two most common traumatic events that can lead to SI joint pain are motor vehicle collisions and falls.[7] Pain is typically located in the gluteal or lower lumbar paraspinals and can be associated with or without radiation to the thigh or the knee.[7] What makes SI joint pain different from other forms of axial pain LBP is that pain typically occurs with transitional movements and can occur while in a seated position.[4]

Physical Therapy and Exercise

Physical therapy (PT) has been used as a conservative treatment to help patients with LBP, and it is believed that PT may decrease the need for invasive and costly interventions.[8] Not many studies have shown benefit for exercise in acute LBP, and in certain situations starting therapy and exercise should be delayed until appropriate analgesia is achieved. PT can be viewed as a continuous process with a focus on developing immediate, intermediate, and long-term goals. These goals are usually determined at the initial evaluation of the patient by the licensed therapist. When ordering PT, the physician should inform the patient of the expectations and goals of therapy, as well as the anticipated duration of therapy. In the initial evaluation, the patient's current pain level and functional limitations are assessed. Initially, the therapist aims to decrease the pain level with a series of modalities, which may include heat, ice, transcutaneous electrical nerve stimulation (TENS), and message. The patient also should be given an exercise program to perform at home, because the number of therapy sessions is limited. Another option is a back school, which focuses on educating the patient on the anatomy of the spine, common causes of back pain, posture, and stability, and may include instruction on gait and balance. There is often emphasis on prevention of positions or activities that can elicit or worsen the pain and other symptoms. Once the patient is able to adequately participate in therapy, the patient's gait and posture are evaluated.[8–10]

According to a review conducted in 2010, TENS failed to provide relief for patients with LBP, so Medicare no longer covers it.[11] However, TENS is often used in combination with other modalities for pain relief early in the therapy process.

The modality of heat has two forms, superficial and deep. Examples of superficial heat include heating pads, warm compresses, and fluid therapy. The goal of superficial heat is to provide muscle relaxation and analgesia. These modalities can also be used at home. Deep heat, which is achieved with ultrasound, shortwave diathermy, and microwave are usually performed under the direction of the therapist. Although a useful treatment, heat can cause injury and often skin hyperpigmentation. Cold therapy is almost exclusively superficial, and is suggested to be superior to heat in the acute setting. It can also play a role in the intermediate to long-term treatment of LBP. Cold therapy for LBP is relatively safe but should be avoided in the extremities of patients with arterial insufficiency and decreased sensitivity in the extremities such as peripheral neuropathy and radiculopathy.[10]

Once patients have developed a general understanding of the principles of their back pain, lumbar stabilization will be emphasized. Various techniques have been described in the literature, but there is a general consensus on including combinations of core strengthening, back strengthening, and stretching. The McKenzie method involves focusing LBP toward the spinal midline. This is done by repetitive motions or sustained postures. Studies have failed to show the benefit of such exercises over flexion and extension exercises. The Alexander technique is a hands-on method to improve balance, posture, and coordination and to break poor habits.

Often persons who are not as active have a tendency to develop LBP, so there is a period of time where therapy can cause some soreness and worsening of pain because muscles that have become weak over time are now being retrained.[9] Although therapy sessions are usually held two to three days per week, the patient is instructed to perform some limited home exercises and stretching on the other days. PT ends when patients have demonstrated the ability to independently perform their exercises and when they are no longer making significant functional gains.

Patients should then transition into a home exercise program, which has been useful for pain in the subacute and chronic periods after the onset of pain. The exact amount or type of exercise that provides the best results has not been determined; more studies need to be conducted. Typical programs involve a combination of core strengthening exercises, aerobic exercises, range of motion, and functional restoration programs. Patients should start aerobic exercises slowly, and gradually increase their frequency and intensity.

In a review of 43 trials, exercise therapy for patients with chronic LBP was slightly superior to no treatment in improving functional outcomes and pain.[9] Incorporation of aerobic activities is recommended, and may include yoga, Pilates, tai chi, and aquatic therapy. Pilates focuses on core strengthening. In a study comparing PT, no treatment, and Pilates, patients had more relief with reduction of pain in chronic LBP with Pilates. Yoga has been shown to provide some benefit to patients with LBP depending on the type of yoga performed. Viniyoga has shown to be superior to typical treatments at 12 weeks, but showed no difference at 26 weeks. Tai chi is a form of Chinese martial arts that involves slow movements, breathing, and meditation. In a study of a 160 patients with LBP, those who performed tai chi had greater relief and functional improvement than those who underwent standard treatment. But the long-term efficacy of tai chi has yet to be studied.[9] Aquatic therapy has been shown to be beneficial in patients with LBP, but has not been shown to be superior to other interventions for chronic LBP. To best determine the most beneficial therapy and exercises for patients with LBP, more studies need to be conducted.

In certain patients, such as those who sustained occupational injuries, further evaluation of work-specific tasks, ergonomics, home and workstation modifications, and work hardening programs may have to be explored to limit the return of pain and prevent further or future injury.

Pharmacotherapy

Several medication treatment options are available for patients with nonspecific LBP. The choice of medication depends largely on the patient's symptoms, the etiology of the pain, the severity of pain, the patient's previous response to medication, the patient's medical comorbidities, and adverse side-effect profiles.[12] Some medications have been shown to be more efficacious in acute LBP versus subacute and chronic pain LBP.

Acetaminophen

The American Pain Society recommends acetaminophen as a first-line pharmacological option for LBP, because of its safety profile. The major concern with acetaminophen is hepatotoxicity. In patients with a history of alcohol abuse or other risk factor for hepatotoxicity, the maximum dose advised is 2 g per day. In patients without such risk factors, the maximum dose is 4 g per day. Acetaminophen does not contain significant anti-inflammatory properties, and has been shown to be inferior to nonsteroidal anti-inflammatory drugs (NSAIDs) in several studies.[13]

Nonsteroidal Anti-Inflammatory Drugs

The NSAIDs exert their anti-inflammatory properties and analgesic effects by blocking cyclooxygenase (Cox) enzymes. They are also considered as a first-line treatment, but they are associated with gastrointestinal and renal adverse effects. Studies have shown that nonselective NSAIDs and Cox-2 inhibitors have been associated with a twofold increase in myocardial infarctions. Naprosyn has the lowest cardiac risk and is available over the counter.[13] No study has shown a significant difference between traditional NSAIDs versus Cox-2 NSAIDs in the treatment of LBP, but traditional NSAIDs cause more side effects.[14] There is no evidence that switching from one NSAID to another provides superior analgesia.

Muscle Relaxants

Muscle relaxants have been shown to be more effective than placebo in patients with nonspecific back pain. Data shows that they typically work better in acute versus chronic pain.[4] In the United States, the muscle relaxants that are approved for musculoskeletal conditions are carisoprodol, cyclobenzaprine, chlorzoxazone, methocarbamol, and orphenadrine. Approved medications for spasticity include diazepam, dantrolene, tizanidine, and baclofen. Muscle relaxants are not considered first-line treatments due to the high prevalence of adverse side effects. They are commonly associated with central nervous system (CNS)-related adverse events including drowsiness, dizziness, fatigue, and headache. No study thus far has shown one muscle relaxant to be superior to another. Carisoprodol should be avoided because of its high potential for abuse and addiction. In 2007, the European Medicines Agency recommended the suspension of all carisoprodol-containing medications. In patients who do not respond to first-line treatments such as acetaminophen or NSAIDs, there has been evidence to suggest that the addition of a muscle relaxant was superior to monotherapy for short-term pain relief.[13]

Antidepressants

The role of antidepressants in the treatment of axial or radicular LBP is controversial. Antidepressants are not considered a first-line treatment due to the lack of evidence of their effectiveness for LBP, and they can be associated with QRS prolongation and arrhythmias. Some antidepressants require laboratory testing to assess therapeutic drug levels and routine electrocardiograms (ECGs). Tricyclic antidepressants (TCAs) have been shown to be superior to serotonin-norepinephrine reuptake inhibitors (SNRIs), which are more efficacious than selective serotonin reuptake inhibitors (SSRIs).[4] Tertiary amines such as amitriptyline and imipramine have a higher risk of adverse events compared with secondary amines such as nortriptyline and desipramine. Some SNRIs such as venlafaxine, duloxetine, and milnacipran have demonstrated some benefit in patients with LBP that may or may not have had a neuropathic component.[13]

Synthetic Opioids

Tramadol, a synthetically derived analgesic, binds to mu-opioid receptors and weakly inhibits norepinephrine and serotonin reuptake. However, it is not recommended as a first-line treatment because of limited evidence of their effectiveness for LBP and the lack of data to suggest an advantage over NSAIDs. Moreover, although not a true opioid, tramadol does entail the potential for abuse. In a review conducted by Chung et al, it was found that tramadol did not have statistically significant pain relief when compared with placebo, but there was improvement in function associated with its use.[4] One must use caution when prescribing tramadol to patients who are also taking an SSRI antidepressant medication because of the potential for developing a potentially life-threatening condition known as serotonin syndrome.[13] Mild symptoms of serotonin syndrome include agitation, confusion, elevated blood pressure or heart rate, diarrhea, and headache. Severe symptoms include fever, arrhythmia, seizures, and unconsciousness.

Opioids

Opioids remain controversial for LBP. They are considered a potent class of analgesics and carry a risk of respiratory depression, abuse potential, and addiction. The more common side effects associated with opioids include constipation, nausea, somnolence, pruritus, and myoclonus. The American Pain Society recommends the usage of opioids in severe, debilitating LBP that is not controlled by either acetaminophen or NSAIDs or when a patient has a high risk of complications on NSAIDs. For acute short-term use, short-acting opioids are generally recommended, whereas long-acting opioids are recommended for long-term use.[13] A review by Chung et al[14] found that opioids were able to provide statistically significant pain relief in patients with chronic nonspecific LBP. Many opioid medications such as hydrocodone and oxycodone are available in forms containing acetaminophen; physicians must counsel patients on their potential for hepatotoxicity, according to the same guidelines as acetaminophen monotherapy.

Glucocorticoids

Although commonly prescribed in an acute setting such as an urgent care or emergency care department, systemic glucocorticoids are not recommended for the treatment of LBP associated with or without radiculopathy because they have not been shown to be more efficacious than placebo.[12]

Antiepileptic Drugs

There is insufficient evidence to support the usage of antiepileptic drugs in LBP. Gabapentin has been efficacious in a few studies for chronic LBP with associated radiculopathy, but it is not approved by the Food and Drug Administration (FDA) for this indication.[14] There is some evidence to suggest that antiepileptic drugs such as gabapentin have a potential to prevent central sensitization when prescribed early in radiculopathy.

Topical Analgesics and Ointments

The benefit of topical analgesics is that they do not entail the risk of systemic side effects. They may be used alone or with other medications. Side effects are typically mild and include allergic reaction or skin irritation. Capsaicin works by depleting substance P from the sensory afferent nerve fibers. There has been some evidence, although not strong, that capsaicin can be useful in the treatment of both neuropathic and musculoskeletal pain. Most patients tolerate capsaicin well. The most commonly reported side effect is an intolerable burning sensation.[11] Lidocaine 5% patches may be another option, but there are no data supporting the utilization of lidocaine for acute or chronic LBP. A few studies have shown its benefit for myofascial pain syndromes. Generally, lidocaine patches are well tolerated.[11]

Alternative Medicine

Herbal Medicine

Short-term studies have shown that herbal preparations such as devil's claw, white willow bark, and cayenne may have a role in the treatment of LBP.[11] A 2014 Cochrane review addressed the usage of herbal medication for LBP. It found that Solidago chilensis Meyen (Brazilian arnica) may improve flexibility when applied twice a day. Capsicum frutescens cream or plaster showed effectiveness in treating chronic LBP in three separate trials, yet it is unclear if it provides relief in acute back pain. Harpagophytum (devil's claw) was found to be better than placebo in providing short-term relief. Another study found that it was equivalent to 12.5 mg of rofecoxib. White willow bark (*Salix alba*) was shown to be better than placebo for short-term improvements in pain and rescue medication. Aromatic lavender essential oil, when applied by acupressure, reduced pain intensity and improved lateral spine flexion and walking time, compared with controls.[15] These studies show promise in utilization of herbal medications, but some of the trials are not of the best quality, and there are few comprehensive large trials.

Acupuncture

Patients often turn to complementary or alternative medicine for the treatment of LBP. An option that patients frequently consider is acupuncture, which is based on the concepts of Chinese medicine. According to the Chinese, there are twelve main meridians in the body, which the *Qi* energy must flow through. Needles are inserted along the meridians to activate the body's natural healing process. Acupuncture exerts its effect by inhibition at the dorsal horn, by activating the descending inhibitory pathways, and by stimulating the release of opioids and serotonin.[16] There are mixed data regarding the efficacy of acupuncture in the treatment of LBP. A 2015 review by Liu et al[17] found that in acute phases acupuncture was inconsistent in its ability to provide relief. But in patients with chronic LBP, acupuncture as an adjunct to conventional therapy provided patients with short-term relief and functional improvement. Better studies need to be conducted before acupuncture can be recommended as a standard of care.

Injections

Another form of conservative management for LBP is steroid injections. Epidural steroid injections are used in patients who have radicular pain and pain secondary to disk herniation, spinal stenosis, postlaminectomy syndrome, and diskogenic pain. The different approaches to injecting epidurals include transforaminal, interlaminar, and caudal. The response to epidural injections varies with the pathology.[18] Typically, steroid and local anesthetics or local anesthetics alone are administered. The steroids exert anti-inflammatory effects. Multiple high-quality randomized controlled trials have shown grade I evidence that supports the utilization of caudal epidurals for lumbar disk herniation, diskogenic pain, spinal stenosis, and postlaminectomy syndrome. A review by Manchikanti et al[18] analyzed several studies for lumbar transforaminal epidurals in patients with disk herniation and lumbar stenosis. They found that there was level I evidence that local anesthetics with steroids or local anesthetics alone provided significant pain relief in patients. There was also grade II evidence in two studies that showed some patients were able to avoid surgery after the injections.

Lumbar facet–mediated pain is treated by intra-articular injections, lumbar medial branch nerve blocks, and sometimes RFA. There are conflicting data regarding the efficacy of such interventions. Facet joint injections have been studied using saline, local anesthetics, and steroids. Injections can be both diagnostic and therapeutic depending on whether or not steroids are utilized. The most recent guidelines by the American Society of Interventional Pain Physicians does not recommend intra-articular injections for therapeutic purposes, but anesthetic-only facet injections may provide diagnostic utility and may aid in spine surgery planning.[6] Medial branch nerve blocks can be diagnostic or diagnostic and therapeutic. Therapeutic medial branch nerve blocks entail administering 1 to 2 cc of a combination of steroid and anesthetic at each nerve. However, for diagnostic injections, only 0.5 cc of anesthetic is used. A diagnostic block confirms the diagnosis of facet-mediated pain; it is also used if therapeutic injections offer only short-term relief and RFA is being considered. After a double-positive diagnostic block, RFA can be performed and may provide patients with longer relief. A diagnostic nerve block is considered successful or positive if there is a reduction in pain by 80%.[6] RFA has been demonstrated to provide significant pain relief in patients for 6 to 12 months, and even for more than 3 years in some patients in a retrospective study conducted by McCormick et al.[19] It should be considered only in patients who demonstrate two positive diagnostic blocks.

Trigger point injections involve dry needling in the muscle and soft tissue. They can be performed with anesthetic or in a combination of anesthetic and corticosteroid. Although they are a nonspecific treatment, there is some evidence to suggest improvement in patients with chronic LBP.[10]

Spinal Cord Stimulators

Spinal cord stimulators (SCSs) are another option for patients who have LBP due to failed back syndrome or who have refractory neuropathic pain despite extensive medical and interventional therapies. Sanders et al[20] performed a retrospective study in patients with failed back syndrome and complex regional pain syndrome who had received SCS, and they found that patients had significant and sustained pain reduction and opioid medication utilization. SCS therapy is used after a successful trial period in which percutaneous stimulator leads (typically two) are placed into the epidural space and connected to an external pulse generator. A successful trial is defined as pain improvement such that the patient reports a reduction in oral analgesic medications, a reduction of pain of at least 50%, and improvement in quality of life and participation in activities of daily living. After a successful trial usually lasting about 1 week, an implantable pulse generator and permanent leads or paddle arrays are placed surgically. The device is then programmed remotely and charged percutaneously. The exact mechanism of spinal cord stimulators is not completely understood.

Chapter Summary

Low back pain is a common cause of pain in the adult and geriatric population and is a major cause of debility. A comprehensive history and detailed neurologic examination is key in understanding LBP, as the differential is broad. In the absence of neurologic compromise, imaging is not necessary, but it should be considered when the diagnosis of LBP is unclear or the patient fails to response to initial treatment. Conservative treatment options include combinations of physical therapy and first-line medications such as acetaminophen and NSAIDs. Physical therapy is a goal-driven process that ultimately educates the patient and develops a long-term home exercise program. If a patient fails to respond to initial treatments, medications such as muscle relaxants, antidepressants, and opioids can be considered. Image-guided injections can be useful not only to aid in the diagnosis of the patient's pain but also to treat pain. Identifying the etiology of LBP is crucial to determine which type of injection should be used. Alternative treatments such as acupuncture, herbal medications, and exercise programs such as yoga and Pilates may also be used to help treat LBP, but they are not considered first-line treatments. Physical therapy is indicated in treating LBP before and after surgery. Spinal cord stimulators can be used in patients with persistent neuropathic pain after surgery.

Pearls

- Acetaminophen and NSAIDs are recommended as first-line oral analgesia.
- Opioids can be considered for acute and severe pain for short-term use.
- Topical ointments can be useful when trying to avoid systemic side effects.
- Physical therapy should be started as soon as tolerated.
- Imaging may be necessary in situations when the diagnosis is unclear or the patient fails to respond to initial treatment.
- Caudal and transforaminal epidural steroid injections have shown benefit in lumbar disk herniation, diskogenic pain, spinal stenosis, and postlaminectomy syndrome.
- Medial branch nerve blocks are recommended for facet-mediated pain.
- Radiofrequency ablation can be considered after two successful medial branch nerve blocks provide > 80% pain relief.
- Alternatives such as acupuncture, tai chi, Pilates, yoga, devil's claw, and arnica have the potential to provide relief in patients, but more studies are needed.

Pitfalls

- Failure to identify the etiology of the patient's complaint may lead to costly and unnecessary procedures.
- Avoid unnecessary imaging.
- Facet intra-articular joint injections are not recommended.
- Avoid using oral glucocorticoids.
- Avoid starting physical therapy in patients with elevated pain levels until appropriate analgesia is achieved to allow for maximal participation.

References

Five Must-Read References

1. Searle A, Spink M, Ho A, Chuter V. Exercise interventions for the treatment of chronic low back pain: a systematic review and meta-analysis of randomised controlled trials. Clin Rehabil 2015;29:1155–1167
2. Natour J, Cazotti LdeA, Ribeiro LH, Baptista AS, Jones A. Pilates improves pain, function and quality of life in patients with chronic low back pain: a randomized controlled trial. Clin Rehabil 2015;29:59–68
3. Izzo R, Popolizio T, D'Aprile P, Muto M. Spinal pain. Eur J Radiol 2015;84:746–756
4. Hooten WM, Cohen SP. Evaluation and treatment of low back pain: a clinically focused review for primary care specialists. Mayo Clin Proc 2015;90:1699–1718
5. Schneider GM, Jull G, Thomas K, et al. Derivation of a clinical decision guide in the diagnosis of cervical facet joint pain. Arch Phys Med Rehabil 2014;95:1695–1701
6. Roy C, Chatterjee N, Ganguly S, Sengupta R. Efficacy of combined treatment with medial branch radiofrequency neurotomy and steroid block in lumbar facet joint arthropathy. J Vasc Interv Radiol 2012;23:1659–1664
7. Cohen SP, Chen Y, Neufeld NJ. Sacroiliac joint pain: a comprehensive review of epidemiology, diagnosis and treatment. Expert Rev Neurother 2013;13:99–116
8. Ojha HA, Wyrsta NJ, Davenport TE, Egan WE, Gellhorn AC. Timing of physical therapy initiation for nonsurgical management of musculoskeletal disorders and effects on patient outcomes: a systematic review. J Orthop Sports Phys Ther 2016;46:56–70
9. Hartigan C, Rainville J, Atlas SJ, Park Lee exercise based therapy for low back pain. Uptodate Waltham, MA (accessed December 2015)
10. Barr KP, Harrast MA. Low back pain. In: Braddom RL, ed. Physical Medicine and Rehabilitation. Philadelphia: Saunders Elsevier; 2007:883–928
11. Becker JA, Stumbo JR. Back pain in adults. Prim Care 2013;40:271–288
12. Chou R, Qaseem A, Snow V, et al; Clinical Efficacy Assessment Subcommittee of the American College of Physicians; American College of Physicians; American Pain Society Low Back Pain Guidelines Panel. Diagnosis and treatment of low back pain: a joint clinical practice guideline from the American College of Physicians and the American Pain Society. Ann Intern Med 2007;147:478–491
13. Chou R. Pharmacological management of low back pain. Drugs 2010;70:387–402
14. Chung JWY, Zeng Y, Wong TKS. Drug therapy for the treatment of chronic nonspecific low back pain: systematic review and meta-analysis. Pain Physician 2013;16:E685–E704
15. Oltean H, Robbins C, Tulder MWV, Berman BM, Bombardier C, Gagnier JJ. Herbal medicine for low-back pain. Cochrane Database Syst Rev 2014;12:CD004504. http://onlinelibrary.wiley.com/doi/10.1002/14651858.CD004504.pub4/pdf

16. Hutchinson AJP, Ball S, Andrews JCH, Jones GG. The effectiveness of acupuncture in treating chronic non-specific low back pain: a systematic review of the literature. J Orthop Surg 2012;7:36
17. Liu L, Skinner M, McDonough S, Mabire L, Baxter GD. Acupuncture for low back pain: an overview of systematic reviews. Evid Based Complement Alternat Med 2015;2015:328196
18. Manchikanti L, Nampiaparampil DE, Manchikanti KN, et al. Comparison of the efficacy of saline, local anesthetics, and steroids in epidural and facet joint injections for the management of spinal pain: A systematic review of randomized controlled trials. Surg Neurol Int 2015;6(5, Suppl 4):S194–S235
19. McCormick ZL, Marshall B, Walker J, McCarthy R, Walega DR. Long-term function, pain and medication uses outcomes of radiofrequency ablation for lumbar facet syndrome. Int J Anesth Anesth 2015;2:28
20. Sanders RA, Moeschler SM, Gazelka HM, et al. Patient outcomes and spinal cord stimulation: a retrospective case series evaluating patient satisfaction, pain scores and opioid requirements. Pain Pract 2015; Aug 27. doi: 10.1111/papr.12340. [Epub ahead of print]

12

Outcome Evaluation in Back Pain Patients

Martin H. Pham, Andre M. Jakoi, Neil N. Patel, and Jeffrey C. Wang

Introduction

Back pain is among the most frequently encountered problems in medicine; 75 to 85% of the population will experience low back pain (LBP) at some point in life, and 1 to 2% of the United States adult population is disabled because of LBP.[1,2] The yearly prevalence of back pain, alone, is estimated to range from 15 to 20% in the United States and from 25 to 45% in Europe, and these data do not include other pathology involving the spinal column.[1,2] Usually the clinical course is fairly benign, with 90 to 95% of patients recovering within several months. The middle-aged adults are the age subset most commonly afflicted with an even distribution between males and females. However, almost every age population has been noted to be affected. The lower back is the primary site of pain in 85% of those who report suffering from back pain.

Because of this significant prevalence of LBP in the general population, it is important to have useful outcome measures to determine the clinical success of the treatment of this condition. Typical measures of success involve domains of pain intensity, functional disability, and work status. Likewise, identifying the prognostic factors that are associated with good outcomes after the treatment of LBP is important for clinical decision making as well as for understanding this complex multifactorial disease. Identifying the prognostic factors also facilitates selecting the appropriate treatment regimens and for managing expectations of outcome in this patient population.

Low Back Pain

Low back pain is the second most common reason (after upper respiratory illness) for all physician visits in the United States. The direct costs associated with these office visits and the indirect costs of time missed from work are considerable. Total incremental direct health care costs due to LBP in the United States were estimated to be $26.3 billion in 1998, and the costs are estimated to increase yearly.[3] In addition, indirect costs related to days lost from work are substantial, with 2% of the U.S. work force compensated for back injuries each year. Couple this with the fact that the 5% of the population that receives back pain disability payments accounts for 75% of the costs associated with LBP, and it is clear to see the significant impact that the diagnosis of LBP has on society.[4]

But back pain is an ambiguous condition that leads to myriad diagnoses, a situation that creates enormous problems in patient management. Acute back pain is defined as pain persisting for 1 month or less; fortunately, most patients have self-limited episodes of acute LBP for which they do not seek medical attention.[1,2]

For those patients who do seek medical care, cessation of symptomatology and return to work are occur in the first month.[5] However, up to one third of patients have reported persistent back pain of at least moderate intensity for more than 1 year after an acute episode, and 20% of those patients have further reported limitations in activity later in life.[6] These patients would be defined as having chronic back pain, which is pain persisting for longer than 2 months.

There is a multitude of options available for evaluation and management of LBP. However, there is little consensus on which evaluation and treatment are most appropriate.[7] Numerous studies have shown differences in the use of diagnostic studies and treatment modalities between clinical specialties, but most of the outcomes were the same.[8,9]

The patient with back pain presents a challenge to the physician. The patient's complaint is a symptom, not a diagnosis. A considerable number of anatomic parts of the lumbar spine have the potential to cause pain. In addition, the spectrum of disease processes that may affect paraspinal structures is broad. More than 85% of patients presenting to their primary care physician who have LBP will not have a reliable diagnosis attributed to a specific disease or spinal abnormality.[10] Compounding this problem are the patients who have spinal pain that is associated with a work-related injury or motor vehicle accident. The extent and intensity of symptoms may be exaggerated by nonphysiological factors, thus further muddling the physician's task in treating patients with back pain, and making it more difficult to identify the entity that is causing the pain and the pathological process producing it.

Unfortunately, in most patients in whom no particular pathological etiology is found, no evidence suggests that labeling with a specific anatomic diagnosis will improve the outcome. Only in a minority of patients who present for initial evaluation does back pain have a specific disorder as its etiology. Malignancy (0.7%), compression fracture (4%), spinal infection (0.01%), ankylosing spondylitis (0.3–5%), spinal stenosis (3%), and herniated intervertebral disk (4%) are the most common diagnosis found on initial evaluation. Although these maladies are regularly seen and manageable pathologies, they make up only a small subset of the diagnoses found and matched with an initial complaint of back pain.[11,12]

It is important to have a practical approach to the assessment of the patient with back pain. A focused history and physical examination are always required, and a thorough neurologic examination is also warranted to determine the level of neurologic involvement. Such an approach facilitates the classification of patients into one of three categories: nonspecific LBP, back pain potentially associated with radiculopathy or spinal stenosis, and back pain potentially associated with another specific spinal cause. Diagnostic triage into one of these categories will aid the physician in subsequent decision making. The location of pain, frequency of symptoms, and duration of pain, as well as any previous symptomology, treatment, and responses to treatment, should all be reviewed. Other systems should be explored as well, such as the possibility of back pain on account of pancreatitis, nephrolithiasis, aortic aneurysm, endocarditis, or viral syndromes. All patients should be evaluated for rapidly progressive or severe neurologic deficits including motor deficits, bladder dysfunction, and fecal incontinence.

Clinicians should also inquire about risk factors for malignancy and infection. In a large, prospective study from the primary care setting, a history of cancer, unexplained weight loss, failure to have back pain improvement after 1 month, and age older than 50 years were each associated with a higher likelihood for cancer. The posttest probability of cancer in patients presenting with back pain increases from 0.7% to 9% in patients with a history of malignancy (excluding nonmelanoma skin cancer). Features predicting the presence of vertebral infection include fever, intravenous drug use, and recent infection.[11] Clinicians should also consider risk factors for vertebral compression fracture, such as older age, history of osteoporosis, steroid use, and low- or high-energy trauma.

Patients with back and accompanying leg pain and a typical history for radicular pain have a high sensitivity but uncertain specificity for herniated intervertebral disk.[13,14] More than 90% of symptomatic lumbar disk herniation occur at the L4-L5 and L5-S1 levels. A focused examination including a neurologic examination that includes the evaluation of strength, reflexes, and sensory distribution should be performed to assess the presence and severity of nerve root dysfunction. A positive result on the straight-leg-raise test has a high sensitivity (91%) but modest specificity (26%) for diagnosing a herniated disk.[15] There is less evidence on the utility of history and examination for identifying lumbar spinal stenosis.[16] The usefulness of pain relieved by sitting for predicting the presence of spinal stenosis ranges from poor to high. Age over 65 years was associated with a positive likelihood ratio of 2.5 and a negative likelihood ratio of 0.33.[17]

Psychosocial factors and emotional distress should be taken into account due to their strong predictors of LBP outcomes. In fact, psychosocial factors and emotional distress have a higher prediction factor for back pain outcomes than do either physical examination findings or severity/duration of pain.[18,19] Assessment of psychosocial factors identifies patients who may have delayed recovery in an effort to tailor interventions specifically. These patient-specific interventions may include intensive multidisciplinary rehabilitation, which has been found to be more effective than standard care in patients with acute or subacute LBP and risk factors for chronic back pain disability.[20] Psychosocial factors that may ultimately predict poorer LBP outcomes include depression, passive coping strategies, job dissatisfaction, higher disability levels, disputed compensation claims, and somatization.[18,19,21]

The pathophysiology of nonradicular LBP is usually indeterminate, and the defining feature of this disorder is its nonspecific etiology. Pain may arise from several sites, including the vertebral column, surrounding muscles, tendons, ligaments, and fascia. Stretching, tearing, or contusion of these tissues can occur after sudden unexpected forces are applied to the spine from either low- or high-energy trauma. Whether muscle spasm is a significant etiology of lumbar spine pain, either as a cause or effect of back injury, has yet to be proven.

The pathophysiology of radicular spine pain and lumbosacral radiculopathy is usually more obvious. Disk herniation through the annulus fibrosis does not in itself produce pain, but compression by the disk on the dural lining around the spinal nerve root sleeve is one explanation for back pain associated with acute disk herniation. This is also likely to contribute to the pain from the spinal nerve compression of arthritic spurs at degenerative facet and uncovertebral joints. Compression can directly stretch nociceptors in dura or nerve root sleeve tissues, but ischemia from compression of vascular structures, inflammation, and secondary edema is also likely to play a role in the causation of pain.

In the initial workup for nonspecific LBP, routine imaging or diagnostic tests are not recommended. There is no evidence that routine plain radiography in patients with nonspecific LBP is associated with a greater improvement in patient outcomes than that with selective imaging.[22] This practice of conservative investigation also decreases unnecessary exposure to radiation. This is best illustrated by the fact that a single plain radiograph (two-view) study of the lumbar spine is equivalent to being exposed to a daily chest radiograph for more than 1 year.[23] Routine advanced imaging such as computed tomography (CT) or magnetic resonance imaging (MRI) is also not associated with improved patient outcomes.[24] Plain radiography is recommended for the initial evaluation of possible vertebral compression fracture in selected higher-risk patients. Little evidence exists to guide optimal imaging strategies for patients enduring more than 1 to 2 months of back pain, although at that juncture it may be a reasonable initial imaging option. But this is not the case with patients with severe or progressive neurologic deficits. Those patients should receive prompt workup with MRI or CT scans to accompany initial imaging studies.

Outcome Measures

The ability to score outcome measures enables the assessment of treatments and of how they improve both functional ability and the subjective experience of pain. Treatment outcomes as measured by patient-reported assessments are not only a reflection of the treatment methods but also of the patient's perception of their treatment. Many factors are involved in the biopsychosocial aspects of medicine. Although pain levels may be similar among patients, the perceived level of suffering can vary widely.[25]

Functional outcome measures for LBP are evaluated with regard to LBP-specific disability. For LBP, this disability is determined by pain that typically interferes with the activities of daily living that involve mobility, dressing, sitting, and standing.[26] Questionnaires are utilized to determine the severity of these disabilities, and are generally considered to be more reliable than taking a history due to the reproducibility of the same question in exactly the same way to every patient every time.

Commonly used functional outcome measures include the Oswestry Disability Index (ODI) and the Roland-Morris Disability Questionnaire (RDQ). The ODI contains 10 items that reference the activities of daily living that could be disrupted by LBP.[27] Each item has six response options ranging from "No problem" to "Not possible" and is scored on a point scale accordingly. The total score is then doubled and expressed as a percentage, with a minimum score of 0 (no disability) and a maximum score of 100 (maximum disability). The RDQ is originally derived from the Sickness Impact Profile and consists of 24 yes/no questions. These focus on physical functions that include walking, bending over, sitting, lying down, dressing, sleeping, self-care, and daily activities. The responses are then summed for a minimum score of 0 (no disability) and a maximum score of 24 (maximum disability). The ODI and RDQ have been found to be valid, reliable, responsive to treatment effects, and applicable in a wide variety of settings.[26] Both evaluative measures are interpreted so that the higher the score, the greater the disability.

In addition to functional measures, pain intensity is also a factor that can be measured to assess the success of treatment. Pain intensity is essentially defined as how much a patient is hurt by the LBP. This is quantitatively measured as an estimate of the patient's perceived severity or magnitude of pain. It is important to keep in mind, however, that despite these quantitative measurements, pain intensity remains a very subjective experience that is determined by the interpretation and assignment of pain by the patient. For the assessment of pain, there is the Numeric Pain Rating Scale (NPRS), Brief Pain Inventory (BPI), Pain Disability Index (PDI), McGill Pain Questionnaire (MPQ), and the Visual Analogue Scale (VAS).[28] The VAS consists of a line with each end indicating the extreme levels of pain, range from "No pain" to "The worst pain I have ever experienced." Points in between correspond to intermediate levels of pain intensity. Patients are asked to select which point along this continuum best represents their pain intensity. Because the VAS continuum line is usually 100 mm long, it has a high number of response categories and can be considered to have as many as 101 response levels. This makes the VAS potentially much more sensitive at detecting differences in pain intensity over time and after treatment regimens. The NPRS is an 11-point scale that instructs patients to rate their pain from 0 to 10. This scale can be expanded to 21 points (rating from 0 to 20) or to 101 points (0 to 100). This pain assessment is easily administered and remains a simple, well-validated, and robust measurement method.[26]

Although the NPRS and the VAS are often considered the "gold standard" for pain, it is important to note that they have not necessarily been validated specifically for patients with LBP. Nevertheless, pain itself may be the most responsive measure after conservative or surgical treatment for LBP, and therefore it remains a critical measurement.[29] Because the NPRS and VAS are so widely used and have been found to reflect the response to treatment, these measures should receive strong consideration for routine use.

The psychosocial aspect of a patient's wellbeing is often overlooked on routine questioning and evaluation for clinical LBP. The recent literature has shown, however, that psychological evaluations play a major role in the ability to anticipate and predict outcomes after initiating treatment for LBP. Psychosocial evaluations include the Fear-Avoidance Beliefs Questionnaire (FABQ), Tampa Scale for Kinesiophobia (TSK), and Beck Depression Inventory (BDI). These three evaluative parameters have been validated and found to be reliable within the chronic LBP population.[29] Most important with respect to the psychosocial evaluation is whether depression is a domain that would change after treatment of the LBP as opposed to requiring separate treatment itself to affect the overall prognosis of the patient.

Because LBP often results in disability that prevents a continued productive positive contribution to society, the measurement of work status is an important indicator of outcome and treatment effect. Work status can be measured as the duration of sick leave in days, which enables using time to return to work as an outcome measure. Practically, it is known that people who return to work are not as productive as before they developed back pain. Future research will be needed to determine reliable ways to measure productivity at work in different sectors.[26]

Prognostic Factors

Identifying prognostic factors that can influence outcomes after the treatment of LBP is important to manage expectations for both patients and providers. Physicians should be knowledgeable about which factors may portend a poor prognosis in order to provide appropriate counseling and to avoid treatments that entail a higher risk of a less than ideal outcome. It is important to note that there are differences in pain intensity, physical disability, and health-related quality of life across different health care sites, and they also vary by patient age, sex, and race.[30] This is important with regard to adjusting patient baseline differences when evaluating factors associated with these outcome measures.

Smoking has been studied extensively in its effect on outcome measures. Former smokers have been found to have somewhat higher levels of physical disability and pain as compared with patients who never smoked.[30] Current smokers reported even higher levels of pain and disability. Smoking has been linked to worse back pain outcomes and greater pain, and those who quit smoking were found to have a reduction in pain that is significantly greater than in those who continued to smoke.[31] Because this is a modifiable risk factor, close attention should be paid to identifying those patients who are current smokers, and appropriate measures taken to counsel these patients about the importance of smoking cessation not just for their overall health, but for the improvement of the LBP that may be a significant factor in their pain and disability.

Age and sex have not been shown to be prognostically associated with decreases in pain or outcome disability at short-term follow-up.[32] There is some conflicting evidence that age and sex are associated with outcome disability over longer follow-up times and when reviewed in younger populations, such that women may report persistent greater disability even after treatment intervention.[33–36] Although some studies show statistical significance, the clinical significance of these differences may not be as large as that for the other prognostic factors discussed here.

It has been shown that less educated patients report worse functioning.[37] Education may be a marker for other factors such as adaptability to stress, access to health care, occupational factors, and behavioral factors. Additionally, it is possible that less educated patients were at a financial disadvantage and delayed seeking care due to concerns of insurance co-pay costs. The psychosocial stress of low incomes associated with lower education brackets may also affect overall health outcomes. Finally, lower education may be an indication of the cumulative effects of social disadvantage on disease burden that is reflected in worse health-related outcome scores.[38]

Studies have also found that even after adjusting for geographic location, education, and pain duration, African-Americans were associated with worse baseline physical disability and pain at presentation for back pain–related care as compared with other ethnicities.[39,40] Similar to education status, this could be a result of a variety of other factors, such as lack of access to health care, lower socioeconomic status, and poorer behavioral coping mechanisms.

Patients with leg involvement or spinal stenosis have reported slightly worse physical disability and pain scores on follow-up than did those with otherwise uncomplicated back pain.[41,42] This may reflect the compressive etiology associated with radiculopathy and lumbar stenosis as compared with the multifactorial etiology of LBP that may respond robustly to a variety of nonsurgical treatments.

Psychosocial factors and occupational changes may also play a part. The impact of psychosocial factors on the development and perpetuation of chronic pain and disability has been widely demonstrated throughout the literature.[43,44] Psychological conditions such as anxiety, depression, and somatic disorders have been shown to have negative effects on treatment outcomes in both operative and nonoperative cohorts of lower back pain patients.[45–47] Fear-avoidance beliefs as measured by the FABQ have also shown a positive association with outcome disability. To this end, the biopsychosocial model was intended for the successful treatment of LBP. Physicians should consider implementing a psychosocial outcomes measure as part of the routine clinical evaluation for patients presenting with LBP. This would enable appropriate counseling measures as well as the consideration of other psychosocial treatments beyond the realm of just the LBP and associated pain and disability.

Workers' compensation (WC) patient cohorts have shown typically worse outcomes when compared with those patients without WC claims.[48–50] They show low return to work, high reoperation rates, and high prevalent opioid dependence even at 2 years postoperatively. The conscious or unconscious exaggeration of symptoms likely plays some role when compensation is involved, which subsequently will manifest as adverse effects on self-reported pain, depression, disability, postrehabilitation outcomes, and return to work status.

With regard to outcomes at 12 months, some studies have found statistically significant associations with unemployment, work absence, high functional disability, high pain intensity, anxiety, and poor self-rated health after adjusting for confounding factors.[51] The strongest associations with poor outcome were with unemployment and high pain intensity. Combining these prognostic risk factors compounded the effect of poor outcome; people with both high pain and high functional disability were seven times more likely to have a poor outcome than people with neither risk factor. Likewise, 78% of patients with poor outcome had both high pain and unemployment at baseline compared with 11% of those with better outcomes. Multivariable regression modeling has shown that unemployment, widespread pain, high level of chronic pain grade, and catastrophizing were significantly associated with disability at 12 months in both acute/subacute and chronic LBP.[52] Catastrophizing and fear of pain have been found in other studies to be predictive of the development or continuation of pain.[53,54] Another study found a poor prognosis for patients who have taken a previous sick leave for LBP, have high baseline disability levels, or high pain intensity, lower education, or perceive themselves as having a high risk of persistent pain.[55] Overall, the baseline level of disability was found to be a large predictor of overall outcome and has explained the largest proportion of variance as compared with other prognostic indicators.

Chapter Summary

Low back pain is the second most common reason for all physician visits in the United States and presents a challenge to the treating physician. A considerable number of anatomic parts of the lumbar spine have the potential to cause pain. In addition, the spectrum of disease processes that may affect paraspinal structures is broad. Therefore, it is of the utmost importance to utilize outcome measures to provide assessments of treatments and how they improve both functional ability and the subjective experience of pain. In addition, identifying prognostic factors that can influence outcomes after the treatment of LBP is important to manage expectations for both patients and providers. This facilitates performing the appropriate workup and determining the appropriate treatment for the underlying and often multifactorial etiology of the LBP.

Pearls

- Low back pain is a very frequently encountered problem with a high prevalence in the adult population.
- Many outcome measures assess the treatment success of LBP by evaluating functional outcome, pain, psychosocial well-being, and work status.
- Smoking, less education, poor psychosocial well-being, workers' compensation, unemployment, and high initial pain intensity and disability are associated with a poor overall outcome in LBP.

Pitfalls

- The treating physician should always be aware of factors that may portend a poor prognosis even in the face of treatment.
- Knowledge of these factors will help both the physician and patient manage expectations as well as help determine the appropriate workup and treatment for the underlying and often multifactorial etiology of the LBP.

References

Five Must-Read References

1. Deyo RA, Mirza SK, Martin BI. Back pain prevalence and visit rates: estimates from U.S. national surveys, 2002. Spine 2006;31:2724–2727
2. Friedly J, Standaert C, Chan L. Epidemiology of spine care: the back pain dilemma. Phys Med Rehabil Clin N Am 2010;21:659–677
3. Luo X, Pietrobon R, Sun SX, Liu GG, Hey L. Estimates and patterns of direct health care expenditures among individuals with back pain in the United States. Spine 2004;29:79–86
4. Frymoyer JW, Cats-Baril WL. An overview of the incidences and costs of low back pain. Orthop Clin North Am 1991;22:263–271
5. Pengel LH, Herbert RD, Maher CG, Refshauge KM. Acute low back pain: systematic review of its prognosis. BMJ 2003;327:323
6. Von Korff M, Saunders K. The course of back pain in primary care. Spine 1996;21:2833–2837, discussion 2838–2839
7. Cherkin DC, Deyo RA, Wheeler K, Ciol MA. Physician variation in diagnostic testing for low back pain. Who you see is what you get. Arthritis Rheum 1994;37:15–22
8. Cherkin DC, Deyo RA, Loeser JD, Bush T, Waddell G. An international comparison of back surgery rates. Spine 1994;19:1201–1206
9. Volinn E, Mayer J, Diehr P, Van Koevering D, Connell FA, Loeser JD. Small area analysis of surgery for low-back pain. Spine 1992;17:575–581
10. van Tulder MW, Assendelft WJ, Koes BW, Bouter LM. Spinal radiographic findings and nonspecific low back pain. A systematic review of observational studies. Spine 1997;22:427–434
11. Jarvik JG, Deyo RA. Diagnostic evaluation of low back pain with emphasis on imaging. Ann Intern Med 2002;137:586–597
12. Underwood MR, Dawes P. Inflammatory back pain in primary care. Br J Rheumatol 1995;34:1074–1077
13. van den Hoogen HM, Koes BW, van Eijk JT, Bouter LM. On the accuracy of history, physical examination, and erythrocyte sedimentation rate in diagnosing low back pain in general practice. A criteria-based review of the literature. Spine 1995;20:318–327
14. Vroomen PC, de Krom MC, Knottnerus JA. Diagnostic value of history and physical examination in patients suspected of sciatica due to disc herniation: a systematic review. J Neurol 1999;246:899–906
15. Devillé WL, van der Windt DA, Dzaferagić A, Bezemer PD, Bouter LM. The test of Lasègue: systematic review of the accuracy in diagnosing herniated discs. Spine 2000;25:1140–1147
16. de Graaf I, Prak A, Bierma-Zeinstra S, Thomas S, Peul W, Koes B. Diagnosis of lumbar spinal stenosis: a systematic review of the accuracy of diagnostic tests. Spine 2006;31:1168–1176
17. Katz JN, Dalgas M, Stucki G, et al. Degenerative lumbar spinal stenosis. Diagnostic value of the history and physical examination. Arthritis Rheum 1995;38:1236–1241
18. Fayad F, Lefevre-Colau MM, Poiraudeau S, et al. [Chronicity, recurrence, and return to work in low back pain: common prognostic factors]. Ann Readapt Med Phys 2004;47:179–189
19. Pincus T, Burton AK, Vogel S, Field AP. A systematic review of psychological factors as predictors of chronicity/disability in prospective cohorts of low back pain. Spine 2002;27:E109–E120
20. Gatchel RJ, Polatin PB, Noe C, Gardea M, Pulliam C, Thompson J. Treatment- and cost-effectiveness of early intervention for acute low-back pain patients: a one-year prospective study. J Occup Rehabil 2003;13:1–9
21. Steenstra IA, Verbeek JH, Heymans MW, Bongers PM. Prognostic factors for duration of sick leave in patients sick listed with acute low back pain: a systematic review of the literature. Occup Environ Med 2005;62:851–860

22. Kendrick D, Fielding K, Bentley E, Kerslake R, Miller P, Pringle M. Radiography of the lumbar spine in primary care patients with low back pain: randomised controlled trial. BMJ 2001;322:400–405
23. Jarvik JG. Imaging of adults with low back pain in the primary care setting. Neuroimaging Clin N Am 2003;13:293–305
24. Gilbert FJ, Grant AM, Gillan MG, et al; Scottish Back Trial Group. Low back pain: influence of early MR imaging or CT on treatment and outcome—multicenter randomized trial. Radiology 2004;231:343–351
25. Daubs MD, Norvell DC, McGuire R, et al. Fusion versus nonoperative care for chronic low back pain: do psychological factors affect outcomes? Spine 2011; 36(21, Suppl):S96–S109
26. Ostelo RW, de Vet HC. Clinically important outcomes in low back pain. Best Pract Res Clin Rheumatol 2005;19:593–607
27. Fairbank JC, Couper J, Davies JB, O'Brien JP. The Oswestry Low Back Pain Disability Questionnaire. Physiotherapy 1980;66:271–273
28. Von Korff M, Jensen MP, Karoly P. Assessing global pain severity by self-report in clinical and health services research. Spine 2000;25:3140–3151
29. Chapman JR, Norvell DC, Hermsmeyer JT, et al. Evaluating common outcomes for measuring treatment success for chronic low back pain. Spine 2011;36(21, Suppl):S54–S68
30. Jarvik JG, Comstock BA, Heagerty PJ, et al. Back pain in seniors: the Back pain Outcomes using Longitudinal Data (BOLD) cohort baseline data. BMC Musculoskelet Disord 2014;15:134
31. Behrend C, Prasarn M, Coyne E, Horodyski M, Wright J, Rechtine GR. Smoking cessation related to improved patient-reported pain scores following spinal care. J Bone Joint Surg Am 2012;94:2161–2166
32. Verkerk K, Luijsterburg PA, Miedema HS, Pool-Goudzwaard A, Koes BW. Prognostic factors for recovery in chronic nonspecific low back pain: a systematic review. Phys Ther 2012;92:1093–1108
33. Bartley EJ, Fillingim RB. Sex differences in pain: a brief review of clinical and experimental findings. Br J Anaesth 2013;111:52–58
34. Fillingim RB, King CD, Ribeiro-Dasilva MC, Rahim-Williams B, Riley JL III. Sex, gender, and pain: a review of recent clinical and experimental findings. J Pain 2009;10447–485
35. Hansson TH, Hansson EK. The effects of common medical interventions on pain, back function, and work resumption in patients with chronic low back pain: A prospective 2-year cohort study in six countries. Spine 2000;25:3055–3064
36. Hägg O, Fritzell P, Ekselius L, Nordwall A; Swedish Lumbar Spine Study. Predictors of outcome in fusion surgery for chronic low back pain. A report from the Swedish Lumbar Spine Study. Eur Spine J 2003;12: 22–33
37. Dionne CE, Von Korff M, Koepsell TD, Deyo RA, Barlow WE, Checkoway H. Formal education and back pain: a review. J Epidemiol Community Health 2001; 55:455–468
38. Lacey RJ, Belcher J, Croft PR. Does life course socioeconomic position influence chronic disabling pain in older adults? A general population study. Eur J Public Health 2013;23:534–540
39. Olsen TL, Anderson RL, Dearwater SR, et al. The epidemiology of low back pain in an adolescent population. Am J Public Health 1992;82:606–608
40. Baker TA, Green CR. Intrarace differences among black and white Americans presenting for chronic pain management: the influence of age, physical health, and psychosocial factors. Pain Med 2005;6:29–38
41. Grotle M, Brox JI, Veierød MB, Glomsrød B, Lønn JH, Vøllestad NK. Clinical course and prognostic factors in acute low back pain: patients consulting primary care for the first time. Spine 2005;30:976–982
42. Tubach F, Beauté J, Leclerc A. Natural history and prognostic indicators of sciatica. J Clin Epidemiol 2004;57:174–179
43. Gatchel RJ. Comorbidity of chronic pain and mental health disorders: the biopsychosocial perspective. Am Psychol 2004;59:795–805
44. Mayer TG, Gatchel RJ, Brede E, Theodore BR. Lumbar surgery in work-related chronic low back pain: can a continuum of care enhance outcomes? Spine J 2014; 14:263–273
45. Main CJ, Wood PL, Hollis S, Spanswick CC, Waddell G. The Distress and Risk Assessment Method. A simple patient classification to identify distress and evaluate the risk of poor outcome. Spine 1992;17:42–52
46. Trief PM, Grant W, Fredrickson B. A prospective study of psychological predictors of lumbar surgery outcome. Spine 2000;25:2616–2621
47. Trief PM, Ploutz-Snyder R, Fredrickson BE. Emotional health predicts pain and function after fusion: a prospective multicenter study. Spine 2006;31:823–830
48. Deyo RA, Nachemson A, Mirza SK. Spinal-fusion surgery—the case for restraint. N Engl J Med 2004; 350:722–726
49. Errico TJ, Gatchel RJ, Schofferman J, et al. A fair and balanced view of spine fusion surgery. Spine J 2004; 4(5, Suppl):S129–S138
50. Fisher CG, Vaccaro AR, Patel AA, et al. Evidence-based recommendations for spine surgery. Spine 2015;40: E309–E316
51. Dunn KM, Jordan KP, Croft PR. Contributions of prognostic factors for poor outcome in primary care low back pain patients. Eur J Pain 2011;15:313–319
52. Grotle M, Foster NE, Dunn KM, Croft P. Are prognostic indicators for poor outcome different for acute and

chronic low back pain consulters in primary care? Pain 2010;151:790–797

53. Leeuw M, Houben RM, Severeijns R, Picavet HS, Schouten EG, Vlaeyen JW. Pain-related fear in low back pain: a prospective study in the general population. Eur J Pain 2007;11:256–266

54. Picavet HS, Vlaeyen JW, Schouten JS. Pain catastrophizing and kinesiophobia: predictors of chronic low back pain. Am J Epidemiol 2002;156:1028–1034

55. Costa LdaC, Maher CG, McAuley JH, et al. Prognosis for patients with chronic low back pain: inception cohort study. BMJ 2009;339:b3829

13

Role of Minimally Invasive Surgery in Back Pain for Degenerative Spine

Roberto Bassani and Elena Serchi

Introduction

The goals of surgery for degenerative diseases are to reduce the pain and disability and to improve the health-related quality of life. Selection of patients is crucial for treatment success. Data from prospective and randomized studies indicate that surgery is effective for the treatment of specific degenerative spine pathologies, such as disk herniation, lumbar radiculopathy, degenerative spinal stenosis, and lumbar spondylolisthesis. Surgery is also appropriate after conservative treatment has failed. More complex spinal disorders are suitable for surgery, although there is a higher risk of adverse events.[1,2]

The recent literature has addressed the issue of morbidity in spine surgery for degenerative pathologies, which increases the risk of an unsuccessful outcome and reduces the cost-effectiveness of treatment. Patients who are smokers and patients who have a large body habitus or diabetes mellitus have an increased risk of morbidity.[3] Another factor that may increase the morbidity of degenerative spine surgery is the approach; a traditional open approach entails soft tissue damage, such as subperiosteal stripping of multiple spinal segments, leading to blood loss, devitalization of paravertebral muscles, and postoperative pain. From this first trigger event, an ongoing pathological chain is generated: postoperative pain leads to prolonged immobility and use of narcotics, increasing the risk of pneumonia, abdominal ileus, and deep venous thrombosis. Biologically, the large devitalized surface caused by retraction and electrocautery predisposes the patient to a deep wound infection, which can result in sepsis, risk of reoperation, and additional prolonged immobility.[4] The degree of iatrogenic soft tissue injury negatively correlates with long-term clinical outcome, and can have mechanical effects (a 30% decrease in lumbar isokinetic strength on flexion testing), electrophysiological effects (15 to 20% of patients experience chronic denervation on electrophysiological testing of paraspinal muscles after open surgery), and biological effects (10 to 15% of patients experience histological and radiological alteration in muscles).[2]

This background explains the current trend in favor of using minimally invasive surgery (MIS) techniques to achieve the same goals as those of an open procedure while limiting surgery-related morbidity.[2] MIS techniques are designed to minimize muscle and soft tissue injury, thus reducing postoperative pain and narcotics consumption, decreasing blood loss, and leading to more rapid mobilization.[4] MIS approaches have been developed to reach most sites of the spine (cervical, thoracic, and lumbar spine), and in the lumbar spine include posterior, lateral, and anterior approaches. With the development of new technology, such as new endoscopic tools and autostatic retractors, MIS techniques are improving rapidly.

Another advantage of MIS techniques is that they enable treating high-risk populations of patients with pain or degenerative pathologies, such as the elderly and the obese, who are not candidates for the traditional open approaches.

High-Risk Patient Populations

Elderly Patients[1]

The overall mortality from spine surgery doubles between the 65- to 69-year age group and the 80-year and older age group, and morbidity increases in parallel with age and is associated with longer hospitalizations and greater complications. In addition, the aging population has numerous comorbidities, such as cardiovascular and renal disease, poor nutritional status, immobility, obesity, and diabetes mellitus, that are associated with higher complication rates particularly due to cardiac and infectious complications. But the aging population has increased disability related to degenerative pathologies of the spine that lead to back pain and radicular symptoms and cause abnormal posture, which in turn can lead to easy fatigability and predispose to falls (due to alterations in vision and weight distribution). Globally, all these conditions lead to reduced mobility, which ultimately compromises the overall medical health status (in particular the cardiopulmonary status) and decondition the patient. The recent literature supports surgical intervention for these conditions among elderly patients, especially with less invasive techniques that are safer than the traditional open procedures with comparable biomechanical patterns.

Obese Patients[5,6]

Obesity, defined as a body mass index (BMI) ≥ 30, is an increasing worldwide problem. Obese patients often suffer from pathologies of the spine, but spine surgery entails higher risks for complications due to medical comorbidities, higher infection rates (the risk is doubled due to the wider skin incision, elevated blood glucose, and poor antibiotic penetration in fat), and more difficult access to the surgical site, often requiring a longer surgical incision, leading to additional tissue injury. To reduce the complications related to tissue dissection, new transmuscular MIS techniques can be applied. These techniques entail an overall complication rate of 21.8%, with a postoperative infection rate of 0.7% (with an open procedure it is 29 to 33%), a higher incidence of intraoperative durotomies (9.4% vs 3 to 5% of microsurgical diskectomies, apparently related to the greater working distance in this particular population), and a reoperation rate of 9.4%.[5]

Anatomic and Biological Factors in Preserving Lumbar Musculature[7]

The paraspinal cutaneous tissue is vascularized by a double arterial network, a median and a lateral one, both arising from the lumbar arteries. A part of the lateral lumbar cutaneous territory is also vascularized by the arterial system that emerges through the thoracolumbar aponeurosis at between 5 and 9 cm lateral to the midline.

Two posterior paraspinal muscle groups are present, both of them attaching caudally and running along the thoracolumbar spine:

1. The deep paramedian transversospinalis muscle group, including the multifidus (MF), intertransversarii (IT), and quadratum lumborum (QL)
2. The more superficial and lateral erector spinae longissimus (Lo) and iliocostalis (IC) (**Fig. 13.1**)

Globally, posterior paraspinal muscles provide motion and dynamic stability of the multisegmented spinal column, among which the MF muscle plays a key role.

Numerous studies have investigated the anatomy, histochemical properties, and radiological imaging of many of these muscles, with the goal of improving clinical and surgical results and reducing muscular iatrogenic trauma.

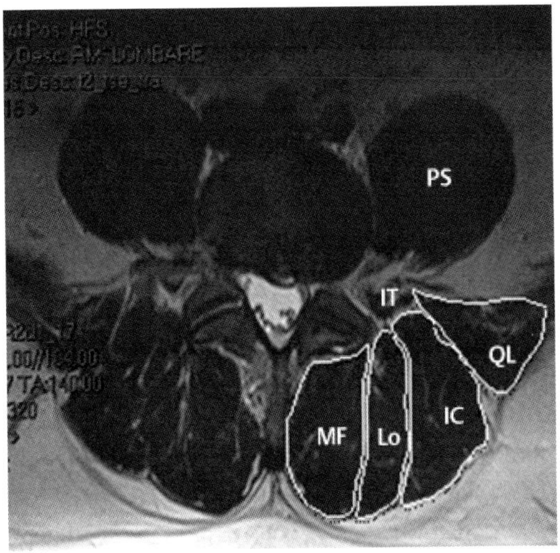

Fig. 13.1 Axial T2-weighted magnetic resonance imaging (MRI) of the L4–L5 disk. MF, multifidus; Lo, longissimus; IC, iliocostalis; IT, intertransversalis; QL, quadratus lumborum; PS, psoas muscle.

The structure, function, and design of the upper and lower extremity muscles are well described, but only a few studies have investigated paraspinal muscles. Studies have evaluated the number and orientation of muscle fibers within a muscle, defined as the "skeletal muscle architecture," in order to predict muscle function. Lumbar spinal muscles were found to have relatively short fibers (~ 10 cm) with moderate-sized physiological cross-sectional areas (~ 10 cm^2), which confirms that their global function is to provide stabilization. Among all paraspinal muscles, the MF muscle stands out as the most extreme example of a muscle designed to stabilize the lumbar spine against flexion; the MF showed a greater cross-sectional area than the other lumbar muscles, This design enables the MF to produce vary large forces over a narrow range of lengths. Another peculiar aspect of the MF among the other paraspinal muscles is the uniqueness of its fiber arrangement: an MF slack sarcomere length of 2.2 μm and an elastic moduli of 35 kPa (kilopascals), indicating biomechanical properties comparable with those of the extremities and the quadriceps muscles. Indirectly, assuming that mammalian muscle generates ~ 250 kPa of stress under conditions of optimal sarcomere length and maximum activation, the MF muscle could direct ~ 60 N of extension force to the spine, which is more than twice the amount that could be generated by any other lumbar extensor muscle.

Morphologically, the MF consists of several bundles that originate from the spinous process, that spread caudally for two to five segments, and then insert into the mammillary process of the facet joints and the iliac crest. Functionally, the MF is divided into two layers: deep (dMF) and superficial (sMF).[6] The dMF is formed by short muscle bundles and a high percentage of type I fibers (i.e., slow oxidative muscle fibers with high mitochondrial content, which differ from type IIa fibers, which are fast glycolytic fibers with low mitochondrial content, and from type IIb fibers, which are fast oxidative fibers with high mitochondrial content), and it seems to provide compressive force and proprioception. The sMF generates an extension force. Electromyography (EMG) studies documented that the dMF is activated to stabilize the spine, regardless of the direction of stress, whereas the sMF is activated in accordance with the direction of the external load.

The MF muscle receives innervation from only the medial branch of the dorsal ramus, with no intersegmental supply (**Fig. 13.2**). This nervous branch is relatively fixed as it runs beneath the fibro-osseous mamilloaccessory ligament, exits the intertransversalis fascia, and finally enters the MF muscle from its cranial side.

Neuroimaging of the lumbar MF muscle with magnetic resonance imaging (MRI, **Fig. 13.3**), computed tomography (CT), and ultrasound assesses its morphology and function, and their possible correlation with pain and disability. Morphology and quantitative measures of the MF muscle are best obtained with MRI. T1-weighted acquisitions are used to measure the cross-sectional area of the muscle, and T2-weighted scans measure the intramuscular adipose tissue. Function assessment is best obtained with ultrasound imaging by measuring changes in MF thickness during submaximal contraction task.

In healthy subjects, the lumbar MF is symmetrical bilaterally and increases its size

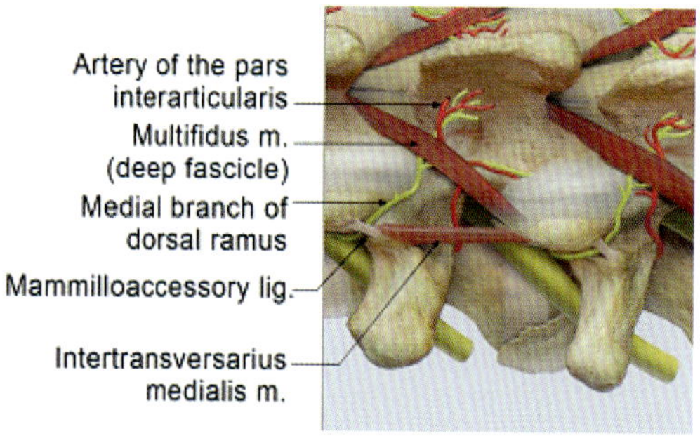

a

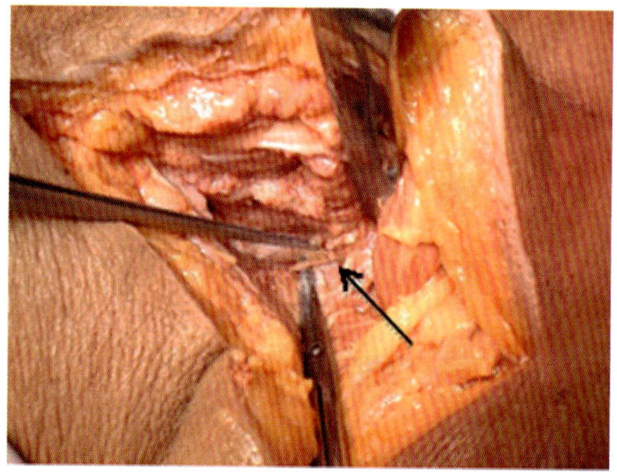

Fig. 13.2 **(a)** Anatomic model of the innervation and vascularization of the paravertebral musculature. **(b)** The medial branch *(arrow)* of the nerve supply to the multifidus.

caudally. The cross-sectional area is larger in males, unrelated to age. The mean adipose infiltration in MF muscle is reported to be between 15% and 29%.

Pathological Changes in the Multifidus Muscle[2,6,7]

Preservation of normal anatomy and functioning of paraspinal muscles, particularly of the MF, is a crucial factor in treating low back pain and preventing the postoperative failed back syndrome. Because the adverse effects caused by iatrogenic muscle damage may potentially persist for several years postoperatively, techniques that cause less damage to the paraspinal muscle should be considered when performing lumbar surgery.

During back pain, both acute and chronic, the size and consistency of the lumbar MF change; specific and localized patterns of atrophy are documented in the MF muscle in

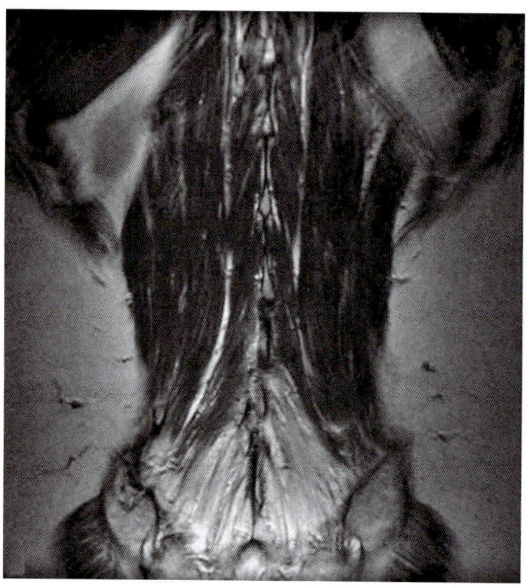

a

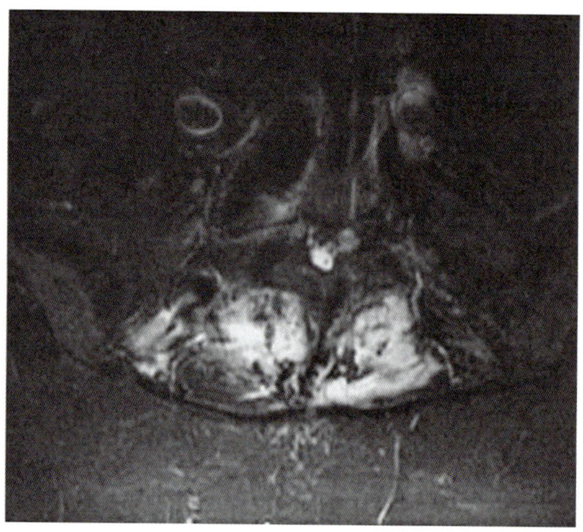

b

Fig. 13.3 Wiltse's approach. **(a)** Postoperative coronal T2 MRI. **(b)** Postoperative axial T2 MRI: no muscular trauma is visible.

chronic back pain, greatest at the L5 disk level, with parallel alteration of the neurocontrol.

Physiological and morphological alterations have been observed in dMF and sMF in patients with recurrent/chronic spontaneous low back pain; the changes in the control of the lumbar MF include decreased activation of the sMF, lack of anticipatory contraction of the dMF, and changes in the composition of muscle fibers. Ultrasonography shows an unclear image of the MF in patients with chronic neck pain. The same applies to the lumbar MF: the boundaries of the different layers are less clear and the fat content is higher. Fatty degeneration of the MF muscle has been studied to determine if there is a correlation between the risk of developing chronic low back pain and failed back surgery syndrome.

The traditional midline open procedure causes the detachment of the MF from the spinous process, which compromises its neurovascular supply (**Fig. 13.2**) and compresses the muscle with prolonged retraction. These factors cause adverse histological and biomechanical changes, resulting in muscle atrophy and consequent decreased force-production capacity of the muscle. Kim et al[2] compared trunk muscle strength in patients treated with open midline posterior spinal instrumentation and in those treated with the paraspinal approach, and found that those treated with a midline paraspinal approach had > 50% improvement in lumbar extension strength, whereas those treated with a midline open procedure had no improvement.

Muscle biopsy specimens from patients undergoing revision spine surgery have revealed a change in the type of fibers that form the paraspinal muscle (selective type II fiber atrophy, as well as widespread fiber-type grouping, a sign of reinnervation), and a higher glycerol concentration in the paraspinal muscles than in the deltoid muscles of the same patients; glycerol is an important component of glycerophospholipid, the basic structure of the cell membrane; when the integrity of a cell membrane is destroyed, glycerol is released into the interstitial fluid. Muscle denervation has been proposed to be the main pathological mechanism leading to muscle atrophy (the nerve supply to the MF is monosegmental, making it especially vulnerable to injury), which often worsens with prolonged retraction.[8] But other authors proposed that injury is induced by a crush mechanism similar to that caused by a pneumatic tourniquet during surgery on the extremities.[9] During the application of self-retaining retractors, elevated pressure leads to decreased intramuscular perfusion. The severity of the muscle injury is affected by the degree of the intramuscular pressure and the length of the retraction time. Muscle biopsies in patients with failed back surgery syndrome showed signs of advanced chronic denervation.[2]

Indirect evaluation of paraspinal muscle damage has been done with neuroimaging. The iatrogenic damage to paraspinal muscles is demonstrable as T2-weighted hyperintensity on MRI that corresponds to muscle edema, denervation, and fatty infiltration that leads to muscle atrophy (**Fig. 13.3**).

Because the MF receives innervation from the medial branch of the dorsal ramus in its cranial part, increased T2 signal due to denervation is usually seen in the caudal part of the MF.[7] The degree of MF atrophy significantly correlates with the level of low back discomfort as measured with Visual Analogue Scale (VAS) scores.[10] Mori et al reported that detection of high T2 signal on MRI after 1 year is valuable as an indicator of paraspinal muscular damage.[11] Progressive reduction of edema up to 1 year after surgery and reinnervation of muscles that were denervated during surgery is associated with recovery of signal intensity on T2 MRI. After 3 years, the T2 signal is reported to be almost at the preoperative level, and its evaluation at this time point after the procedure may be less valuable.

Soft tissue trauma can have widespread regional and systemic effects that laboratory tests can demonstrate. Serum creatine phosphokinase (CPK) peaks on postoperative day 1 and subsequently declines, reaching preoperative values 1 week after surgery. Because an increased CPK level is associated with gender and individual muscle volume, the CPK ratio is usually compared instead of its absolute value. Kim et al found that levels of creatine CPK, aldolase, proinflammatory cytokines (interleukin [IL]-6 and IL-8), and anti-inflammatory cytokines (IL-10 and IL-1 receptor antagonist) in patients treated with open surgery were increased severalfold compared with the levels in patients treated with the MIS. Some studies found the CPK ratio to be lower in the paraspinal approaches versus the open midline surgeries, whereas other studies found no difference in postoperative CPK ratio levels between MIS and open surgery, and the authors thus concluded that muscle injury was directly related to the muscle retraction time during surgery.[12]

Posterior Surgical Approaches to the Lumbar Spine

Minimally Invasive Diskectomy[3,12]

The first pain generator in the spine is the intervertebral disk, which is where degenerative failure begins. The first description of the pathophysiology of sciatica was made in 1934 by Mixter, and many refinements in diagnosis and treatment techniques of the herniated disk have been made subsequently. Numerous MIS techniques have been developed to treat a degenerated disk, preserving notable structures, such as the musculature and soft tissue, from iatrogenic injury. Among these techniques are percutaneous chemonucleolysis, nucleotomy, percutaneous laser disk decompression, and percutaneous endoscopic/microscopic diskectomy.

Chymopapain chemonucleolysis, which enzymatically dissolves the nucleus, resulted in satisfactory treatment in 72% of patients, but the technique has progressively fallen into disfavor because of the reported complications of back pain and stiffness in 20 to 40% of cases, which is sometimes intractable for months, anaphylaxis in 1% of patients, and cauda equine syndrome and acute transverse myelitis in one case each.

Nucleotomy is indicated only for patients with a contained disk. The technique is based on a direct puncture of the annulus to the retroperitoneum to let the nucleus pulposus extrude on the opposite side from the spinal canal. The reported success rate was 72%, but the technique has not been widely accepted, because of potential vascular and nerve damage and the risk of infection in the disk space. The technique is contraindicated in previously operated patients in obese patients and in L5-S1 disk for its specific anatomy.

Laser diskectomy is indicated to obtain reduction in intradiskal pressure due to tissue absorption activity and ablation delivery of the laser, and in contained disks (i.e., prolapsed, not herniated). But few controlled studies are reported in the literature, although there are anecdotal reports of satisfactory results in 60 to 85% of patients. The technique has not been widely accepted.

Surgical Diskectomy[3]

Microsurgical diskectomy is the first MIS procedure of spine surgery for degenerative pathology. Although more refined techniques have been developed subsequently, microsurgical diskectomy is still the gold standard of care.

Microscopic and endoscopic diskectomy are basically the same procedure, differing only in the type of magnification used; under direct visualization of the herniated disk (increasing the safety and efficacy of the procedure) the sequestered fragment is removed and decompression of the annulus is possible.

Soft tissue retraction during the surgical procedure is widely reported in the literature to cause a regional ischemia, even after short microdiskectomy in young patients. Among recent technical refinements, the transmuscular tubular diskectomy has reduced muscle trauma. Despite a clear perception of better clinical results, a prospective randomized multicenter study failed to demonstrate that tubular diskectomy compared with conventional microdiskectomy results in a statistically significant improvement in the clinical outcome scores. A possible explanation is that the standard microsurgical diskectomy is defined as an open approach, but the surgical incision and muscles dissection are very small (usually 1 to 3 cm), and can be performed in an MIS technique.

Technique (Transmuscular Approach)

The patient is placed in the prone position with the abdomen free and the spine flexed to aid exposure of the interlaminar space. Under fluoroscopic control, a needle is used to localize the disk level. The entry point is 1.5 to 2 cm off the midline and can be checked under fluoroscopy (on the medial border of the anteroposterior [AP] projection of the pedicles). A small linear longitudinal incision is made, and a guidewire is directed toward the inferior edge of the superior lamina. Through the skin incision, sequential cannulated dilators are inserted over the wire, with the initial dilator directed to the region between the spinous process and the facet complex, just above the inferior edge of the lamina. Magnification is obtained with the microscope or endoscope. The laminar edge is identified, and a medial facetectomy is accomplished. Once the nerve root has been identified, it is retracted medially, and the herniated disk is then removed.

Far Lateral Disk Diskectomy

The protrusion of the herniated disk is most commonly located in the preforaminal space, but it can occur in different areas along the perimeter of the annulus. The extrusion of the herniated disk in the extraforaminal space occurs in 7 to 12% of cases, but it leads to the same symptom of radiculopathy as does any other nerve root conflict situation. Conservative treatment is commonly tried first, along with injection of steroids in the extraforaminal area.

Surgical treatment is achieved via a more obliterative approach (monolateral laminectomy and arterectomy) or via an MIS transmuscular approach, described by several authors, that is better known as the far lateral or Wiltse approach.[13] This approach is reported to be safe and effective, and it avoids the risk of secondary spinal instability. But it may be especially tricky to perform it at the L5-S1 disk if the L5 vertebra is impacted; at higher levels this is not a problem. This surgical approach is very anatomic but it is technically demanding and is not recommended for surgeons who lack expertise in using it for more typical disk herniations.

Technique

The patient is positioned prone. The affected disk level is checked under fluoroscopy, and a linear longitudinal skin incision is made 4.5 to 5 cm off the midline (the exact position is determined by the AP X-ray projection, at the lateral border of the pedicles). Once the muscular aponeurosis is exposed, the fascia is incised to locate the passage between the MF and the longissimus, which is then dissect with a finger to palpate the transverse process of the vertebra. An autostatic retractor is positioned (Beckman, Williams, or Taylor models) and fixed to the operating table. Bony structures are detached and used as anatomic landmarks (upper vertebra isthmus, upper and lower vertebrae joint bone, and lower vertebra transverse process), and the intertransverse fascia is exposed. It is important to search for the perforating branch of the dorsal branch of the lumbar artery and coagulate it by bipolar forceps, because it is a landmark for the nerve root under the fascia. The safer area is the lower part of the fascia near the lower vertebra transverse process; this is where the fascia is coagulated and cut and then removed. It is not necessary to remove all the intertransversalis fascia but at least remove its medial half. The nerve root is located transversally going from the upper medial aspect of this area, downward and laterally. It may be flattened by the herniated fragment, and mistaken for the hernia. It is essential not to attempt to remove the hernia before having properly visualized the nerve root. Once the root is identified, it may be protected with a nerve retractor and the herniated disk can be safely removed (preferably proceeding from the shoulder of the nerve root). The disk need not be removed. At end of the procedure, it is mandatory to check along the canal and along the root, using an oblique hook.

Minimally Invasive Treatment of Synovial Cysts[4]

Among degenerative lumbar pathologics causing pain, synovial cysts are a rare condition (incidence 0.8%) referred to as degenerative arthropathy of the facets joints. The first-line treatment is percutaneous aspiration or steroid injection (may require a multiple injection, with 75% response rate), but surgery might be recommended in cases of recurrence or intractable pain (immediate symptomatic improvement in > 90%). The laminectomy and partial medial facetectomy can be achieved through a transmuscular MIS tubular retractor system aided with a microscope or endoscope.

Percutaneous Pedicle Screw Fixation

Degeneration of the spine not only often affects the disk but also determines the extent of the deformity and instability, and the extent of bone and ligaments causing stenosis. In most of these conditions, pain and disability are present and after an attempt at conservative treatment (including percutaneous injections) surgery is often recommended (decompression and fusion).

Fusion is achieved with an internal fixation, usually using pedicle screws with or without interbody cages. There have been numerous reports in the literature on this subject.

Fixation of the lumbar spine can be performed in an MIS fashion with a percutaneous approach, eliminating the need for a large midline incision and significant paraspinous muscle dissection.[5] (The advantages of muscle preservation were earlier in the chapter.) The procedure was first described by Magerl,[14] and it has continued to evolve. But all versions of the procedure use a small paramedian skin incision and position the screws under fluoroscopy. The risk of malpositioning a pedicle screw without direct anatomic vision is low (despite an obvious learning curve) and is reported to be as low as that with open surgical procedures (6.6%, with none requiring surgical revision).[15]

The rod is then inserted and connected to the screws as in open procedures, but the technique of rod insertion differs, as does the instrumentation used.

In degenerative pathologies, is often recommended to add an internal fusion with an interbody cage to the posterior screw and rod fixation, as this improves stability and provides long-lasting fusion. As in open procedures, interbody fusion is achieved with two cages, positioned through a preforaminal working corridor, such as with posterior lumbar interbody fusion (PLIF), or by using one longer cage and one transverse cage, positioned through a transforaminal working corridor, such as with transforaminal lumbar interbody fusion (TLIF).

Both the PLIF and TLIF techniques can be realized in an MIS fashion (**Fig. 13.4**). In both cases the patient is positioned prone, with the operating table accessible to X-ray for the latero-lateral (LL) and AP projections.

Minimally Invasive Posterior Lumbar Interbody Fusion[16]

Open PLIF has the following disadvantages: a 0.3 to 2.4% risk of posterior extrusion of the graft, a 0.5 to 4% risk of retraction injury to the nerve roots, as well as epidural fibrosis and chronic radiculitis, dural tears, and simultaneous destabilization of anterior and posterior columns because PLIF requires the most extensive destabilization of posterior elements (soft tissues, ligaments such as the interspinous ligament complex, leading to the loss of flexion strength and delayed spinal stability, loss of strength in the facets, and extensive laminectomy). Overall clinical failure of open PLIF is reported to be 16%; most authors believe that this failure is directly correlated with the degree of iatrogenic paraspinal muscle injury and with an increased incidence of postoperative failed back syndrome.

Both open and MIS PLIF are reported to achieve 25% restoration of intervertebral disk height, and some degree of retrolisthesis correction is obtained via ligamentopexis; segmental lordosis improved by 29% on average, and foramina volume increased of 20%.

Technique

The skin incision is made 1 cm lateral to the exact projection of the pedicle to achieve the correct angulation for accurate screw positioning. The position and trajectory of each pair of

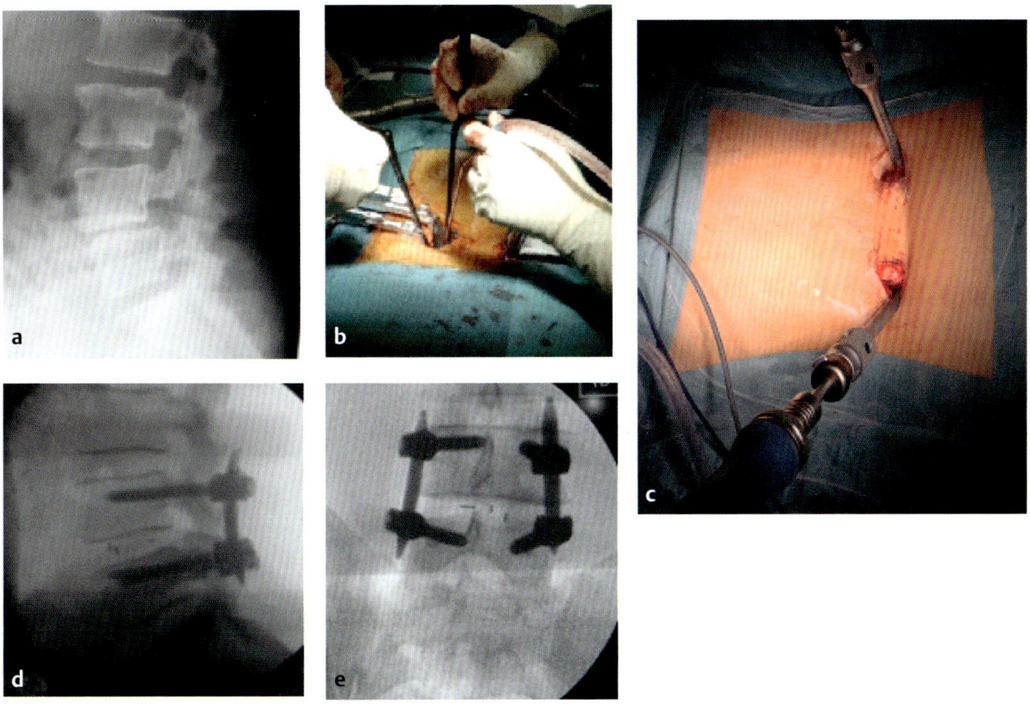

Fig. 13.4 (a) Preoperative sagittal X-ray showing degenerative L4-L5 listhesis. **(b,c)** Intraoperative view of the small skin incision and working channel. **(d,e)** Postoperative lateral and anteroposterior (AP) X-ray showing the pedicle screws and intervertebral cage.

pedicles is checked with LL and AP fluoroscopy. Two small paramedial transmuscular incisions (similar to the Wiltse approach described for the far lateral disk diskectomy, above) are made; they are used for both screw positioning and a minimally invasive PLIF-type decompression (hemilaminotomy, flavectomy, facetectomy, or foraminotomy) on each side. With the aid of the microscope or endoscope, the root and dural sac is recognized and retract medially. The external aspect of the annulus is identified on both sides, and an aggressive diskectomy is performed to prepare the intervertebral disk space for placement of the interbody grafts. The appropriate size (especially height and lordosis) are calculated on preoperative lateral radiographs and checked on LL projection during the procedure (disk height is suggested to be as similar as possible to that of the upper and lower level disk); in the L5-S1 segment, extra care should be taken with addressing the lordosis. The correct positioning of the cages is checked with both lateral and AP projections. It is of particular importance to assess the height of the selected cage (cage height should be similar to that of the closer normal disk) and the position in the ventrodorsal direction (the cage must be anterior to the spinal canal; the more anterior it is, the more lordotic an angle is obtained). After the insertion of the cages, the rods are inserted and the system is closed in compression, according to the instrumentation system used. A posterolateral bone fusion also can be added in this MIS approach.

Minimally Invasive Transforaminal Lumbar Interbody Fusion[16]

As compared with the PLIF approach, The TLIF approach is less destructive of bone structures and requires less exposure of nervous structures. Its MIS variant, which was first described in 2002, has gained widespread popularity in the treatment of degenerative lumbar diseases.

In 2015, Khan et al[16] presented an updated meta-analysis of the MIS approach as compared with open approaches. They reported a statistically significant decreased operative blood loss (in 22 studies), decreased postoperative need for narcotic pain relief (in 15 studies with follow-up > 1 year, and in 10 studies with follow-up < 6 months; no difference was found in early VAS scores, but a significant difference was found in late VAS scores), statistically significant shorter hospital stays (in 18 studies, with an MIS group mean hospital stay of 1.3 days), similar patient-reported outcome (in 15 studies with follow-up > 1 year, and in eight studies with hollow-up < 6 months; no differences in both early and late outcome), and similar radiographic outcome (no statistically significant fusion rates differences in 20 studies). But, as with all MIS procedures, this procedure entailed a steep learning curve for the surgeons, longer operative times (in 20 studies, no statistical difference), and longer fluoroscopic times (in eight studies, statistically significant difference; 38.2 seconds more radiation times in the MIS group). Complications in MIS and open TLIF were reported in 25 studies; there were lower risks in MIS, but it depended on the surgeon's experience (relative risk 0.65 comparing MIS TLIF with open TLIF, with a 95% confidence interval of 0.50 to 0.83). Khan et al believe that the decreased rate of complications with MIS TLIF is due to decreased tissue damage and decreased blood loss, as these two factors are strongly correlated with postoperative infection rate, which is decreased in MIS procedures. Interestingly, a new subpopulation of patients can benefit from these findings, as MIS TLIF procedures may now be appropriate for obese patients and elderly patients, groups that were previously considered to be at high risk.

Technique

Patient positioning and insertion of the screw are identical to those for the MIS PLIF procedure, as are cage selection and positioning. The main difference is that the cage is inserted through a monoportal corridor obtained from a monolateral complete arterectomy and subsequent diskectomy and disk preparation for the graft. The cage shape for TLIF is different from that for PLIF: it is longer than those used for the PLIF approach, because it has to cover the entire disk space in laterality, and it can be straight or banana-shaped. At the end of cage insertion, AP and LL fluoroscopy views must be obtained; in TLIF, the cage is positioned across the midline (on the AP view). The considerations regarding cage height and lordosis are the same as for the PLIF procedure.

Anterior and Lateral Approaches to the Lumbar Spine

The major benefit of an MIS procedure is that it is muscle-sparing. By definition, anterior and lateral approaches to the lumbar spine must be consider of pivotal interest for MIS procedures in the degenerative spine.

Minimally Invasive and Laparoscopic Retroperitoneal Approach[17–21]

The traditional transperitoneal open approach is an invasive procedure in which considerable trauma to abdominal muscles and abdominal organs (in particular the small bowel) is caused in order to gain access to the surgical target area. Consequently, as with other surgical approaches for spine pathologies, attempts to perform mini-open or pure laparoscopic approaches have been made and developed over the years. The retroperitoneal corridor has been demonstrated to be largely superior to the transperitoneal approach, eliminating the risk of small-bowel obstruction and postoperative intraperitoneal and abdominal adhesions. A purely laparoscopic approach was first used by general, vascular, and urologic surgeons for a variety of conditions, and in recent years it has been applied to spine pathologies. More commonly a mini-open muscle-sparing retroperitoneal approach is used because it achieves a decreased morbidity associated with incising the oblique musculature during a flank approach but provides enough space to perform a proper interbody fusion.

Anterior approaches to the lumbar spine are technically challenging with a steep learning curve, especially a purely laparoscopic approach, because the retroperitoneal space is a small cavity.

A purely laparoscopic technique is reported for single-level pathologies, in which the minimally invasive retroperitoneal approach provides access to any level of the lumbar spine and enables reaching even multiple levels during the same procedure. The goal of an anterior or lateral approach to the disk is to achieve restoration of disk height and fusion of the treated spinal unit (**Fig. 13.5**). Stability obtained through an anterior or lateral fusion is higher (spinal stiffness increased by 80%) than with a posterolateral fusion (spinal stiffness increased by 40%).

The efficacy of the anterior approaches is well documented in the literature,[17,19,20] as is the safety of the technique; there is very little blood loss (10–100 mL), no operative vascular or neurologic injuries (such as retrograde ejaculation in men), reduced postoperative pain, and shorter hospitalization (mean of 3.4 days). The advantage of anterior approaches is that they facilitate obtaining a complete diskectomy without affecting the facet joints of the vertebra directly above, as often happens in the posterior approach.

Indications[22] (Table 13.1)

This approach is appropriate for lumbar disk pathologies causing back pain that are unresponsive to a minimum of 6 months of conservative treatment, with degenerative changes in the disk demonstrated with preoperative MRI, such as collapsed disk and Modic changes. It is not universally accepted that a provocative diskography indicates the need for surgery. The literature reports that patients with a grade 1 spondylolisthesis can also be treated via an anterior approach, and many revision cases can benefit with this surgical approach, too. A relative contraindication for this approach is patients who had previous abdomen surgery.[19]

Technique

Mini-Laparotomy

Before surgery, it is important to identify on MRI or CT the location of the aortic bifurcation relative to the disk space. The bowel is prepared the night before surgery. Because it is not possible to ascertain the rate of presacral nerve injury leading to retrograde ejaculation and

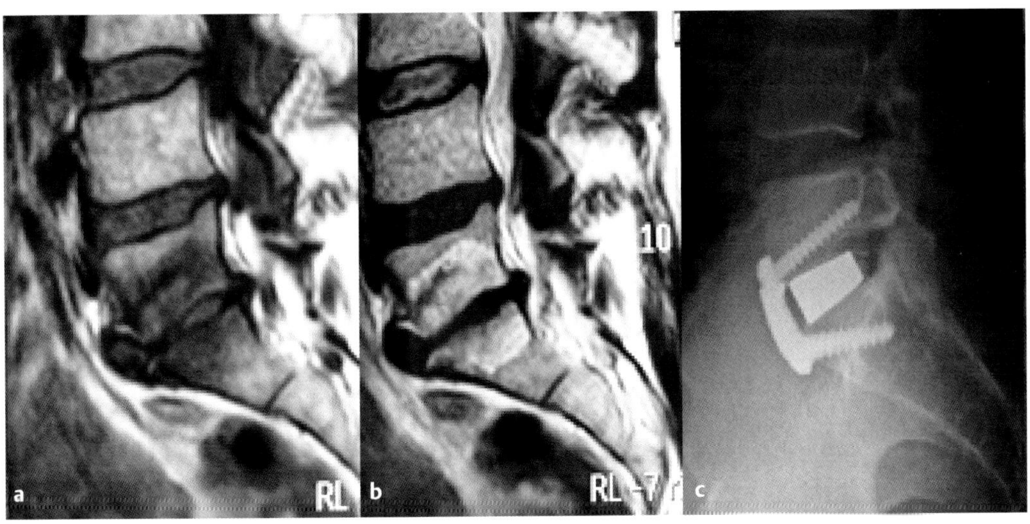

Fig. 13.5 L5-S1 diskopathy treated with an anterior arthrodesis (cage and anterior plating). **(a,b)** Preoperative sagittal T1 and T2 MRI. **(c)** Disk height is restored.

Table 13.1 Indications for Anterior Lateral Interbody Fusion (ALIF) and for Arthroplasty

	Indication for ALIF	Indication for Arthroplasty
Patient/clinical	Psychosocial and working factors (greater impact on back pain disability than biomedical or biomechanical factors) and evaluation of other pain-generating syndrome such as fibromyalgia No contraindications to anterior approach Understanding possible complications	
Patient/anatomy	Any lumbar level	DDD at L4-L5 and/or L5-S1
	No major concerns regarding deformity on the preoperative workup Preoperative imaging: • Whole spine standing X-ray: including sacral tilt, pelvic tilt, pelvic incidence, and global lordosis to characterize sagittal balance • MRI: to evaluate the DDD and eventual herniated disk	No deformity on the preoperative workup (no scoliosis, spondylolisthesis, or fracture) Preoperative imaging: • Whole spine standing X-ray: including sacral tilt, pelvic tilt, pelvic incidence, and global lordosis to characterize sagittal balance (some studies found that DDD patients generally do not have abnormal sagittal balance, and others reported improved balance post-TDR) • CT: no osteophytes, no sclerosis of end plates; check bony alignment, check posterior intervertebral joints • MRI: to evaluate the spinal canal, space for neural structures, bony alignment and facet joints, and to provide direct assessment of neural and disc structures • *Note:* intervertebral disk height of 4 mm is considered the minimum height to perform a disk prosthesis (disk height < 4 mm, with or without scarring, and thickening of annulus fibrosis with osteophytes indicate osteoarthritis)

Abbreviations: CT, computed tomography; DDD, degenerative disk disease; MRI, magnetic resonance imaging; TDR, total disk replacement.

infertility, male patients should be informed of this risk.

The surgery is performed with the patient in the supine position, with extended legs, in a 20- to 30-degree Trendelenburg position to enable a more perpendicular approach to the disk and to retract the intestines toward the diaphragm and away from the lumbosacral region. Some authors recommend keeping the patient's legs abducted, with the surgeon standing in front of the patient's pelvis, but recent studies recommend placing the patient in the standard supine position without abduction of the legs, with the surgeon standing at the side of the patient.

The mini-open muscle-sparing retroperitoneal approach is performed via a small transverse 3- to 5-cm medial skin incision (for L5-S1, which remains under the underwear line) or through a small belly incision ("perinavel Bassani" incision; **Fig. 13.6**), and provides direct visualization and access to any lumbar disk space. The whole procedure is performed through a 270-degree round incision with the use of a 30-degree angled, 10-mm endoscope. This provides the best view on a high-definition monitor at a higher magnification for all the surgical steps, entailing less invasiveness and improved accuracy.

The anterior rectus sheath is divided 1 cm superiorly and 1 cm inferiorly at the lateral border of the rectus muscle (**Fig. 13.7**) which is retracted toward the midline to expose the posterior sheath (above the arcuate line) and the arcuate line (or preperitoneal space). At this point, the arcuate ligament is cut (**Fig. 13.8**).

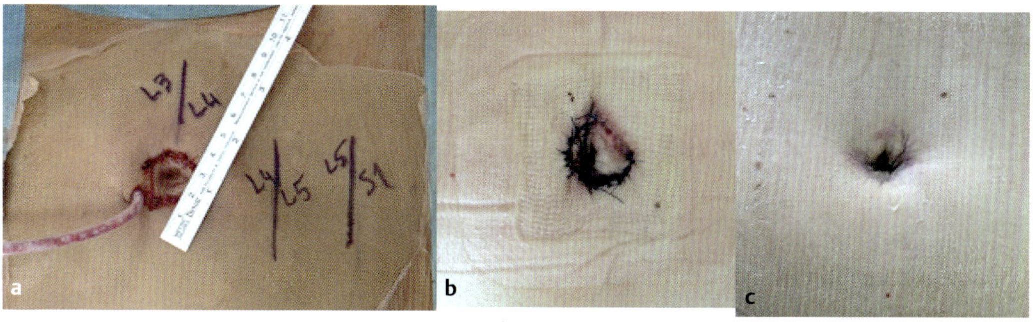

Fig. 13.6 Perinavel Bassani incision. **(a)** The multilevel approach through a Bassani incision. Note the theoretical transverse incisions for a mini-laparotomy. **(b)** The incision 3 weeks after surgery. **(c)** The incision 3 months after surgery.

This enables widening the working space and facilitates visualization of the deep structures. The posterior rectus sheath–arcuate line is divided in a vertical direction, and the preperitoneal space is identified. The line is then extended bluntly, and the peritoneum is separated medially to expose the retroperitoneal space. After identification of the psoas muscle, the left ureter (**Fig. 13.9**), peritoneum, and abdominal contents are mobilized across the midline. The anterior aspect of the lumbar column is then visible and the level to treat can be identified. The position of the ureter (**Fig. 13.9**) must constantly be noted; the right upper ureter courses over the right iliac artery and vein (**Fig. 13.10**) and can be identify by peristalsis associated with probing this structure, whereas the left ureter lies deep to the sigmoid colon in the retroperitoneal space. The middle sacral vein is used to identify the midline (**Fig. 13.10**).

After the insertion of deep retractors, the large vessels are visualized and mobilized (**Fig. 13.11a,b**). For the L4–L5 disk, the aorta, cava, and common iliac veins and arteries are retracted laterally from left to right after the ligature of the iliolumbar veins. The L5-S1 disk

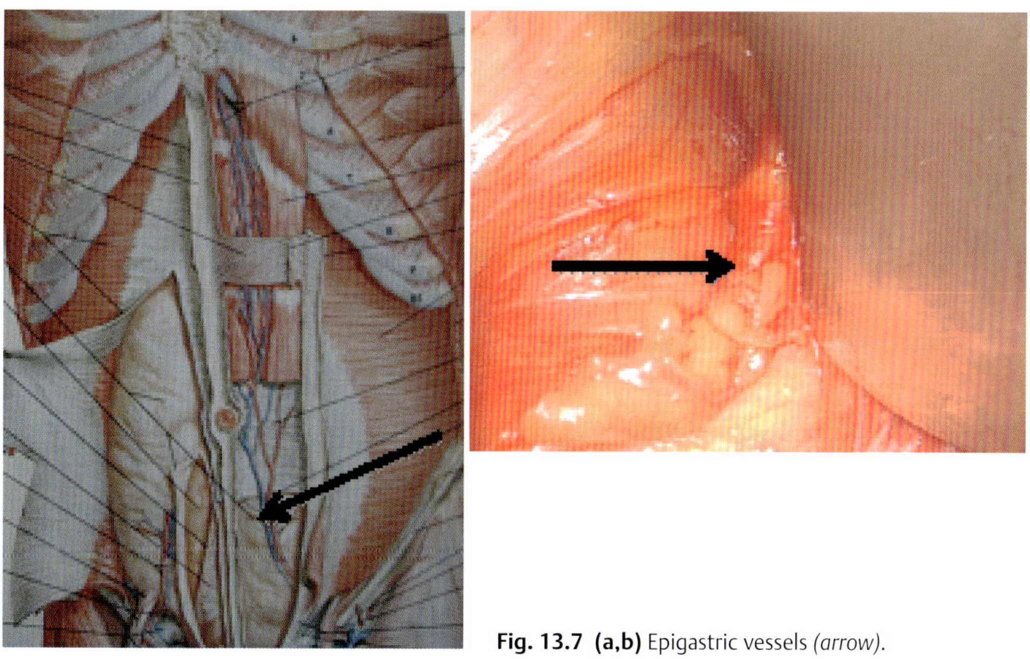
b

a

Fig. 13.7 **(a,b)** Epigastric vessels *(arrow)*.

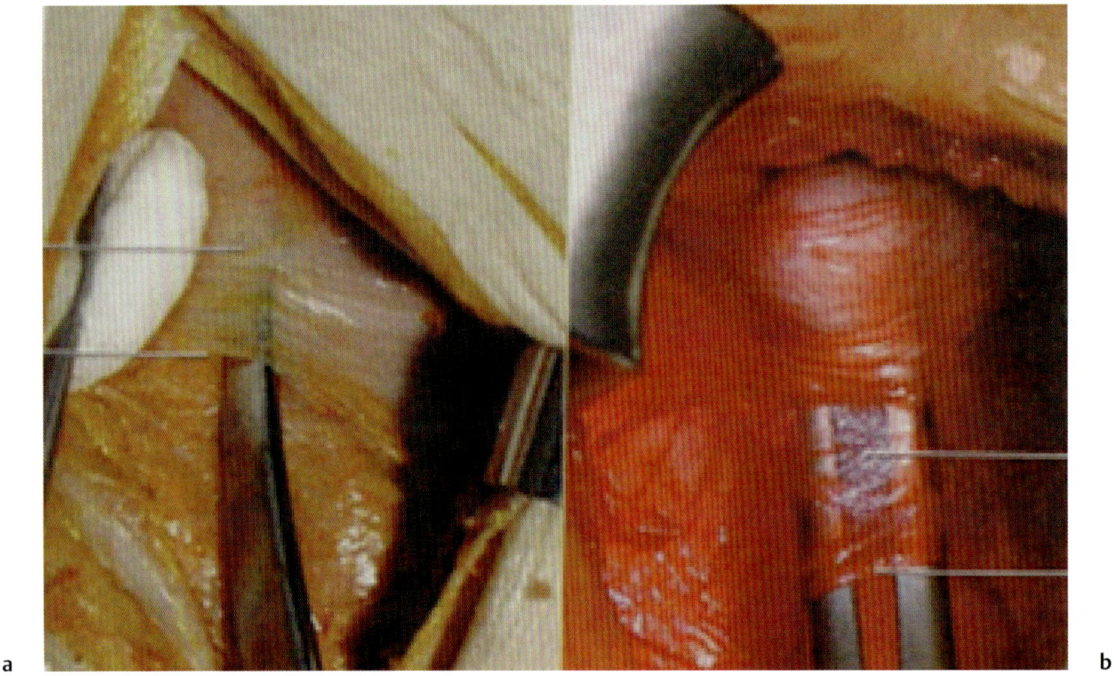

Fig. 13.8 (a,b) The arcuate line.

is located below the aorta and the cava bifurcation into the two common iliac arteries and veins. These vessels are then retracted on both sides to expose the disk, and the middle sacral vessels are coagulated with a bipolar forceps or ligated. Approaching the L5-S1 level, the median sacral artery and vein must be identified and ligated with vascular clips, avoiding the use of electrocautery to preserve the median sacral plexus (correlated to retrograde ejaculation), which is displaced laterally by blunt dissection. Approaching all other lumbar levels, segmental vessels must be identified, dissected free from the underlying bone, ligated with hemoclips on both two edges, and transected.

After the complete exposure of the disk, the retractors are fixed to the bony surface through dedicated pins. This very stable configuration

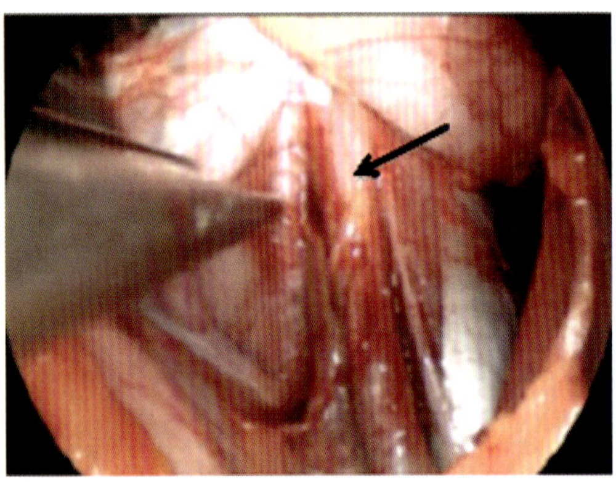

Fig. 13.9 The ureter *(arrow)*.

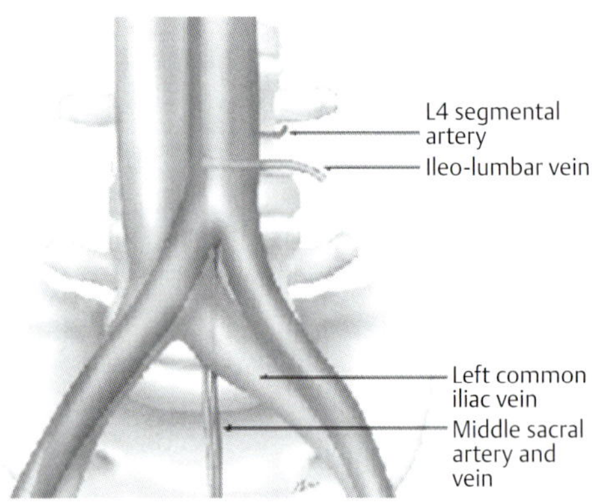

Fig. 13.10 Arterial and venous system and their relation to the L4-S1 spine.

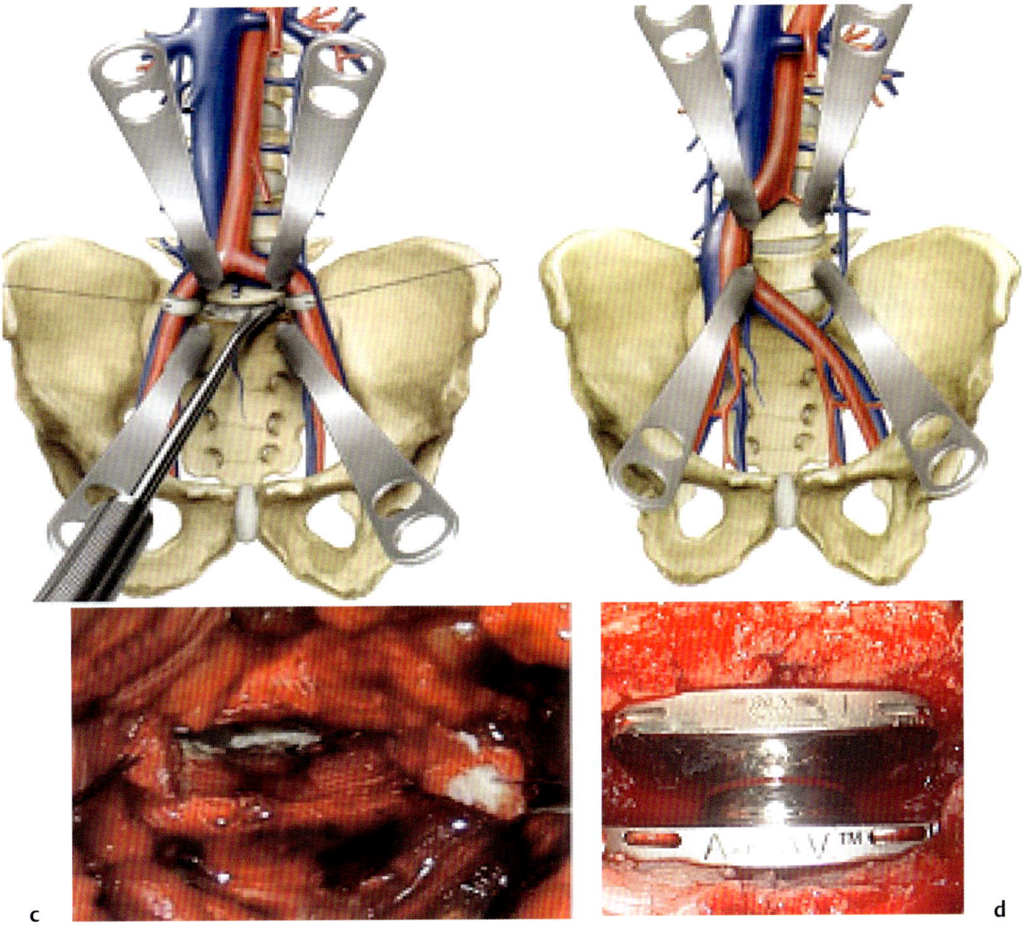

Fig. 13.11 The surgical approach for a disk prosthesis is identical to that described for anterior interbody fusion. **(a)** Exposure of L5-S1. **(b)** Exposure of L4-L5. **(c)** Intraoperative image after disk removal. Note the posterior aspect of the annulus. **(d)** The prosthesis in situ.

avoids the risk of soft tissue or vascular injury due to the implant of the pins. A ring is then placed to connect the handles of the retractors, to achieve a 360-degree stability to keep the surgical field wide open.

The disk is exposed and, under endoscopic view and magnification, two horizontal cuts are performed with a scalpel on the anterior longitudinal ligament, corresponding to the upper and lower limits of the disk. A vertical incision is then performed on the midline, and the anterior ligament is detached from the midline laterally. This procedure results in two flaps that are preserved to be sutured together after the cage implant. The disk is then removed, and the end plates are prepared by scraping off the cartilaginous layer, obtaining a complete diskectomy. Then the intervertebral cage (usually packed with cancellous bone graft) is inserted (**Fig. 13.12a**) and checked with LL fluoroscopy projection. Increasingly sized templates are then implanted in the intervertebral space, to find the proper fit. Finally, the definitive cage is implanted and, depending on the system used, the cage is screwed into the intervertebral disk space or an anterior plating is recommended (**Fig. 13.12b**). Mechanically, a cage with an anterior plate gains the same stiffness as a cage with posterior fixation (four pedicle screws).

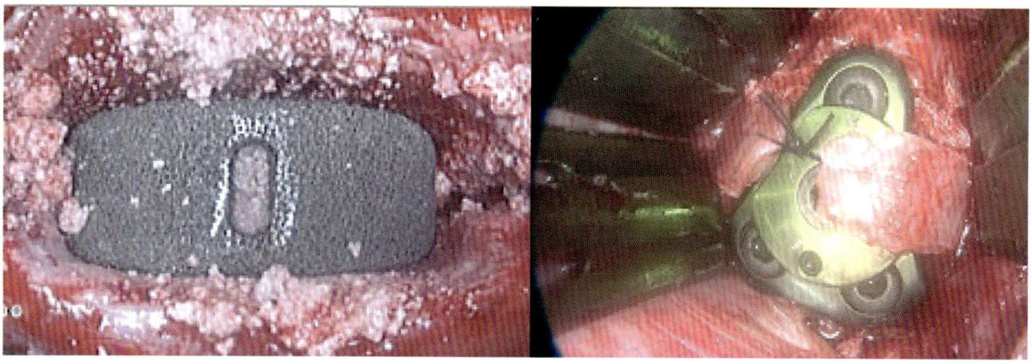

Fig. 13.12 (a) Intraoperative image of the cage insertion, with the cage in place. **(b)** The anterior plating.

Laparoscopy

Laparoscopy requires the use of CO_2 insufflation to transform the virtual retroperitoneal space in a real cavity, and the 0-degree laparoscope can be used rather than the 30-degree angled laparoscope. The patient is placed supine in a 20- to 30-degree Trendelenburg position. The first portal (for placement of the video channel) is inserted through the umbilicus; then, up to four additional working portals are placed under direct visualization. These portals can include a 10-mm umbilical port for a 10-mm, 0-degree camera; a right lower quadrant, 5-mm working port; a left lower quadrant, 5-mm working port; a left lower quadrant, 10-mm dissecting instrument port; and an 18-mm, end-organ docking port in the suprapubic area cranial to the bladder.

L5-S1

The suprapubic port must be in alignment with the L5–S1 intervertebral space using intraoperative fluoroscopy. The small intestine is packed into the upper portion of the abdomen with retraction. The sigmoid colon mesentery is approached from the right side, and accurate identification of the ureters and the aortic bifurcation is achieved. The sigmoid mesentery is incised longitudinally, and the median sacral artery is identified. A suture is passed through the abdominal wall in the left lower quadrant and sutured through the transected distal end of the sigmoid mesocolon, thus suspending the colon to the left side and exposing the space between the aortic bifurcations.

Prevertebral vessels (median sacral artery and vein for L5–S1 level, and segmental vessels for other lumbar levels) must be identified, dissected from the periosteum, clipped on both sides, and then cut.

The disk is exposed and the complete diskectomy is achieved. Then the disk end plates are prepared and the intervertebral cage (usually packed with cancellous bone graft) is inserted and checked with LL fluoroscopy projection. Depending on the system used, the cage is screwed into the intervertebral disk space or an anterior plating is recommended.

L4-L5

As in the laparoscopic approach, it is mandatory to check the bifurcation of the great vessels to assess the feasibility of the procedure. The exposure can be obtained by reflecting the iliac artery and vein to the right when the bifurcation is at the L4–L5 disk level or by placing it below the bifurcation in patients with a high bifurcation at the L3–L4 level. The operative setup is identical, with five portals positioned (the fifth portal is higher than the L5–S1 suprapubic port and is in line with the L4–5 disk space). The intestines are packed into the superior aspect of the abdomen, and the bifurcation of the aorta is identified. The posterior peritoneum (overlying the lumbar spine and great vessels) is elevated in the midline and incised along the medial border of the sigmoid mesocolon. The inferior mesenteric vessels and the left ureter are identified and retracted to the left. The superior hypogastric plexus is dissected until the L4–5 disk space is identified. The midline disk space is verified with C-arm fluoroscopy and a pin. Once the midline is identified, the procedure is identical to the one at the L5–S1 interspace.

Lumbar Disk Replacement (Nucleus Prosthesis and Total Disk Replacement)[10]

Spine surgeons have gained experience with, and confidence in using, anterior approaches to the lumbar spine over the last two decades. The clinical outcome with anterior lumbar interbody fusion (ALIF) is good, but there is a long-term risk of developing adjacent-level disease. The exact incidence of adjacent-disk disease has not been determined because most of the findings in the literature come from older, noninstrumented, posterolateral fusions, which was not an ideal technique, and pertain to local sagittal unbalance. Moreover, over time, a concern is that the modern and more rigid constructs may lead to even higher rates of adjacent-segment disease.

The first goal of an arthroplasty procedure is to *remove* the diseased intervertebral disk tissue that is considered to be the generator of diskogenic pain. Removal of the diseased disk is also accomplished in fusion surgery with interbody fusion techniques, either through anterior (ALIF) or posterior approaches (PLIF and TLIF). Posterolateral fusion techniques alone do not remove disk tissue but rely on immobilization of the tissue for relief of pain.

The second goal is the restoration of disk height, as in the ALIF procedure. The restoration of disk height is necessary to the achieve enough space for positioning the implant itself, to increase the height of the intervertebral foramen, to improve the sagittal alignment, and to diminish the contact forces between the facet joints (pain generator). Furthermore, when accomplished through an MIS procedure (small anterior incision in the absence of posterior surgery or bone grafting techniques), the functional recovery rates for patients are higher and occur sooner.

Both these goals can be achieved with other procedures[10] (e.g., ALIF), but the real difference is that the goal of spinal arthroplasty is to replicate or augment the function of the normal spinal elements, by taking into consideration both the quantity and the quality of motion that occurs across the replaced joint.[23] This is the key theoretical advantage of arthroplasty over fusion surgery; we do not actually know whether adjacent-disk disease can be prevented if the correct technique is performed, with the proper amount of disk material removed, and disk height and motion restored or maintained.

The surgical approach is identical to that described above, and the indications and preoperative workup are summarized in **Table 13.1**.

Artificial Disk Prostheses

Artificial disk prostheses come in two forms: a nucleus prosthesis and a total disk prosthesis.

Nucleus Prosthesis

A nucleus prosthesis was designed to replace only the nucleus pulposus, and it relies on a normal or minimally disrupted annular structure and vertebral end plates. A nucleus prosthesis does not directly restore biomechanical function of the annulus fibrosus, facet joints, or the vertebral end plates, but indirectly restores their function by reestablishing the proper mechanics of load transfer from one vertebra to the next. Therefore, designs for nucleus prostheses do not have components for the annulus fibrosus or the vertebral end plates, and can be inserted via a posterolateral or a posterior approach (**Fig. 13.13**). The current designs of the nucleus prosthesis have four different approaches to reproduce the biomechanical effect of incompressible hydrostatic pressure within the nucleus cavity: (1) a cavity filled with fluid, gel, oil or soft polymer; (2) a solid body in the disk space; (3) hydrophilic polymer in various shapes, sizes, and amounts; and (4) injection of biomaterial into the nucleus cavity for in-situ polymerization.[24]

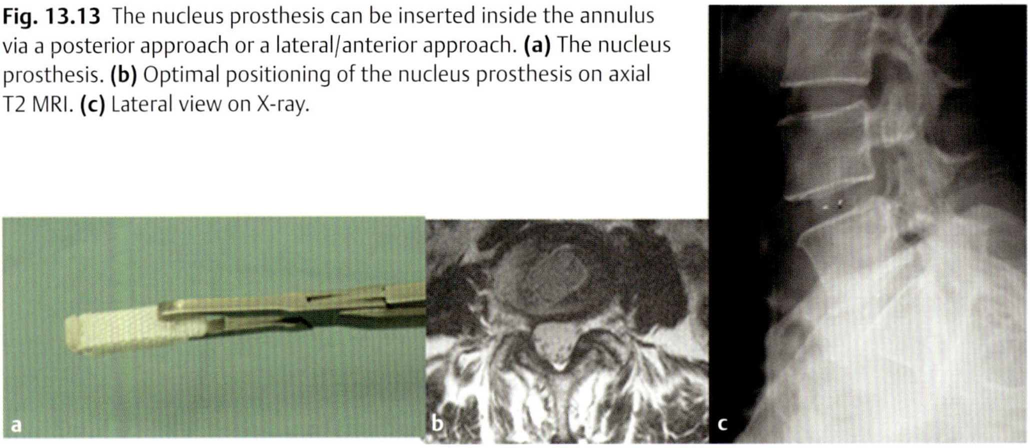

Fig. 13.13 The nucleus prosthesis can be inserted inside the annulus via a posterior approach or a lateral/anterior approach. **(a)** The nucleus prosthesis. **(b)** Optimal positioning of the nucleus prosthesis on axial T2 MRI. **(c)** Lateral view on X-ray.

Reports on biomechanical tests of the prosthetic disk nucleus (PDN) device showed that it produced some degree of stabilization and distraction.[25] Clinical trials of the Ray nucleus replacement show a positive effect in patients with degenerative disk disease,[10] with an 80% reported improvement of symptoms and returned to employment, whereas the remaining 20% had complications, such as implant migration, extrusion, vertebral end-plate changes (**Fig. 13.14**), or subsidence and infection.[10]

Some of these complications with the hardware can be related to the prostheses design, such as a small contact surface area at the interface between the nucleus prosthesis and the vertebral end plates, producing an abnormal stress concentration leading to radiological changes in the vertebral end plates and subsidence. Uncontrolled and excessive lateral wall bulge of nucleus prostheses with a thin-walled fluid-filled balloon or cavity can be a contributing factor for prosthetic migration during compression bending. Another area of concern with nucleus prosthesis is postimplantation stability within the disk. Implanted prosthesis should be stable throughout the range of motion (ROM) during compression-bending and compression-torsion. Abnormal movement of the implanted prosthesis within the disk during the ROM could cause harmful effects on the annulus. Proper "fitting" or interlocking at the interface between the nucleus prosthesis and the annulus can prevent this "loose-fitting" problem.

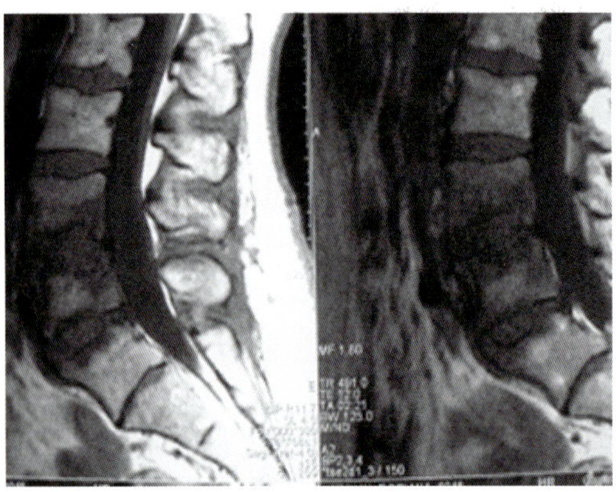

Fig. 13.14 Adverse reaction of the end plates in a nucleus disk prosthesis.

Design criteria for the nucleus prosthesis are of pivotal importance to prevent these problems, and should include methods for proper load transfer from the vertebral body to the annulus fibrosus through the prosthetic nucleus and for primary stabilization of prosthesis itself within the disk.[24]

Total Disk Prosthesis

The total disk prosthesis is intended to replace all three component structures of a painful and dysfunctional disk (the nucleus pulposus, the

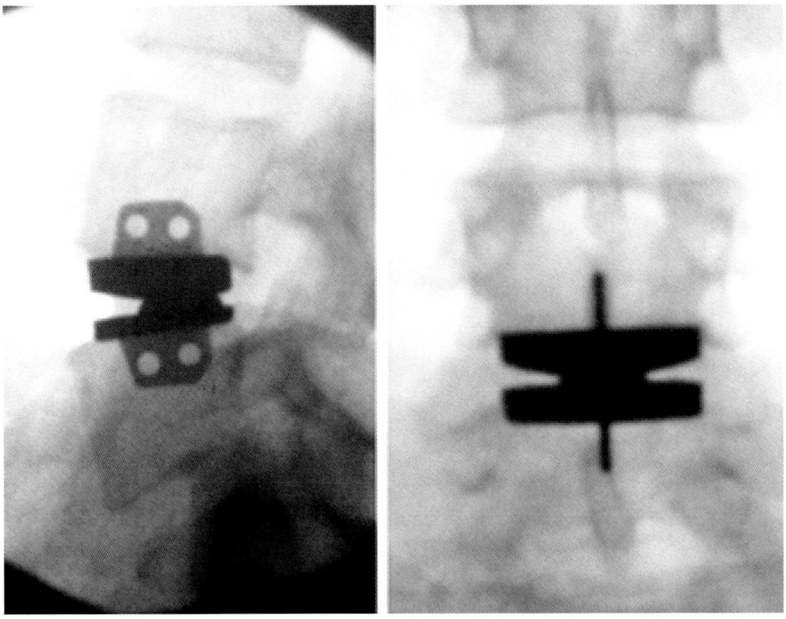

Fig. 13.15 **(a)** Latero-lateral (LL) and **(b)** AP X-ray of an implanted disk prosthesis.

annulus fibrosus, and the vertebral end plates), restoring the function of the disk for motion, stiffness, and stability. Any significant deviation can cause abnormal and harmful effects on the facet joints within the same segment and on the adjacent levels. Various adverse effects of spinal fusion on the adjacent level were reported in clinical and biomechanical studies.[10,23]

The surgical technique of disk exposure and preparation is identical to that described for the ALIF technique (**Fig. 13.11**). Correct positioning of the prosthesis is crucial and must be checked at the end of the procedure with fluoroscopy (both lateral and anterior projections, **Fig. 13.15**). Total disk prostheses can be further divided into two subgroups: total disk prosthesis for motion, and total disk prosthesis for motion and shock absorption. Subcategories for total disk prosthesis for motion include unconstrained and constrained. Subcategories for total disk prosthesis for motion and shock absorption include a fluid-filled cavity, springs, a fiber-reinforced composite, and an elastomeric polymer.[24]

The goal of using the total disk prosthesis is to provide an appropriate ROM (quantity), appropriate patterns of motion (quality), and appropriate stiffness in compression, bending, torsion, and stability. A total disk prosthesis with adequate amounts of motion but with abnormal patterns of motion can be as deleterious as a lack of motion to the surrounding structures. Another reason for accelerated adjacent-level degeneration after spinal fusion is increased stiffness of the fusion construct; the stiffer the construct, the higher the incidence of next-level problems shortly after fusion.

The postoperative stability of the total disk prosthesis, both immediately after surgery and long term, is very important for successful results. Failure to maintain stability could cause subsidence, migration, loosening, and abnormal or excessive motion at the interface between the device and the vertebral end plate. Many designs have various interlocking mechanisms for the immediate and a long-term postoperative period. Revision or removal of the prosthesis might be required for a failed disk prosthesis. No specific considerations for the replacement or revision of the prosthetic designs of total disk prostheses have been identified. Problems of removal or revision surgery for the current designs include the following:

1. Anterior surgical approach through a previous surgical scar
2. Removal of all components of the prosthesis, creating a large area of dead space with loss of a significant amount of bone
3. Lack of designs for revision prostheses

Lateral Retroperitoneal Approach[26]

The lateral retroperitoneal approach provides a different corridor for removal of the intervertebral disk and for achieving an interbody fusion as solid as that with an anterior approach. This surgical corridor is demanding but the learning curve is less steep than with a pure anterior approach. The advantages of this approach are as follows: there is no need for manipulation of the common iliac vein and artery; the approach facilitates exposure of the lumbar spine; the approach does not violate the anterior and posterior ligaments; drilling, reaming, tapping, and cage insertion are directed toward the contralateral psoas muscle instead of the neurologic structures, which obviates the risk of small-bowel obstruction and intraperitoneal adhesions; and the approach entails a lower incidence of retrograde ejaculation. The disadvantages of this approach are as follows: a large mass of the psoas muscle containing lumbosacral nerve roots may have to be mobilized laterally, and at the L4–L5 level it may be necessary to remove part of the iliac crest. The possible complications of this approach are genitofemoral nerve palsy, psoas hematoma, lumbar sympathectomy, peritoneal perforation, thrombophlebitis, and urinary retention.

Technique

The patient is placed in the right lateral decubitus position on a radiolucent operating table capable of flexing near its midportion (a left-sided approach is preferable to a right-sided approach because it is easier to dissect the aorta) (**Fig. 13.16**).

The operating table is tilted (under fluoroscopic control to achieve a parallel projection of the vertebral end plates of the level to be approached) and flexed to increase the distance between the ribs and the iliac crest (excessive breaking of the table is contraindicated to avoid too much tension of the psoas muscle) (**Fig. 13.16**).

This approach is usually performed through a single or a double incision. In a single incision, the direct lateral incision is the working portal, which provides better cosmesis, but adhesions between the peritoneum and the abdominal wall may place the peritoneum and its contents at risk. A double incision tech-

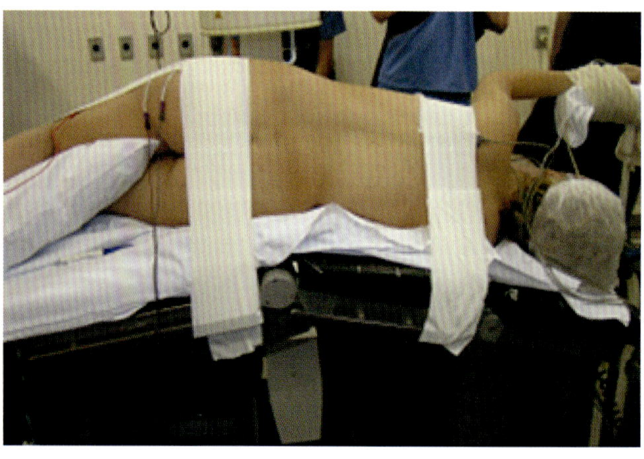

Fig. 13.16 Patient positioning for a minimally invasive surgery (MIS) lateral approach to the lumbar spine.

nique includes a direct lateral incision and a posterolateral incision that is used to gain access to the retroperitoneal space. This incision guides the safe passage of the dilators and retractor system through the retroperitoneal space.

In the single-incision technique, the incision is centered above the projection of the center of the disk space or over the targeted vertebra in the midaxillary line. If two levels are to be treated, then the direct lateral skin incision is made halfway between the two target levels; for multilevel procedures, multiple skin incisions are required. Once the 4-cm skin incision is made and the subcutaneous tissue are incised, blunt dissection of the obliquus externus and internus abdominis and the transversus abdominis muscle is performed following the orientation of the muscle fibers. Under the final layer of fascia, epidural fat is seen, which represents the retroperitoneal space. Using the surgeon's finger the peritoneum is released from the psoas and abdominal wall, enabling the abdominal contents to fall forward and away from the operative field (the transversalis fascia, perinephric fascia, and retroperitoneal contents are retracted anteriorly). Then the surgeon's finger reaches and palpates the anatomic structures; the psoas muscle is just lateral to the vertebral body and disk space, and, posteriorly, the transverse processes of the lumbar spine. The initial dilator is introduced through the main incision (**Fig. 13.17**).

In the double-incision technique, the posterolateral incision is used for the surgeon's finger to guide the safe introduction of the dilator through the retroperitoneal space and onto the lateral surface of the psoas. Fluoroscopy confirms that the initial dilator is centered over the disk space of interest. The nerves of the lumbar plexus (subcostal, iliohypogastric ilioinguinal, and lateral femoral cutaneous) can be encountered during the transpsoas muscle dissection. Anatomic studies have shown that they are most often found in the posterior third of the muscle, and that the lumbar plexus migrates from a dorsal to ventral location from the L1–2 down through the L4–5 disk space. The genitofemoral nerve, which supplies sensory innervation to the femoral triangle and the cremaster muscle in males and the skin of the mons pubis and labia majora in females, lies on the anterior surface of the psoas. The safe passage through the muscle is at the junction of the anterior and middle thirds. To prevent harming any nerve structure, EMG monitoring is recommended.

The dilator is located right over the disk on which a radiolucent blade is placed and docked on the lateral aspect of the disk space (**Fig. 13.18a**). The retractor should not be expanded

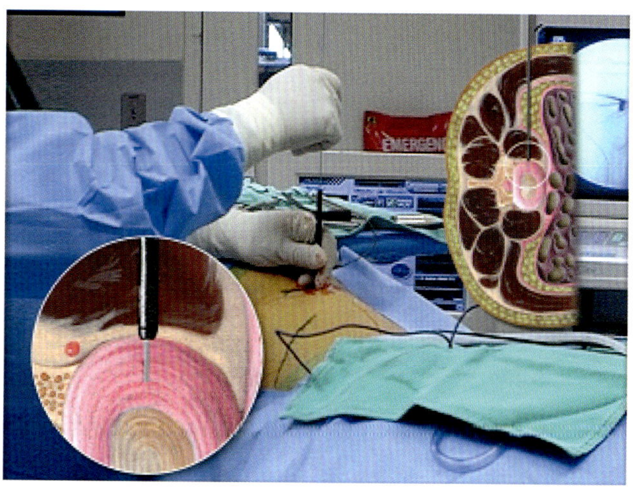

Fig. 13.17 Initial dilatator positioning inside the lateral aspect of the annulus.

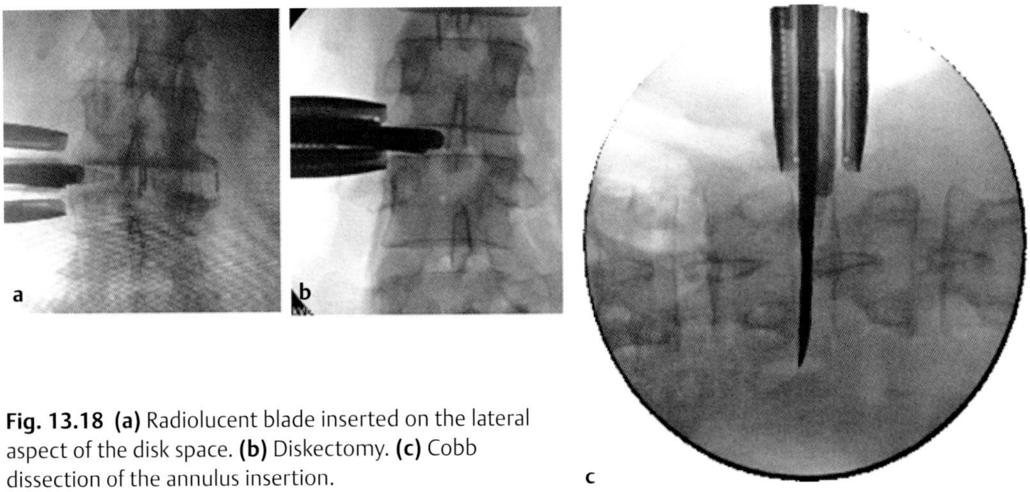

Fig. 13.18 (a) Radiolucent blade inserted on the lateral aspect of the disk space. (b) Diskectomy. (c) Cobb dissection of the annulus insertion.

past the midportion of the vertebral body, to minimize the possibility of segmental vessel injury.

A lateral annulotomy on the side of the approach is performed followed by a complete diskectomy (**Fig. 13.18b**); the contralateral annulus is released by passing a Cobb elevator completely across the disk space, while the anterior and the posterior annulus are preserved (**Fig. 13.18c**).

The definitive cage is chosen with the appropriate trials (**Fig. 13.19**). An appropriate lateral-to-lateral cage length covers the maximum amount of the disk space. After cage implantation, distraction is released. The retractor is removed slowly under visual control for any bleeding.

The table is returned to the neutral position for closing, and particular attention must be paid on the suture of the fascia over the external oblique.

Stand-alone extreme lateral interbody fusion (XLIF) is an off-label use in these cases, so a uni- or bilateral percutaneous pedicle-screw fixation in the same position, or in the prone position, is performed (**Fig. 13.20**)

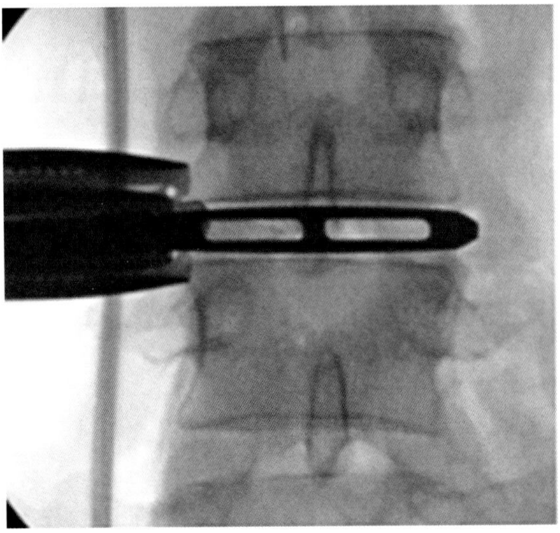

Fig. 13.19 Cage trial on AP X-Ray: intraoperative check.

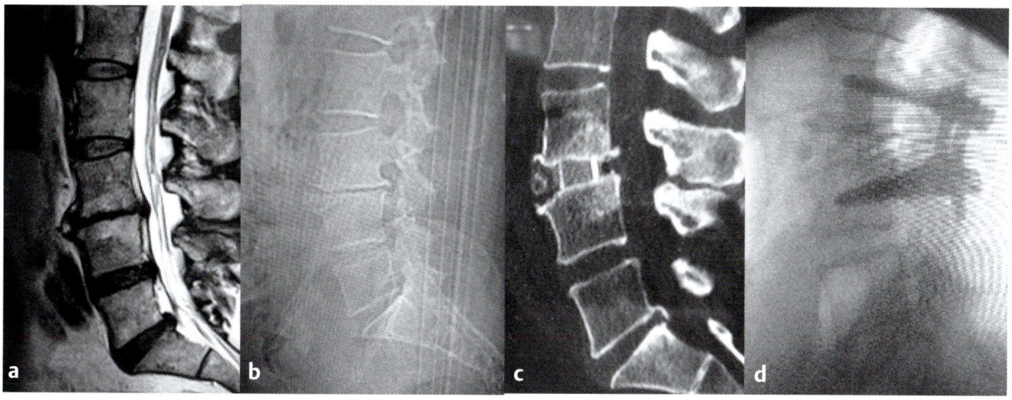

Fig. 13.20 **(a)** Preoperative T2 sagittal MRI showing an L3–L4 diskopathy. **(b)** Preoperative lateral X-ray view. **(c)** Computed tomography (CT) sagittal view after cage insertion, demonstrating the efficacy of the extreme lateral interbody fusion (XLIF) approach to achieve height restoration of the disk space. **(d)** Final X-ray showing lateral control after posterior MIS screw insertion.

Chapter Summary

Degenerative spine pathology is the most common problem encountered in the adult lumbar spine, and it entails high social costs. The results of surgery are often poor, for reasons that are only partially understood. One factor related to persistent postoperative pain is trauma to muscles. MIS is a muscle-sparing approach. Nowadays, almost any level or pathology of the lumbar spine can be treated with an MIS technique, as posterior, anterior, and lateral approaches have been developed. This chapter described the indications for and the technique of each surgical approach.

Pearls

- Understand the philosophy of MIS and the basic biological principles of a muscle-sparing approach to the lumbar spine.
- Be familiar with different approaches and instrumentation for treatment of degenerative spine diseases affecting the lumbar spine.
- Select the approach that entails the minimum trauma.
- Be familiar with the indications for surgery, the site of pathology, and the biomechanical implications of instrumentation and amelioration of sagittal balance.

Pitfalls

- MIS can treat many of the degenerative pathologies of the lumbar spine with some advantages (reduced postoperative pain due to less muscle trauma, less blood loss, and a lower infection rate) but also some disadvantages: long and steep learning curve, higher dose of intraoperative X-ray, less room for the arthrodesis (small approaches).
- Some MIS approaches are particularly indicated for high-risk subgroups (obese and elder patients), but obese patients are particularly challenging in anterior and lateral approaches (the preoperative BMI is one of the selection criteria for surgery).
- High-risks patients are those with vasculopathies (especially for anterior lumbar MISS approaches) and those who had previous abdominal approaches.
- We strongly suggest working in a multidisciplinary team (mandatory during the learning curve) to avoid the most dangerous complications affecting the vessels and the ureter.

References

Five Must-Read References

1. Shamji MF, Goldstein CL, Wang M, Uribe JS, Fehlings MG. Minimally invasive spine surgery in the elderly: does it make sense? Neurosurgery 2015;77(Suppl 4):S108–S115
2. **Kim CW, Siemionow K, Anderson DG, Phillips FM. The current state of minimally invasive spine surgery. J Bone Joint Surg Am 2011;93:582–596**
3. **Arts MP, Brand R, van den Akker ME, Koes BW, Bartels RH, Peul WC; Leiden-The Hague Spine Intervention Prognostic Study Group (SIPS). Tubular diskectomy vs conventional microdiskectomy for sciatica: a randomized controlled trial. JAMA 2009; 302:149–158**
4. Sandhu FA, Santiago P, Fessler RG, Palmer S. Minimally invasive surgical treatment of lumbar synovial cysts. Neurosurgery 2004;54:107–111, discussion 111–112
5. Khoo LT, Palmer S, Laich DT, Fessler RG. Minimally invasive percutaneous posterior lumbar interbody fusion. Neurosurgery 2002;51(5, Suppl):S166–S181
6. Cole JS IV, Jackson TR. Minimally invasive lumbar discectomy in obese patients. Neurosurgery 2007;61: 539–544, discussion 544
7. Wallwork TL, Stanton WR, Freke M, Hides JA. The effect of chronic low back pain on size and contraction of the lumbar multifidus muscle. Man Ther 2009;14:496–500
8. Kim CW, Siemionow K, Anderson G, Phillips FM. The current state of minimally invasive spine surgery. J Bone Joint Surg 2011;96(6):882–886
9. Kawaguchi Y, Matsui H, Gejo R, Tsuji H. Preventive measures of back muscle injury after posterior lumbar spine surgery in rats. Spine 1998;23: 2282–2288
10. **Wei J, Song Y, Sun L, Lv C. Comparison of artificial total disc replacement versus fusion for lumbar degenerative disc disease: a meta-analysis of randomized controlled trials. Int Orthop 2013;37:1315–1325**
11. Mori E, Okada S, Ueta T, Itaru Y, Maeda T, Kawano O, Shiba K. Spinous process-splitting open pedicle screw fusion provides favourable results in patients with low back discomfort and pain compared to conventional open pedicle screw fixation over 1 year after surgery. Eur Spine J 2012;21:745–753
12. Arts MP, Brand R, van den Akker ME, Koes BW, Bartels RH, Peul WC. Tubular discectomy vs conventional microdiscectomy for sciatica: a randomized controlled trial. JAMA. 2009; 302(2):149–158
13. Wiltse LL, Spencer CW. New uses and refinements of the paraspinal approach to the lumbar spine. Spine 1988;13(6): 696–706
14. Dick W, Kluger P, Magerl F, Woersdörfer O, Zäch G. A new device for internal fixation of thoracolumbar and lumbar spine fractures: the "fixateur interne". Paraplegia 1985; 23(4):225–232
15. Wang MY, Anderson DG, Poelstra KA, Ludwing SC. Minimally invasive posterior fixation. Neurosurgery 2008;63:A197–A203
16. Khan NR, Clark AJ, Lee SL, Venable GT, Rossi NB, Foley KT. Surgical outcomes for minimally invasive vs open transforaminal lumbar interbody fusion: an update systematic review and meta-analysis. Neurosurgery 2015;77:847–874, discussion 874
17. **Bassani R, Sinigaglia A, Lamartina C. Video-assisted minimally invasive lumbar total disc replacement. Eur Spine J 2011;20:2282–2283**
18. Kim DH, Jaikumar S, Kam AC. Minimally invasive spine instrumentation. Neurosurgery 2002;51(5, Suppl):S15–S25
19. Liu JC, Ondra SL, Angelos P, Ganju A, Landers ML. Is laparoscopic anterior lumbar interbody fusion a useful minimally invasive procedure? Neurosurgery 2002;51(5, Suppl):S155–S158
20. Bassani R, Cecchinato, R, Morselli C, Berjano P, Lamartina, C. Video-assisted anterior retroperitoneal approach to the lumbar spine. A minimal invasive technique improved by the use of endoscopic camera to treat lumbar spine diseases. International Journal of Clinical Medicine 2016;7:94–100
21. **Bassani R, et al. A new technique for anterior retroperitoneal approach to the lumbar spine: the perinavel approach. Technique description and literature review. (under publication)**
22. Büttner-Janz K, Guyer RD, Ohnmeiss DD. Indications for lumbar total disc replacement: selecting the right patient with the right indication for the right total disc. Int J Spine Surg 2014;8:12
23. Crawford NR. Biomechanics of lumbar arthroplasty. Neurosurg Clin N Am 2005;16:595–602, v
24. Lee CK, Goel VK. Artificial disc prosthesis: design concepts and criteria. Spine J 2004;4(6, Suppl): 209S–218S
25. Jacobs WC, van der Gaag NA, Kruyt MC, et al. Total disc replacement for chronic discogenic low back pain: a Cochrane review. Spine 2013;38:24–36
26. Berjano P, Gautschi OP, Schils F, Tessitore E. Extreme lateral interbody fusion (XLIF®): how I do it. Acta Neurochir (Wien) 2015;157:547–551

14

Back Pain and Sagittal Alignment

Pedro Berjano

Introduction

Every degenerative case is a deformity case too. In the past, degenerative conditions in the lumbosacral spine were attributed to nerve compression, motion in worn or swollen joints, or segmental instability; these were considered the only causes of pain and disability. Alignment received little attention as a potential means of reducing pain and disability. Sagittal alignment has been demonstrated to be an independent predictor of pain and disability in adult patients with spinal deformity.[1–3] Moreover, adjacent-segment degeneration has been attributed mainly to stiffness of the fused segments, with consequent overload at the boundaries of surgical fusion. Adjacent-segment failure following spinal fusion is frequently observed in patients treated for lumbar degenerative segment disease, and it is often expressed initially as hyperextension at the upper adjacent level, leading to the intuitive idea that compensation for lower lumbar hypolordosis could be the mechanism for accelerated degeneration of the adjacent level. Several published studies provide some support for this idea. More recent studies have shown that improving sagittal alignment in surgery for degenerative conditions can increase the clinical benefit that patients perceive. When treating degenerative conditions, the surgeon should always consider spinal alignment and implement a reasonable strategy to restore it.

This chapter discusses degenerative conditions of the lumbar spine in relation to issues of alignment. Basic concepts of sagittal alignment, findings from the literature on the impact of alignment restoration, and technical tips to improve alignment when performing spinal fusion are presented.

Sagittal Balance

A person whose spinal alignment results in minimal requirements of energy to sustain the upright position is considered to be sagittally balanced. Alternatively, a person whose trunk's shape requires exerting great effort to remain upright is considered to be imbalanced. Therefore, sagittal balance is in effect the composite product of spine shape, body mass distribution, and the forces from the stabilizing muscles. Individuals with good alignment require little effort to stand and to walk. For slight deviations from the best possible alignment, standard muscle activity enables an effective, comfortable upright position and walking. But greater deviations in alignment require increased muscle effort, in some instances resulting in decreased function and pain. Individuals with better muscular functional reserve (in terms of muscle power and endurance) can compensate for higher degrees of misalignment with little or no impairment of function and with little or no increase in pain. In contrast, those with lower muscle reserve have poorer function and increased pain for the same degree of misalignment.

A Constant Battle: Loss of Lordosis and Compensatory Efforts

Life events can have kyphosing effects on the spine, such as disk degeneration, muscle deterioration, and changes in bone shape (i.e., due to fractures). These effects reduce lumbar lordosis and increase thoracic kyphosis progressively as the person ages.

A person with sagittal misalignment stands upright by compensating for the misalignment, which entails assuming an unnatural position. When some lordosis at one or a few lumbar segments is lost, the first adjustment usually consists of hyperextension of the adjacent levels. Increasing deformity, for example with loss of lordosis along the entire lumbar spine, can be compensated for by extension of the intact thoracic spine. But these modalities of active extension require increased muscle effort. An additional contribution to compensation can be obtained by posterior rotation of the pelvis around the hip joints (pelvic retroversion), which can be measured by the increase of pelvic tilt. In patients with extreme sagittal deformity, the most energy-consuming compensatory mechanism of knee flexion may be elicited, greatly decreasing the endurance of the patient (**Fig. 14.1**).[4]

How Can Sagittal Balance and Compensation Be Measured?

The knowledge we have gained about sagittal balance and its influence on clinical outcomes

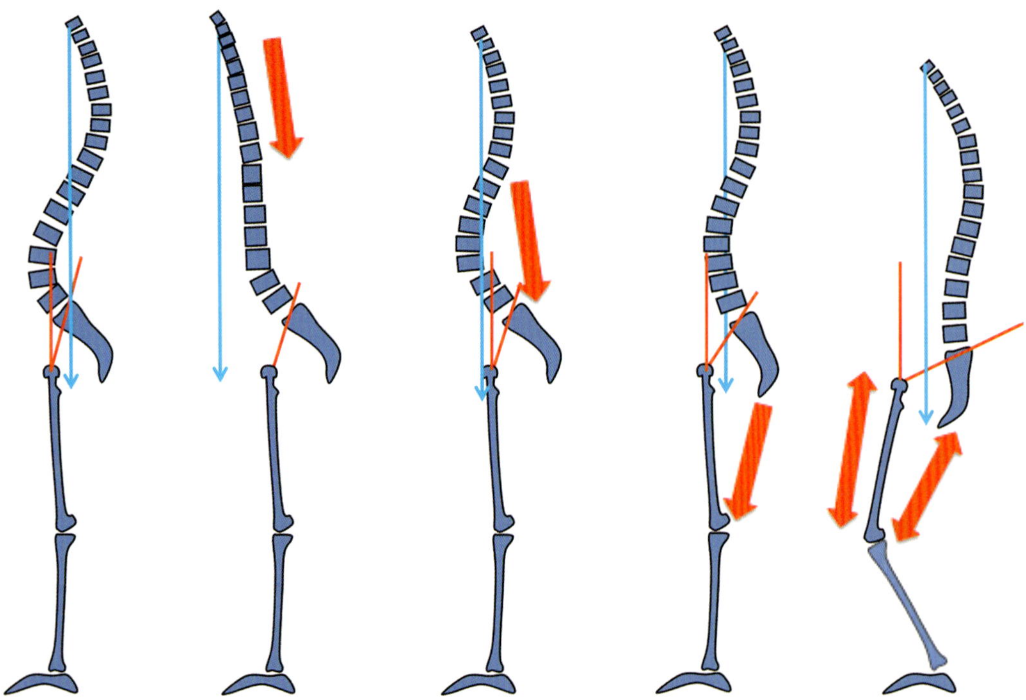

Fig. 14.1 Compensatory mechanisms exhibited in patients with varying loss of lumbar lordosis or thoracic kyphosis. **(a)** A normal spine. **(b)** Active extension of the thoracic spine, resulting in hypokyphosis. **(c)** Active extension of adjacent lumbar segments, resulting in atypical distribution of lumbar lordosis. **(d)** Pelvic retroversion with increased pelvic tilt. **(e)** Knee flexion resulting in an additional increment of pelvic tilt and posterior translation of the trunk mass.

has been derived by evaluating the sagittal alignment of the spine in full-spine standing lateral radiographs that included the pelvis. The position of the arms has an influence on how the alignment of the spine presents in radiographs. It has been shown that positions of the fingers to the clavicle position or the hands crossed in front of the pelvis introduce little variation in the alignment of the spine, and thus they are preferred during radiographic evaluation.[5]

C7 Plumbline and the Sagittal Vertical Axis

Although some earlier work has demonstrated that the degree of forward displacement of the C7 plumbline correlates with health-related quality of life (HRQoL) (see Why Is Sagittal Balance Important?, below), a milestone was represented by the 2010 paper by Schwab et al,[3] which confirmed that three main sagittal parameter measurements correlate with outcomes in adult deformity patients: sagittal vertical axis (SVA), pelvic tilt (PT), and lumbar lordosis–pelvic incidence mismatch (LL-PI).

The SVA is the length of displacement from the C7 plumbline to the posterior angle of S1. Greater anterior displacement of the C7 plumbline correlates with more severe sagittal misalignment. Adolescents frequently have a negative SVA (a posterior C7 plumbline), young adults usually have a neutral SVA, and elderly people tend to have a positive (anterior) SVA. However, the more positive the SVA, the greater the patient's pain and disability and the poorer the function. The SVA threshold to distinguish between patients with better and worse HRQoL is around 50 mm. SVA is a measurement of the degree of efficiency of the global upright trunk position that a patient can achieve.[3]

Pelvic Tilt

Another important parameter to examine is pelvic tilt (PT), which measures the retroversion of the pelvis in the standing position. The PT is related to the pelvic incidence (PI), which measures the inclination at which the sacrum articulates to the pelvis (**Fig. 14.2**). This PI angle can vary greatly among persons with balanced spines, from 30 to 90 degrees. PI has a positive correlation with the curvature of the spine. In general, a balanced spine with a larger PI exhibits both greater lumbar lordosis (LL) and greater thoracic kyphosis. Conversely, a balanced spine with a smaller PI has a smaller LL and smaller thoracic kyphosis.[6]

In spite of the striking variability in PI, the pelvis tends to align itself economically to achieve a rather vertical "magic line" (see below).

The angle of the PT is defined by the intersection of a vertical line with a second line that links the midpoint of the sacral end plate and the midpoint of the bifemoral line (the line drawn through the center of both femoral heads). We now abbreviate the latter line (from the midsacrum end plate to the middle of the bi-coxofemoral axis) and simply refer to it as the "magic line." Of course this nickname is not based on any scientific property or characteristic, but it conveys the idea that this line can "magically" provide intuitive information on the amount of PI and pelvic retroversion present in a specific patient's X-rays. A rather vertical magic line demonstrates that the patient has little or no pelvic retroversion, whereas a more inclined magic line is an expression of increasing pelvic retroversion. Similarly, the angle formed by the magic line and the S1 end plate implies the amount of pelvic incidence. Patients with a very high pelvic incidence tend to have a magic line nearly parallel to the S1 end plate, whereas in patients with decreasing values of PI, the line is more perpendicular to the S1 end plate.

Experimental work in asymptomatic individuals has shown how the PT tends to increase in normal individuals as the PI increases.[6] But although the PI can vary between 30 and 90 degrees in asymptomatic persons, the PT increases correspondingly from a few degrees to 21 degrees, and in very infrequent cases with the highest values of PI reaching as great as 24 to 25 degrees. Thus, asymptomatic individuals very seldom have a PT greater than 21 degrees.

An increase of PT is accompanied by an increase in the pelvic torque, which is the torsion moment of the body weight, mainly applied

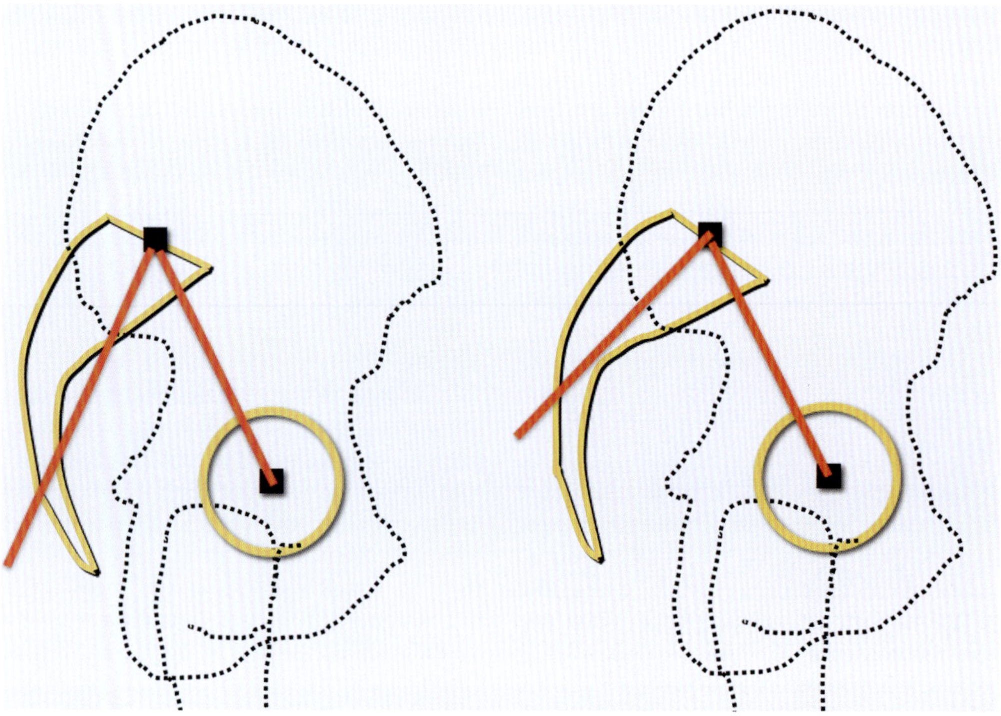

Fig. 14.2 **(a)** Low pelvic incidence due to less forward inclination of the sacrum in the pelvis. **(b)** The sacrum has more forward inclination within the pelvis, corresponding to high pelvic incidence.

to the pelvis at the sacrum, and the ground reaction force, mainly applied to the pelvis at the acetabula (**Fig. 14.3**). Therefore, as PT increases, an increase in compensatory muscle effort ensues to stabilize the pelvis and keep the person upright. More balanced spines exhibit a smaller PT (with a more vertical magic line and a smaller pelvic torque).

Pelvic Incidence–Lumbar Lordosis Mismatch

Asymptomatic individuals have a substantial correlation between the PI and the total lordosis,[6] and the total LL usually equals or exceeds the PI. Patients with too few degrees of LL compared with PI have poor clinical outcomes in terms of pain and disability.[3] One recent study suggests that patients undergoing surgery to fix sagittal malalignment obtained good postoperative alignment when their LL exceeded PI by 10 degrees. In the same study, patients with an adequate distribution of LL (i.e., with two thirds of LL between L4 and S1 and no thoracolumbar junction hyperkyphosis) obtained satisfactory postoperative alignment if their LL was superior to the PI.[7] It is the author's experience that accepting a postoperative value of LL that is inferior to the PI significantly increases the risk of sagittal malalignment, except for patients with PI > 70 degrees, in which case LL > PI – 10 degrees can be sufficient.

Distribution of Lordosis

Lordosis is not distributed equally all along the lumbar spine. We know that in normal subjects, approximately two thirds of LL is located between the superior end plate of L4 and

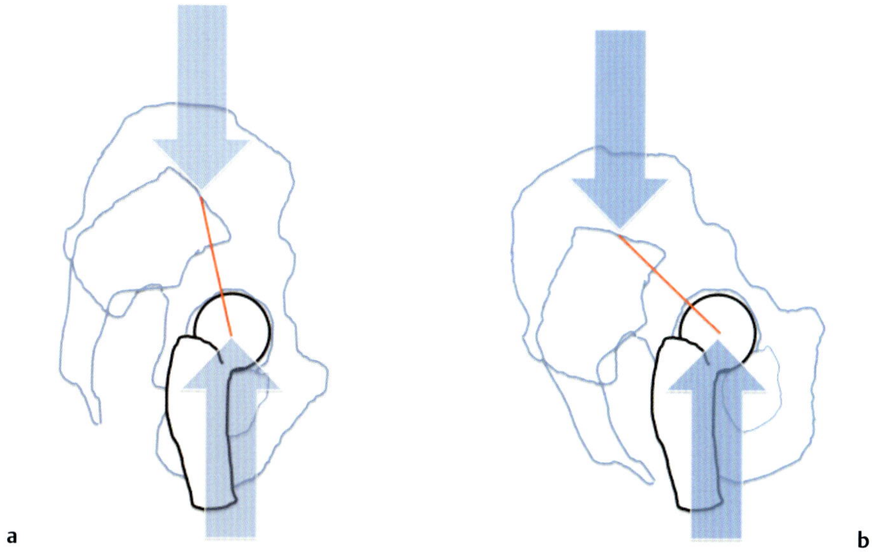

Fig. 14.3 (a) With a low pelvic tilt angle (relatively vertical "magic line," in *red*) the axis of the trunk weight load on the sacrum and that of the ground reaction force on the hip joint are close to each other, resulting in low pelvic torque. **(b)** Increasing pelvic tilt (relatively horizontal "magic line," in *red*) makes the distance between the forces increase, resulting in higher pelvic torque. Between these two drawings the torque increases by about fourfold.

S1. Some individuals with a loss of lordosis between L4 and S1, due to degeneration of the lower lumbar disks, compensate with increased lordosis in the upper lumbar spine, resulting in a normal amount of global lordosis. However, this normal lumbar lordosis is the result of active extension that requires increased muscle effort and can potentially lead to increased pain and decreased function. Although the two-thirds rule has clear clinical utility and is widely used, a more refined approach is available. In a study of 160 volunteers, Roussouly et al[8] defined four types of sagittal alignment, based on the variables of pelvic incidence, length of lordosis, sacral slope, and distribution of lordosis. Their classification can be useful to help determine what could have been the original distribution of lordosis in a given patient and to interpret the patient's adaptation to pathological changes. One recent study suggests that in patients with higher values of PI, the contribution of L4-S1 to total lordosis tends to be lower.[9]

Why Is Sagittal Balance Important?

Sagittal Alignment and Clinical Outcomes

There is substantial evidence in the literature regarding the correlation of sagittal alignment with HRQoL. Mac-Thiong et al[10] demonstrated that the displacement of the C7 plumbline is an important indicator of HRQoL by showing a very strong correlation between increasing anterior displacement of the C7 plumbline and increasing spinal malfunctioning measured by Oswestry Disability Index (ODI) scores. In adult scoliosis patients with and without prior surgery, Glassman et al[11] found that pain and HRQoL measures from the Scoliosis Research Society's SRS-22 questionnaire, the Short Form SF-12 questionnaire, and ODI assessments all correlated with changes in SVA, whereas coronal imbalance (lateral displacement of the C7 plumbline from the center of the sacrum) did not correlate with variations in HRQoL scores. Furthermore, the correlation persisted when controlled for by age. HRQoL scores are also improved with sagittal plane correction in patients without scoliosis.[12] Lastly, Schwab et al[3] established groundbreaking correlations among SVA, PT, PI-LL, and both pain and ODI scores.

The above-mentioned evidence is derived from studies of patients with deformity. It can be demonstrated that similar, albeit more subtle, correlations can also be found in patients with degenerative spine conditions. There is also anecdotal evidence indicating that if sagittal alignment is not considered when planning and performing surgery, it can lead to poorer results and earlier failure. Kim and colleagues[13] provide an excellent example in patients with degenerative spondylolisthesis and stenosis. In this study, sagittal alignment was not considered in the surgical planning before performing posterior interbody fusion, making the resulting changes in PT random. Although all patients' Visual Analogue Scale (VAS) and ODI outcome scores improved, a greater margin of improvement was seen in patients whose PT was decreased, reflecting postoperative improvement of lumbar alignment with a decrease of pelvic compensation.

Sagittal Alignment and Adjacent-Segment Degeneration

Patient Studies

In a study by Heo et al,[14] 378 patients whose spondylolisthesis at the L4-L5 or L4-S1 level was treated with fusion were followed for a minimum of 2 years. The authors found that nearly 25% of the patients exhibited clinically symptomatic adjacent-segment degeneration (ASD) between 5 and 10 years postprocedure, although only 33 patients (8.7%) underwent a subsequent fusion extension surgery on the adjacent L3-L4 segment in this period. They also found that two of the most important risk factors for the incidence of clinically symptomatic ASD following fusion were low overall lordosis and low lordosis in the instrumented segments.

Immediately postoperatively, the amount of lumbar lordosis was greater in patients who did not develop clinically symptomatic ASD. A third parameter found to correlate with a low risk of clinically symptomatic ASD was having interbody fusion (IBF) rather than posterolateral fusion (PLF). This decreased risk can be explained by the fact that the IBF technique enables the surgeon to better maintain lumbar lordosis and can therefore achieve better sagittal alignment than with PLF.[14]

Kumar et al[15] measured the C7 sagittal plumbline and sacral slope immediately postoperatively in a cohort of patients who underwent fusion for lumbar degenerative conditions. Patients with normal sagittal alignment immediately postoperative had the lowest incidence of ASD when compared with patients having poor postoperative sagittal alignment. Furthermore, the authors recommended following patients with postoperative sagittal malalignment for at least 5 years because of the enhanced risk of ASD.

Jackson et al[16] conducted a radiographic comparative study of 100 asymptomatic volunteers and 100 patients suffering from low back pain (LBP). The authors found smaller amounts of overall lumbar lordosis in the LBP patients, as well as a tendency to have greater proximal segment lordosis and less distal segmental lordosis, indicating the occurrence of proximal compensation for distal degenerative loss of lordosis.

Park et al[17] studied patients with isthmic spondylolisthesis and found that patients with a better (smaller) postoperative PT had a lower incidence of ASD, again confirming the importance of sagittal alignment in patient outcomes.

Sagittal alignment has been shown to influence the incidence of some distinct modalities of spinal pathology. In a retrospective study by Barrey et al,[18] patients with higher PI were found to be more predisposed to developing degenerative spondylolisthesis (DS). The phenomenon can be explained by higher amount of lordosis in these patients, causing increased compressive stress and accelerated degeneration in their lower lumbar facet joints and higher shear forces in the lower lumbar disks, finally resulting in wear and vertebral slip.

In a prospective controlled study, Aono et al[19] arrived at a similar conclusion by correlating greater PI with a greater likelihood of DS.

Lastly, a radiological study by Lazennec and collaborators[20] that focused on the importance of considering the pelvis when planning for surgery of the lumbar spine found that sacral tilt (ST) was strongly correlated with postfusion pain.

Experimental Studies

Umehara et al[21] first demonstrated how the intraoperative kneeling position with 90 degrees of hip and knee flexion results in hypolordosis of the fused segments. They then attempted to shed light on the biomechanical effects of a hypolordotic lumbar spine in a cadaveric study in which they mimicked the hypolordosis created by the approach that entails 90 degrees of hip and knee flexion. They found that decreased lordosis in the instrumented segments significantly increased the load across the posterior column and increased the lamina strain in the adjacent levels, which could explain the greater propensity for ASD to manifest in patients with a loss of lordosis.

In another cadaveric study, Akamuru and colleagues[22] aimed to understand how different sagittal alignments affect the movement of adjacent segments. They found that when compared with a baseline specimen, hypolordotic fusion caused greater flexion-extension movement in the cranially adjacent segments and that fusion in a nonanatomic hyperlordotic conformation induced greater flexion-extension motion in the caudally adjacent segments.

An experimental in vivo study by Oda et al[23] aimed to learn more about the effects of kyphosis on the biomechanics of adjacent segments. The authors found that fusion in kyphosis was able to induce ASD. They reported that kyphosis increased the lamina strain and produced significant degeneration in the superior adjacent segments, and they therefore deduced that hypolordosis of the lumbar spine may cause facet joint arthritis, leading to ASD in the upper adjacent segments.[23]

How to Improve Sagittal Alignment

Preoperative Planning

In the previous sections we presented DATA supporting the importance of alignment in patients undergoing spinal fusion. Surgical planning and execution in patients undergoing spinal fusion for degenerative conditions should include an attempt to optimize sagittal alignment to increase the clinical benefit from the procedure and to minimize the risk of ASD.

As each patient's spinopelvic parameters are unique, planning the surgical intervention should ideally include full-spine, standing lateral radiographs. Nonetheless, standing lumbar radiographs that include the hip joints have been shown to be effective in measuring PI, PT, LL, and lower LL, which are some of the most important parameters required for evaluating sagittal alignment and in screening for sagittal malalignment.[24] Planning should include an assessment of PI, LL (globally and for each segment), as well as a calculation of the ideal LL (again, globally and for each segment). No universal agreement exists on the best formula to predict ideal LL. One suggested calculation[25] (derived from studies on normal subjects) is LL = 0.54 PI + 32.56. An approximation to this formula is yielded by the rule LL = PI + 10 degrees, which is fairly accurate for patients in the midrange of PI; subjects with very low PI may need slightly more lordosis than PI + 10 degrees, whereas patients with the highest values of PI need a lesser amount of lordosis than PI + 10 degrees. Regarding the distribution of lordosis along the lumbar spine, the clinician should classify the patient's morphology according to Roussouly et al's[8] types and thus decide the ideal extension of the lordosis and its distribution; again, a practical rule, valid for most patients in the midrange of PI, is to place two thirds of the total lordosis between L4 and S1.

Surgical Procedure

Patient Positioning

After determining the LL goals for the patient, surgical positioning should be considered, as it will affect the potential results one can achieve. Different modalities of prone positioning result in different degrees of lordosis in the patient. As demonstrated by Umehara et al,[21] different types of kneeling positions (**Fig. 14.4a**), although effective in reducing abdominal pressure and epidural bleeding, put the spine into flexion and should be avoided in surgical interventions that aim to attain fusion.

One study by Benfanti and Geissele[26] found that as little as 20 degrees of hip flexion on the operative table on a Wilson frame reduced the LL by 25%. Conversely, with extension of the hips, the preoperative LL was maintained (**Fig. 14.4b,c**).

Interbody Cages and Surgical Approach

Long posterior instrumentation for sagittal deformity can provide and maintain substantial correction until fusion is achieved. Multiple anchors and a long lever arm of the instrumentation explain the good ability of long constructs to provide correction. As a general rule, posterior instrumentation from the lower thoracic spine to the sacrum/pelvis can provide a correction similar to that obtained preoperatively in a fulcrum-extension supine radiograph. Facetectomies or posterior column osteotomies can increase the correction by some degrees per osteotomy level. In case of severe spinal

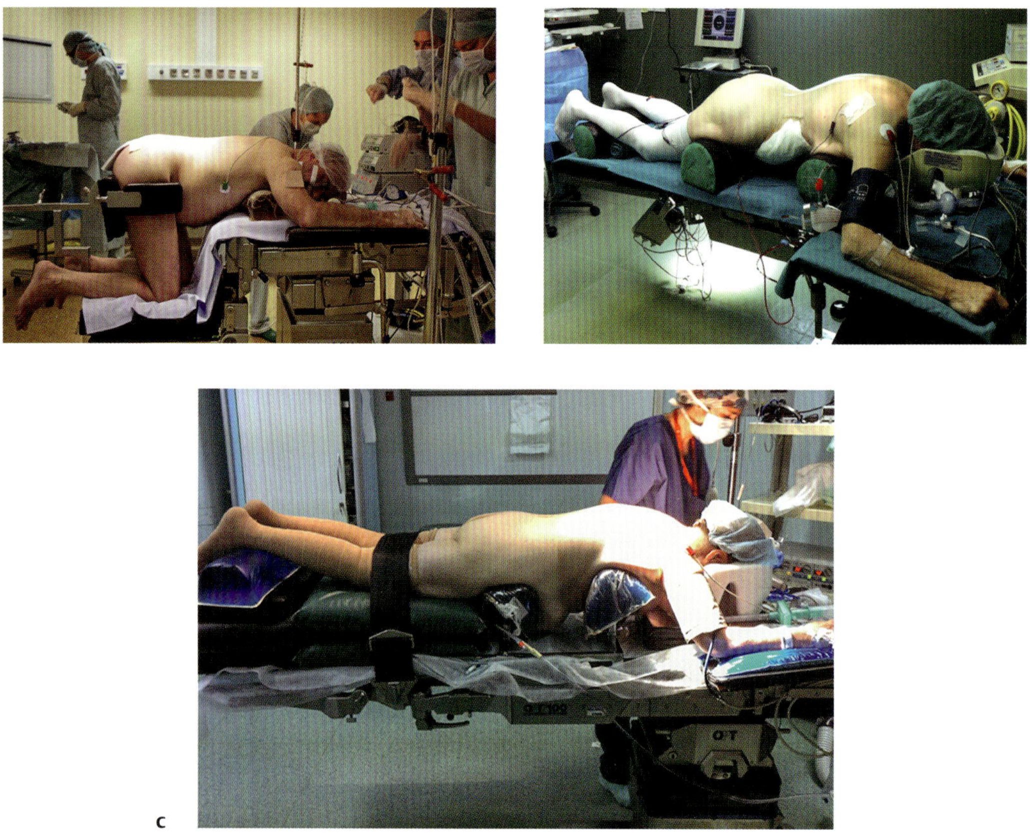

a b c

Fig. 14.4 Patient positioning options. **(a)** Knee–chest position causes an extreme reduction in the lower lumbar lordosis. **(b)** Twenty degrees of hip flexion substantially reduces the lower lumbar lordosis. **(c)** Full hip extension permits the surgeon to maintain and even increase the lumbar lordosis.

stiffness or correction goals much superior to that observed in fulcrum extension films, three column osteotomies[27] (or more recently anterior release techniques[28]) can be used.

Conversely, in short-segment lumbar or lumbosacral fusions for degenerative disease, sagittal plane correction is difficult to achieve and maintain with the use of posterior instrumentation alone. Sagittal realignment at levels with degenerated disks requires restoration of their anterior height, resulting in "empty" space in the anterior column. The distracted, degenerated disk has virtually no resistance to compressive loads, and as a result the posterior instrumentation has a high risk of failure. Interbody cages provide anterior support, filling the gap in the disk space and preventing its collapse. In addition, their implantation itself can provide correction (limited by the length of the annulus fibrosus and of the anterior longitudinal ligament [ALL]), provided that the integrity of the end plates is preserved.

For all these reasons, and for their contribution to fusion mass, interbody cages are a valuable tool in short-segment fusion for degenerative disease when sagittal alignment needs to be restored.

Still, placement of interbody cages is not per se a guarantee of sagittal plane restoration. In fact, high posterior lumbar interbody fusion (PLIF) cages implanted in the posterior part of the disk space can paradoxically be kyphosing. When using interbody cages, the surgeon should consider the technical tips provided in the following subsections to facilitate obtaining the desired sagittal correction and final alignment.

Cage Position

Cages placed in the posterior margin of the disk have a kyphosing effect. Cages in the anterior half of the disk have a lordosing effect (**Fig. 14.5a**).

Cage Height

The higher the cage, the greater the lordosing or kyphosing effect provided by the position of the cage (**Fig. 14.5b**). Too a high cage can be impossible to implant without end-plate violation, which results in postoperative loss of correction due to yielding of the end plate and subsidence.

Cage Length

A shorter, high, anterior cage provides the best opportunity for lordosis restoration after posterior compression through the pedicle screws. Increasing cage length, although providing a larger contact area, restricts the ability of posterior compression to restore the segmental lordosis (**Fig. 14.5c**).

Anterior Longitudinal Ligament Length

This parameter cannot be anticipated by planning, except in those cases that show anterior opening in extension-fulcrum films. Intuitively, a segment with a contracted ALL does not allow for increase of the anterior length of the disk space, thus limiting the ability to correct hypolordosis via posterior interbody approach.

Surgical Approach

Anterior approaches such as anterior lumbar interbody fusion (ALIF) directly release the ALL and annulus, providing the opportunity for larger restoration of the lordosis. The study of Hsieh et al[29] showed how in the upper lumbar spine TLIF and ALIF provide similar lordosis, whereas in the lower lumbar spine TLIF can actually reduce the lordosis and ALIF provides a substantial increase of lordosis. Direct lateral anterior approaches provide excellent correction of the coronal degenerative deformity just by cage implantation. They also provide some restoration of the sagittal profile. One study has shown that the average correction in the sagittal plane at each level is ~ 4 degrees; similarly to posteriorly implanted cages, the more anterior the cage position, the greater the final lordosis.[30] In preoperatively kyphotic disks, proper cage placement usually increases the

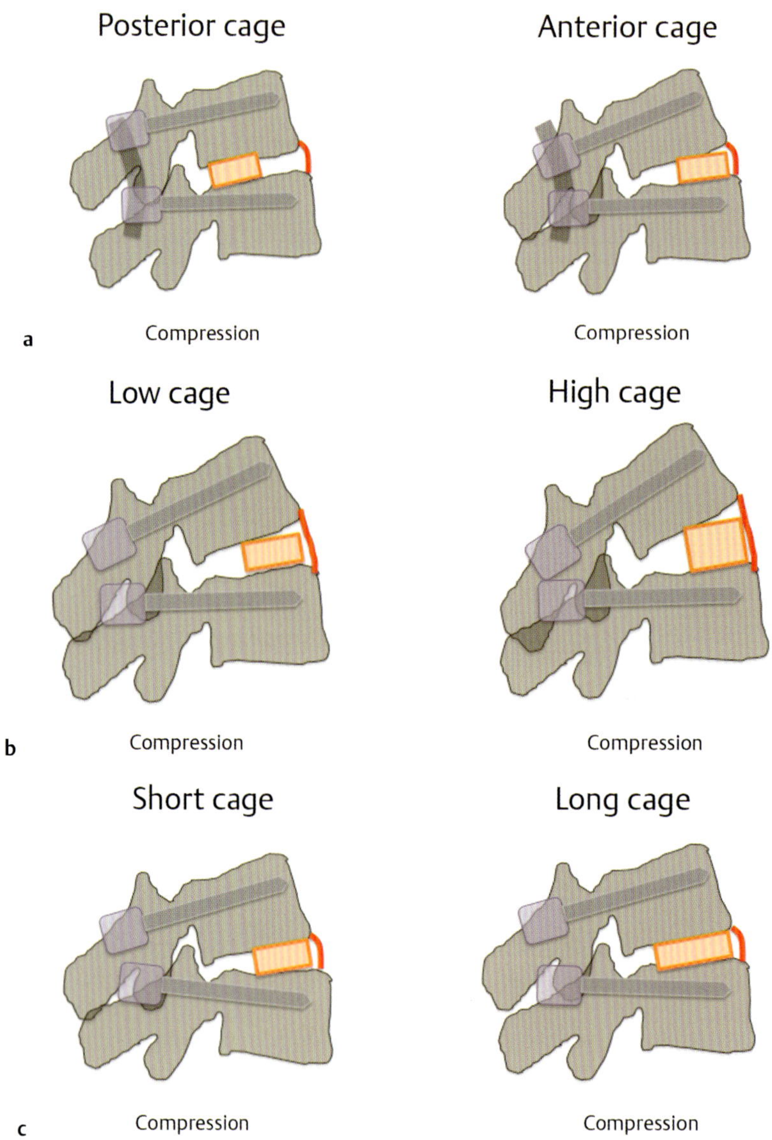

Fig. 14.5 **(a)** A posterior cage distracts the disk space posteriorly and may therefore block compression, limiting the capacity to increase lordosis. An anterior cage distracts the disk space anteriorly, which can be further compressed into lordosis. **(b)** A higher, anteriorly placed cage has a greater lordosing effect than a lower cage. **(c)** A shorter cage placed anteriorly leaves more unsupported disk space posteriorly, with a greater chance of increasing lordosis by posterior compression. A long cage has a similar effect to that of a posterior one, limiting the ability to close the posterior disk space in lordosis.

lordosis substantially, whereas in lordotic disks the capacity to increase lordosis and correct sagittal imbalance is more limited.[31] Recently, techniques for ALL release from a lateral approach have been described, and have demonstrated the ability to provide increases of lordosis in the range of what is achieved with pedicle subtraction osteotomies (**Fig. 14.6**).[28]

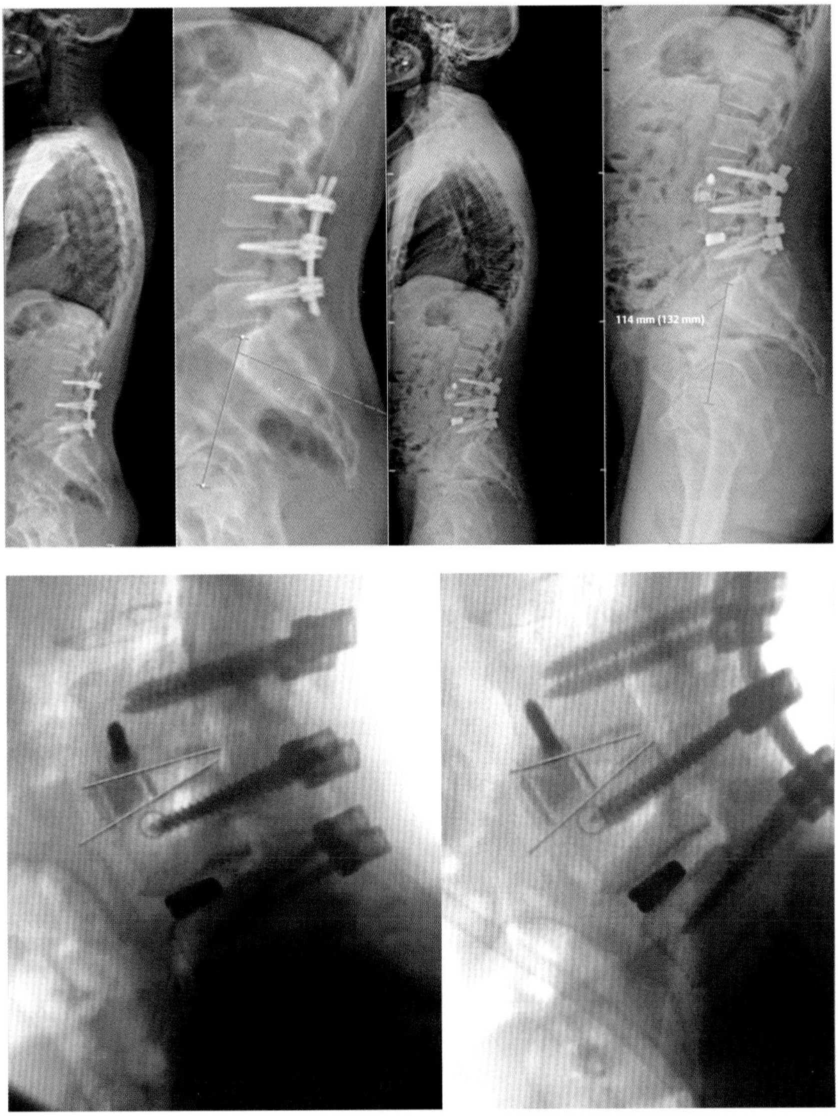

a

b

Fig. 14.6 **(a)** Standing radiographs of a 45-year-old man who underwent L3–L5 fusion for low back pain following the diagnosis of degenerative disk disease. His symptoms did not resolve, and pain and disability progressed over time. One year postoperatively, the patient showed a lack of lordosis in the instrumented levels and compensatory increased lordosis in the upper lumbar spine (*two left images*; see the anterior opening of the L1-L2 and L2-L3 disks). Surgery consisted of posterior implant removal (a fusion mass was confirmed at both levels), anterior interbody fusion at L4-L5, and anterior longitudinal ligament (ALL) release plus interbody fusion at L3-L4, both by a lateral transpsoas approach. The third posterior stage in the same day consisted of a posterior column shortening osteotomy through the fusion mass at L3-L4 and compression through pedicle screw instrumentation. Postoperatively pain resolved, and alignment was improved with a reduction of pelvic tilt (see postoperatively a more vertical "magic line"), an increase of lordosis in both instrumented levels (at L4-L5 the posterior fusion showed elastic enough), and a decrease of lordosis in L1-L2 and L2-L3 *(two right images)*. **(b)** Intraoperative detail of the case in **a.** After anterior release of ALL and interbody cage (secured with one lateral screw), the patient has only a modest increase of lordosis, below the planning target. After posterior column osteotomy and compression, the segmental lordosis is further increased by 10 degrees, matching the planning target.

Anatomic Level

Patients with large pelvic incidence may require relatively larger degrees of lordosis at the L5-S1 space. Due to its trapezoidal shape, and the restraint of the posterior longitudinal ligament, posterior annulus, and lateral annulus, the highest cage that can be implanted from a posterior TLIF or PLIF approach is frequently too low to adequately distract the anterior part of the disk. ALIF does not face these restrictions and can more reliably restore lordosis.

Posterior Compression

Independent of all the parameters mentioned above, posterior compression after cage implantation is an essential maneuver. Posterior compression preloads the cages with compressive forces, increasing stability and the potential for fusion, and shortens the posterior column, acting on the cage as a fulcrum, thus enhancing lordosis. In subjects with an intact ALL, interbody cages placed too far posteriorly should be avoided, as they will prevent effective posterior shortening by compression.

Chapter Summary

Degeneration of lumbar segments is often associated with loss of segmental or regional sagittal alignment, consisting of the loss of physiological lordosis. Different compensatory mechanisms are automatically recruited by the patient to maintain the upright position. These compensatory mechanisms require active, constant muscle contraction that can result in increased energy expenditure, fatigue, and pain. Although elimination of the classic pain generators (nerve compression, painful segmental movement, and instability) provides substantial clinical benefit, addressing the sagittal deformity during surgical correction of segmental degeneration is an opportunity to increase the rate of improvement, and it will likely reduce the probability of developing adjacent-segment degeneration. Knowledge of the different spinal sagittal shapes and calculation of the ideal sagittal alignment based on the individual's pelvic incidence are key in establishing sagittal alignment goals during surgical planning. Proper use of interbody cages and posterior instrumentation enables satisfactory correction of segmental malalignment in most degenerative cases.

Pearls

- Lateral standing films including the hip joints are helpful for sagittal assessment and planning.
- Calculation of alignment goals should include length of lordosis (based on Roussouly's types), distribution of lordosis, and total lordosis, compared to pelvic incidence.
- Anteriorly placed PLIF or TLIF cages provide more lordosis.
- ALIF cages provide significantly more lordosis in the lower lumbar spine than cages through a posterior approach.
- Intraoperative measurement of sagittal alignment is essential to avoid insufficient correction.

Pitfalls

- Long, high, and posteriorly placed PLIF or TLIF cages have a kyphosing effect, especially in the lower lumbar segments.
- Patient positioning for fusion surgery with any degree of hip flexion significantly reduces the lumbar lordosis and can result in postoperative worsening of sagittal alignment as well as a much greater likelihood of adjacent segment degeneration.
- End-plate violation can cause cage subsidence with postoperative loss of sagittal correction.

References

Five Must-Read References

1. Glassman SD, Berven S, Bridwell K, Horton W, Dimar JR. Correlation of radiographic parameters and clinical symptoms in adult scoliosis. Spine 2005; 30:682–688
2. Rose PS, Bridwell KH, Lenke LG, et al. Role of pelvic incidence, thoracic kyphosis, and patient factors on sagittal plane correction following pedicle subtraction osteotomy. Spine 2009;34:785–791
3. Schwab F, Patel A, Ungar B, Farcy JP, Lafage V. Adult spinal deformity-postoperative standing imbalance: how much can you tolerate? An overview of key parameters in assessing alignment and planning corrective surgery. Spine 2010;35:2224–2231
4. Lamartina C, Berjano P. Classification of sagittal imbalance based on spinal alignment and compensatory mechanisms. Eur Spine J 2014;23:1177–1189
5. Aota Y, Saito T, Uesugi M, Kato S, Kuniya H, Koh R. Optimal arm position for evaluation of spinal sagittal balance. J Spinal Disord Tech 2011;24:105–109
6. Vialle R, Levassor N, Rillardon L, Templier A, Skalli W, Guigui P. Radiographic analysis of the sagittal alignment and balance of the spine in asymptomatic subjects. J Bone Joint Surg Am 2005;87:260–267
7. Berjano P, Langella F, Ismael M-F, Damilano M, Scopetta S, Lamartina C. Successful correction of sagittal imbalance can be calculated on the basis of pelvic incidence and age. Eur Spine J 2014;23(Suppl 6): 587–596
8. Roussouly P, Gollogly S, Berthonnaud E, Dimnet J. Classification of the normal variation in the sagittal alignment of the human lumbar spine and pelvis in the standing position. Spine 2005;30:346–353
9. Anwar HA, Butler JS, Yarashi T, Rajakulendran K, Molloy S. Segmental pelvic correlation (SPeC): a novel approach to understanding sagittal plane spinal alignment. Spine J 2015;15:2518–2523
10. Mac-Thiong JM, Transfeldt EE, Mehbod AA, et al. Can C7 plumbline and gravity line predict health related quality of life in adult scoliosis? Spine 2009;34:E519–E527
11. Kim MK, Lee SH, Kim ES, Eoh W, Chung SS, Lee CS. The impact of sagittal balance on clinical results after posterior interbody fusion for patients with degenerative spondylolisthesis: a pilot study. BMC Musculoskelet Disord 2011;12:69
12. Heo Y, Park JH, Seong HY, et al. Symptomatic adjacent segment degeneration at the L3-4 level after fusion surgery at the L4-5 level: evaluation of the risk factors and 10-year incidence. Eur Spine J 2015;24: 2474–2480
13. Kumar MN, Baklanov A, Chopin D. Correlation between sagittal plane changes and adjacent segment degeneration following lumbar spine fusion. Eur Spine J 2001;10:314–319
14. Jackson RP, McManus AC. Radiographic analysis of sagittal plane alignment and balance in standing volunteers and patients with low back pain matched for age, sex, and size. A prospective controlled clinical study. Spine 1994;19:1611–1618
15. Park JY, Cho YE, Kuh SU, et al. New prognostic factors for adjacent-segment degeneration after one-stage 360 degrees fixation for spondylolytic spondylolisthesis: special reference to the usefulness of pelvic incidence angle. J Neurosurg Spine 2007;7:139–144
16. Barrey C, Jund J, Noseda O, Roussouly P. Sagittal balance of the pelvis-spine complex and lumbar degenerative diseases. A comparative study about 85 cases. Eur Spine J 2007;16:1459–1467
17. Aono K, Kobayashi T, Jimbo S, Atsuta Y, Matsuno T. Radiographic analysis of newly developed degenerative spondylolisthesis in a mean twelve-year prospective study. Spine 2010;35:887–891
18. Lazennec J-Y, Ramaré S, Arafati N, et al. Sagittal alignment in lumbosacral fusion: relations between radiological parameters and pain. Eur Spine J 2000;9: 47–55
19. Umehara S, Zindrick MR, Patwardhan AG, et al. The biomechanical effect of postoperative hypolordosis in instrumented lumbar fusion on instrumented and adjacent spinal segments. Spine 2000;25:1617–1624
20. Akamaru T, Kawahara N, Tim Yoon S, et al. Adjacent segment motion after a simulated lumbar fusion in different sagittal alignments: a biomechanical analysis. Spine 2003;28:1560–1566
21. Oda I, Cunningham BW, Buckley RA, et al. Does spinal kyphotic deformity influence the biomechanical characteristics of the adjacent motion segments? An in vivo animal model. Spine 1999;24:2139–2146
22. Berjano P, Damilano M, Bozzaro M, Pejrona M, Cecchinato R, Lamartina C. Standing lateral lumbar spine and pelvis (SLLP) radiograph: a screening, reduced radiation method, for sagittal imbalance. Eur Spine J 2013;22(Suppl 6):S842–S846
23. Aurouer N, Obeid I, Gille O, Pointillart V, Vital JM. Computerized preoperative planning for correction of sagittal deformity of the spine. Surg Radiol Anat 2009;31:781–792
24. Benfanti PL, Geissele AE. The effect of intraoperative hip position on maintenance of lumbar lordosis: a radiographic study of anesthetized patients and unanesthetized volunteers on the Wilson frame. Spine 1997;22:2299–2303

25. Berjano P, Lamartina C. Classification of degenerative segment disease in adults with deformity of the lumbar or thoracolumbar spine. Eur Spine J 2014; 23:1815–1824
26. Berjano P, Cecchinato R, Sinigaglia A, et al. Anterior column realignment from a lateral approach for the treatment of severe sagittal imbalance: a retrospective radiographic study. Eur Spine J 2015;24(Suppl 3):433–438
27. Hsieh PC, Koski TR, O'Shaughnessy BA, et al. Anterior lumbar interbody fusion in comparison with transforaminal lumbar interbody fusion: implications for the restoration of foraminal height, local disc angle, lumbar lordosis, and sagittal balance. J Neurosurg Spine 2007;7:379–386
28. Kepler CK, Huang RC, Sharma AK, et al. Factors influencing segmental lumbar lordosis after lateral transpsoas interbody fusion. Orthop Surg 2012;4: 71–75
29. Costanzo G, Zoccali C, Maykowski P, Walter CM, Skoch J, Baaj AA. The role of minimally invasive lateral lumbar interbody fusion in sagittal balance correction and spinal deformity. Eur Spine J 2014;23 (Suppl 6):699–704

15

Patients with Multiple Surgeries

Claudio Lamartina and Carlotta Martini

Introduction

A growing issue among spine surgeons is the management of the increasing number of symptomatic spine patients who have had multiple surgeries for treatment-resistant pain that has contributed to an unacceptable quality of life.

There are several possible explanations for this phenomenon:

1. The progressive aging of the population and the subsequent increasing number of surgeries for degenerative spine, even on the same patient
2. A propensity for spine surgeons to recommend spine surgery rather than conservative measures
3. The difficulty in identifying pain generators, as a result of the widespread emphasis on imaging techniques. Diagnosis should be based on both a clinical evaluation and imaging.

Revision surgery is a more and more frequent procedure in spine units; these patients tend to be older, thus adding risks related to comorbidities. From a psychological point of view, patients who have experienced repeated surgeries frequently feel hopeless and have a negative attitude toward surgery, making it difficult for surgeons to determine which patients are appropriate for surgery. Patients' expectations are often unrealistic, as their pain has been of long duration and spine surgery is complex.

Revision surgery is frequently performed by a different team. Thus, patients expect the new surgeon to clear up the errors committed by several previous surgeons, which is unrealistic.

This chapter discusses the issues related to managing patients who have had multiple surgeries, and presents an illustrative case.

Case Presentation

A 58-year-old woman with mechanical low back pain and claudication was referred to a spine surgeon, who performed a clinical and radiological evaluation (**Fig. 15.1**), based on which the surgeon determined that the patient was a candidate for an L3–L4 decompression and L3–L4 translaminar screw, using the Magerl technique. The aim of the surgery was to decompress and stabilize the spine. The patient's pain was relieved by the surgery, but 1 year later the symptoms returned, worse than before. The patient was unable to walk more than 50 m, after which pain increased in her lower back, buttocks, and proximal legs, bilaterally. X-rays demonstrated a hypermobility of the L4-L5 disk (**Fig. 15.2**), and the surgeon decided to widen the decompression to L5, and to perform a fusion, including the previously operated segment and extending to the new unstable segment (**Fig. 15.3**). A pedicular screw is the technique of choice, with posterolateral fusion.

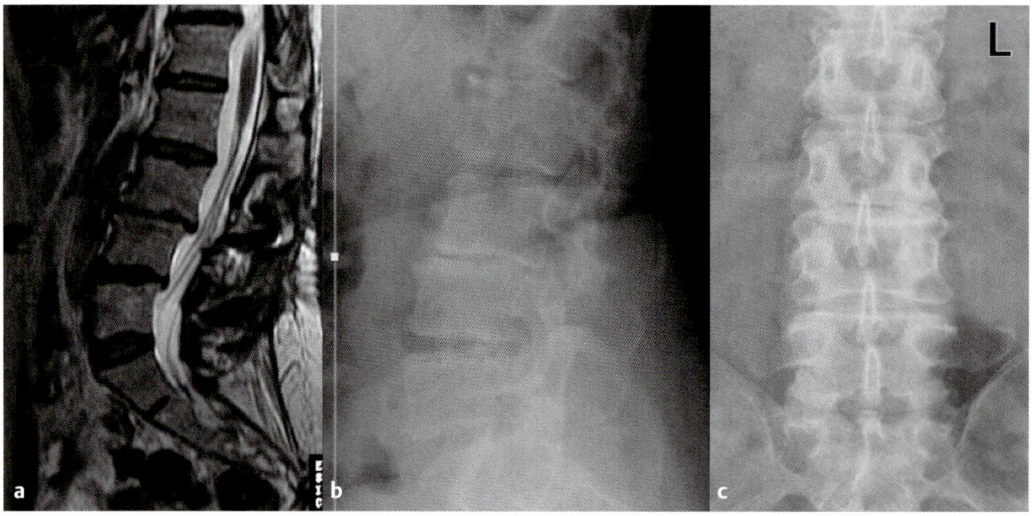

Fig. 15.1 Magnetic resonance imaging (MRI) scan **(a)** and X-rays of the patient in the presented case before the surgical procedure **(b,c)**. The values of lumbar lordosis measured on MRI sagittal cut and on the X-ray are different. The trick is to determine if the patient is standing or not. The L3-L4 disk space is degenerated and flat, and L1-L2 and L2-L3 are in lordosis (Roussouly type 2 or 3). L4-L5 is slightly hyperlordotic. The lordosis distribution is not respecting the rule of two thirds in L4-S1 and one third in L1-L4.

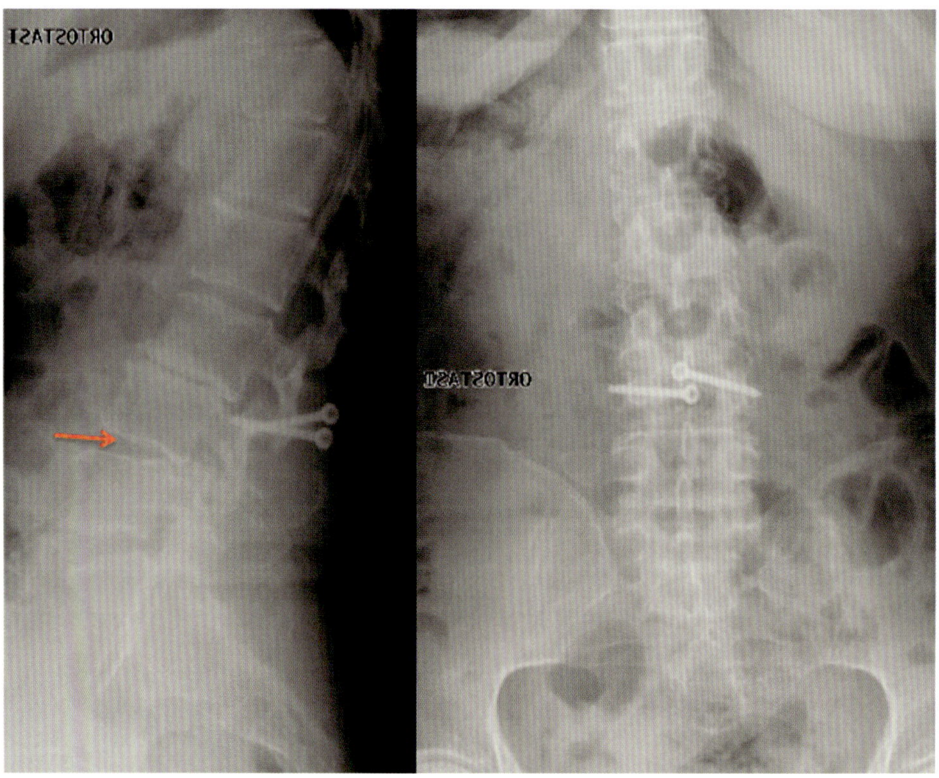

Fig. 15.2 After first surgery, L4-L5 retrolisthesis is present, and the L3-L4 space is flat and fixed with a translaminar Magerl screw.

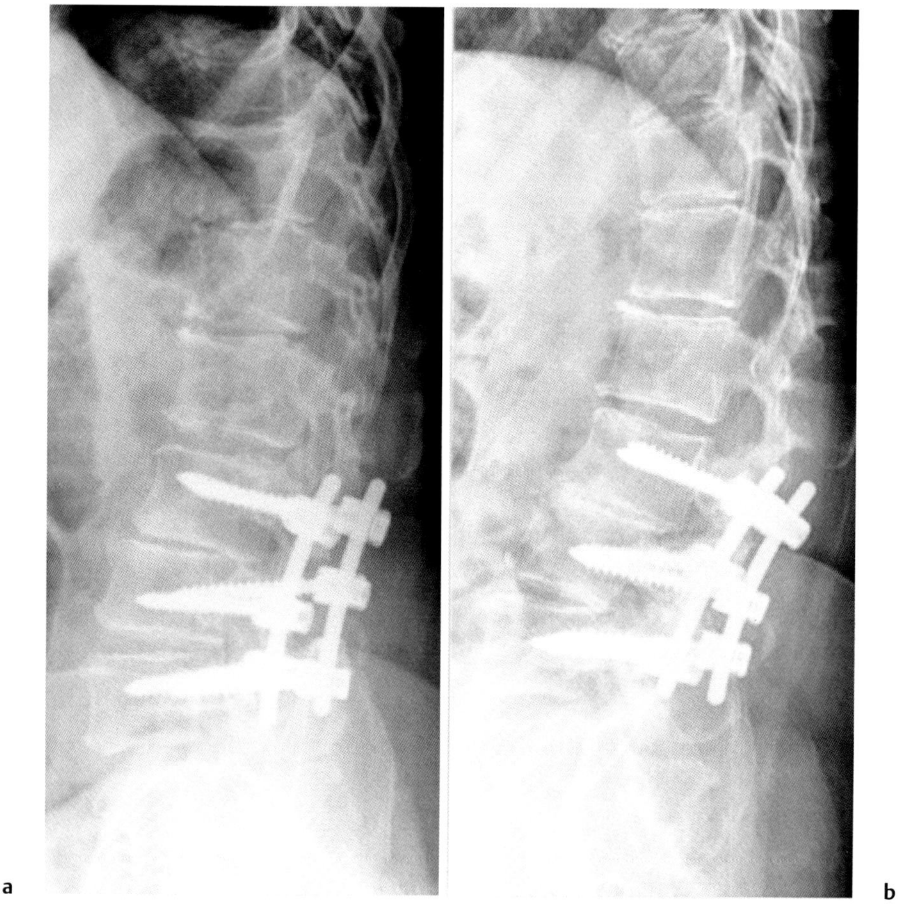

Fig. 15.3 (a) After the second surgery, the decompression area is widened, and the fusion is extended, covering L3–L5. L3-L4 is a little more lordotic in the early follow-up, but this small gain is lost at 1-year follow-up **(b)**. L4-L5 is fused in a lordotic position.

The patient's relief from pain was once again short-term as well as inconsistent. One year later, her pain returned to the preoperative level. The surgeon then decided on conservative treatment, with physiotherapy, multimodal analgesia, and clinical observation. But after another year, the clinical situation had dramatically worsened, as the patient was completely unable to stand or walk for more than few seconds without pain. The patient experienced almost continuous pain that was relieved only by lying down. The first surgeon referred her to a second surgeon.

The second surgeon performed a clinical evaluation, and found a pathological sagittal alignment. The patient's knees were maintained in a flexed position, her pelvis was retroverted, and thoracic kyphosis was nearly absent. On the frontal plane, a moderate coronal deformity was noted. The surgeon updated the imaging with new whole-spine X-rays with the patient in the standing position to assess the sagittal alignment (**Fig. 15.4**). The X-rays demonstrated a lack of lumbar lordosis (LL), proximal junctional kyphosis (PJK) in the thoracolumbar area, a high pelvic tilt (PT), a low sacral slope (SS), and a sagittal vertical axis (SVA) > 5 cm. Because the SS was close to 0 degrees, the pelvic incidence (PI) was nearly equal to the PT.

The surgeon decided to revise the previous surgery, extending the previously instrumented area to T10 cranially and to the ileum caudally. The revision was done with a double approach,

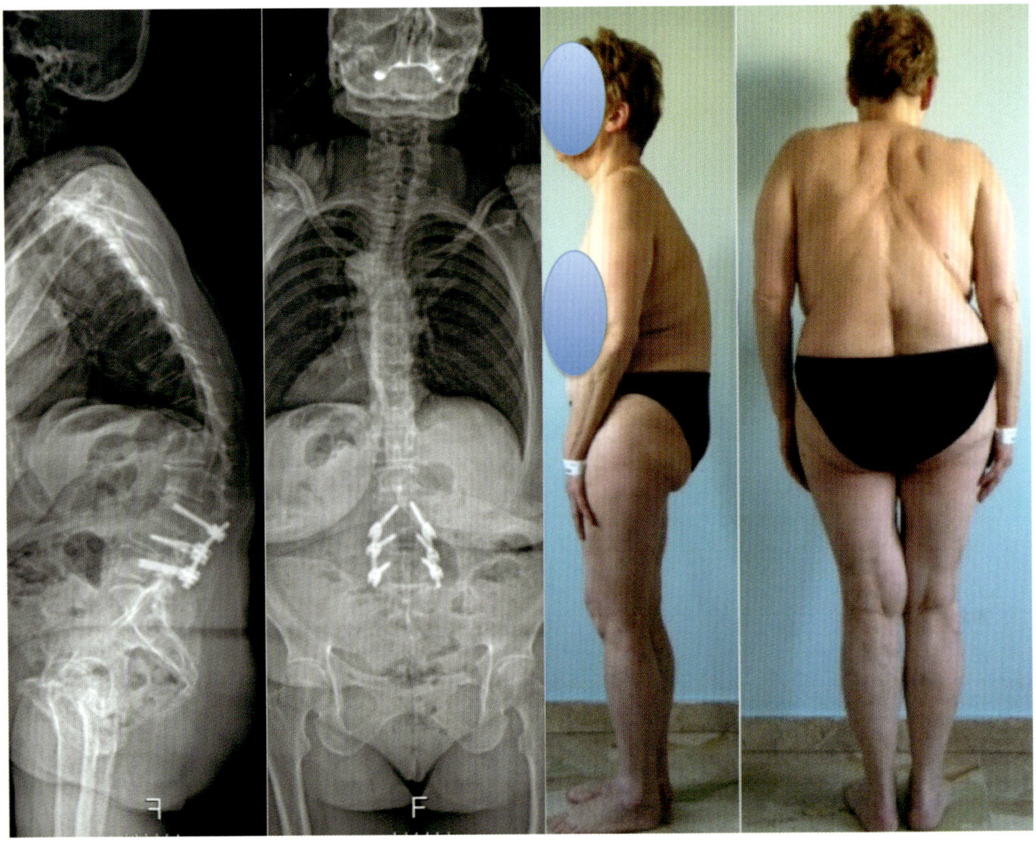

Fig. 15.4 Radiographic and clinical global assessment of the patient before the last revision surgery. A proximal junctional kyphosis in the thoracolumbar area is present, together with close to a 0-degree sacral slope and a consequent high pelvic tilt (equal to pelvic incidence). Neck hyperextension, a flattened thoracic kyphosis, a retroverted pelvis, and flexed knees are clearly visible in the clinical photos.

lateral and posterior. Multilevel extreme lateral interbody fusion (XLIF) cages were implanted at the L1-L2, L3-L4, and L4-L5 levels. At the L2-L3 level, to restore the required lordosis, a hyperlordotic 30-degree cage was implanted, the anterior longitudinal ligament was resected, and the anterior column realignment (ACR) technique was performed. Posterior instrumentation from T10 to the ileum was also performed. Postoperatively, the patient's condition improved; she was quickly mobilized and was able to stand without experiencing additional pain (except for the expected wound-related pain). The sagittal alignment improved, and she demonstrated normal knee extension, a physiologically normal thoracic kyphosis, improved LL, and a more natural neck and head position.

The radiographic results, together with a clinical photo, are shown in **Fig. 15.5**. The patient's improved condition has continued even at the 3-year follow-up.

Case Discussion

Clinical Examination

When a patient with multiple surgeries presents to a new physician, it is important to determine the patient's chief complaint; if it

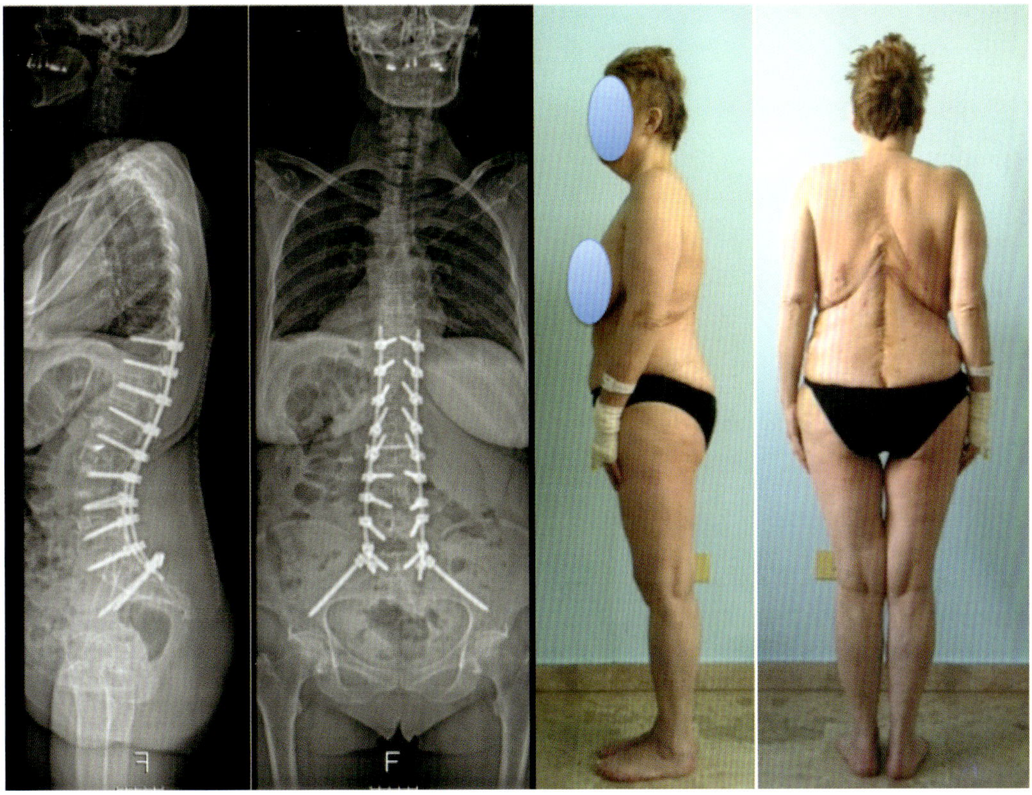

Fig. 15.5 Postoperative radiographic and clinical global assessment of the patient. The fusion area is extended from T10 to the pelvis. Lumbar lordosis and thoracic kyphosis are restored, reproducing the hypothesized Roussouly type 2 that the patient belongs to. All the aforementioned compensatory mechanisms are no longer present in the X-rays and clinical photos.

is back pain, then the pain generator needs to be identified. After a physical examination is performed, imaging with X-rays, magnetic resonance imaging (MRI), or computed tomography (CT), as well as evocative diskography and facet block should help to identify the pain generator and provide additional information. Then the decision of whether to manage the patient conservatively or surgically needs to be made.

In only 15% of patients does low back pain have an organic cause.[1] In the remaining 85%, the cause is unclear. Socioeconomic factors have to be carefully evaluated, and the yellow, blue, and black flags need to be identified (see Chapter 2).

In addition to complaining of back pain, many patients, including the patient in our case presentation, complain of the inability to walk autonomously for more than a limited distance. The ability of the surgeon to differentiate this kind of disturbance from neurogenic claudication is crucial. The case presented above was an example of a patient given a misdiagnosis. When asked about symptoms, during the interview before the last revision surgery, the patient did not describe the typical neurogenic claudication. Rather, her pain was a burning tenderness, radiating from the lumbar region downward to both legs and upward to the dorsal region, starting after walking for a few minutes and remitting with passive extension of the trunk or bed rest. This is quite different from the standard neurogenic claudication, which classically has a different pain quality and remits with trunk flexion or sitting.

We believe that neurogenic claudication should have been the first diagnosis, but the back pain that ensued and persisted after the first surgical procedure was a different matter, as we shall explain.

Imaging

The importance of the evaluation of spinopelvic alignment is widely accepted and evidence-based.[2–4] The clinical workup, as described above, and appropriate imaging are fundamental. The routine use of standing, full-spine, plain X-rays is changing the indications for surgery, as demonstrated by a sample of spine surgeons who answered a blinded questionnaire from the AOSpine organization.[5]

We believe that a possible explanation for the failure of the presented case is hidden in the very first imaging (**Fig. 15.1**). If we carefully review the alignment of the lumbar vertebrae, we can see a nonphysiological distribution of LL. It has been reported that LL in an asymptomatic healthy population has a constant distribution along the lumbar spine: two thirds between L4 and S1, and one third between L1 and L4. This is a simple measurement that anyone can perform on a plain standing lumbar spine X-ray film, as in **Fig. 15.1**.

Additionally, in a standing X-ray, even if the femoral heads are not visible in the field of view and we cannot measure PI and PT (**Figs. 15.1, 15.2, 15.3**), the SS is clearly visible. This is a highly informative parameter, especially if it has a very low value. An SS close to 0 degrees (vertical sacrum, as in **Figs. 15.3b** and **15.4**) means that PT is high (pelvic retroversion). The base concept for the understanding of this deduction is in the fundamental equation:

$$\text{PI (Constant)} = \text{PT} + \text{SS}$$

If SS is 0 degrees, PI is equal PT, whereas the ideal PT is 0.37(PI) – 7 (Vialle formula[6]). It has been demonstrated that high PT values are correlated with pelvic compensation and poor clinical outcomes. In the presented case, we can see that SS is lower in **Fig. 15.2** than in **Fig. 15.1**. Our interpretation is that after the first surgery, the patient started to compensate actively with pelvic retroversion. The compensation was caused by a loss of mobility and lordosis at the fused level. So the lumbar spine was flatter and less able to fight this forced alignment with the spinal segments.

We know that a normal, flexible spine, has the ability to compensate for the alteration of the expected curves at the different levels.[7,8] This is known for the lumbar and thoracic spine, and under evaluation for the cervical spine.[9]

The ability to compensate is proportional to the degree of deviation from the normal values of curves, and it is limited by any type of fixation, be it artificial or autologous. Whenever the spine is not able to compensate, there are several different mechanisms by which the human body tries to maintain horizontal gaze.[10] Pelvic retroversion is the first mechanism, followed by joint movements in the lower limbs. Compensation mechanisms are sometimes so evident and so obvious that it is sufficient merely to observe the undressed patient; imaging is unnecessary. But the compensation mechanisms are not routinely evident. Most often they are hidden, or are in a very early phase of development, so it is important for the surgeon to recognize the possibility that compensation mechanisms are developing.[8]

All these considerations can be evaluated with a simple standing lumbar spine X-ray and by observing the patient. It certainly could have been possible in the presented case. Thus, in the evaluation of a multi-operated spinal patient, the gold standard is the full-spine standing X-ray.

Correctly measured and reliable spinopelvic parameters enable the surgeon to classify the patient in the correct Roussouly type, and consequently to plan the surgical strategy, aiming to reconstruct a physiological, patient-specific, final alignment.[10]

Further examination of the patient's imaging can also lead to a diagnosis of proximal junctional kyphosis in **Figs. 15.3b** and **15.4**, after the instrumented fusion at L3–L5. As we know from the literature, proximal junctional kyphosis is secondary to under- or overcorrection of LL, to an incorrect distribution of lordosis on the lumbar spine, and to a final excessive PT resulting after surgery.[11] Identification of a proximal junction problem should be suggestive of an alignment-related problem, and thus should lead to a careful evaluation of the whole spine.

Surgery

The presented case demonstrates some of the critical issues in reviewing a patient's previous surgery. A new surgeon has to rely on his or her personal experience and the previous surgeon's report. Thus, it is important for surgeons to share knowledge and ideas, and to report their unavoidable mistakes.

Surgical indications in low back pain are controversial. Patients often undergo multiple surgeries because of unclear indications for the first surgery, which begins a vicious circle in which patients never have a chance to heal and additional surgeries are performed, often worsening the situation in a negative progression.

Surgical indications should be one of the first issues to be discussed with the patient. It is important to strictly define what spine surgery can do effectively. In the vast majority of cases, there are just three effective surgical functions:

1. Decompression
2. Fusion
3. Deformity correction

Successful spine surgery always aims to accomplish one or more of these functions. The surgeon has to be clear in his or her mind about the aim of the surgery. If the aim is not on this list, the outcome is unpredictable.

In the majority of cases, the aim of surgery is fusion. To reduce nonunion rates, instrumentation is useful. Instrumentation without fusion has a very limited indication, such as for Chance fractures, in which instrumentation in compression promotes the fracture's healing.

Nowadays, patients are overwhelmed by the availability of medical information on the Internet and in the media. The surgeon should review the information the patient has acquired, and correct any misimpression the patient has, so that the patient does not harbor unrealistic expectations.

A widespread belief among spine degenerative patients is that the greater the pain, the greater the need for surgical intervention. Patients should be informed that this is not true, and given the reason in a fairly detailed way. High preoperative pain levels are related to a worse outcome[12] in every type of spine procedure for degenerative conditions. This fact should be discussed with the patient, together with the low ability of surgery to correct a previous medical error.

Additionally, a thorough description of the surgical risks and possible complications should be presented to patients, to pave the way for their providing their informed consent. Also, patients believe that more extensive surgery results in better outcomes. This misimpression also needs to be corrected, and patients should be told that the more complex the surgery, the greater the risk of complications.

Furthermore, nearly all patients ask for minimally invasive surgery because they read about it on the Internet. This request could lead many surgeons to reduce the goals of the surgery, leading to the potential need for further revisions, when in fact an open procedure could provide definitive treatment without the need for further revisions.

The complication rate in revision surgery for adult spinal deformity is also significantly related to the surgical unit's experience.[13] This is an evidence-based fact that confirms the importance of the surgeon's knowledge and experience. Good results are not easily obtained, so patients who need highly specialized spine surgery should be carefully selected.

The presented case demonstrated all these concerns. Every patient presents a unique scenario, but the most important factors for the surgeon are to observe the patient, review the imaging, do a careful clinical examination, and clearly explain the aims of surgery.

Case Resolution

We believe that the aim of the surgery in the presented case should have been the correction of the sagittal deformity, which could have eliminated the need for the compensatory mechanisms that were responsible for the patient's complaints.

The patient was not able to stand for more than few minutes or walk for more than a short distance without suffering a burning pain in the low back, radiating to the dorsal region and to the proximal lower limbs. This kind of pain is secondary to a sagittal deformity. The sagittal deformity was responsible for the recruitment of compensatory mechanisms to maintain horizontal gaze. The compensatory mechanisms in this case were flattening of thoracic kyphosis, pelvic retroversion, knee flexion, and neck hyperextension (**Fig. 15.4**). All compensatory mechanisms require muscular effort and produce pain.

Once the surgical aim has been defined, a surgical plan is developed, based on the patient's anatomy. In this process the starting point is the patient's PI, in this case 30 degrees, measured for the first time on X-rays (**Fig. 15.4**). Studies have demonstrated that the expected LL can be calculated from the following formula[14–16]:

$$\text{LL expected} = \text{PI} \pm 10 \text{ degrees}$$

In the case of low values of PI, 10 degrees should be added; in the case of high values of PI, 10 degrees should be subtracted. This is a useful formula in that it provides a numerical target value, but the correct expected LL of a patient is not just the result of a formula. Age is another variable that affects surgical planning.[14,17]

In the presented case, the PI was 30 degrees, which is a low value, so the expected LL should be at least 40 degrees. The patient is a Roussouly type 2, a "harmonious flat back,"[10] as LL is long and the L1-2-3 disk spaces are in lordosis (**Fig. 15.1**).

The variation in spinopelvic parameters in the presented patient over time is demonstrated in **Table 15.1.** Interestingly, the global LL value was constantly decreasing with time, and each surgical procedure worsened it, together with the SS. Consequently, the PT increased.

The loss of upper LL, driving the lower compensation of disks L4-L5 and L5-S1 (**Fig. 15.2**) should be our main surgical target. Our surgical plan should address this area specifically, and the restoration of a harmonic angular proportion, including the thoracolumbar kyphosis, would be the goal of surgery in order to have a successful and durable result.[18]

The surgical plan, then, is to achieve a final LL of more than 40 degrees, with two thirds of it in L4-S1 and one third in L1-L4. Thus, we need at least 15 degrees of lordosis in L1–L4, starting from 35 degrees of kyphosis, which means a global correction of more than 50 degrees within L1 and L4. There are several ways to obtain this result. Our choice is to use lordotic cages in L1–L4 with a hyperlordotic cage in L2-L3 to obtain a single-level 30-degree correction by anterior column realignment,[19] with a double-approach procedure (lateral first, posterior second). The remaining correction of 20 degrees has been distributed on two levels, 10 degrees each on L1-L2 and L3-L4.

The fusion area (T10 to the ileum) involves the thoracolumbar area, as the main surgical target was the high lumbar area and the thoracolumbar junction, as well as the ileum for a

Table 15.1 Spinopelvic Parameters as Seen in the Presented Case

	Fig. 1	Fig. 2	Fig. 3a	Fig. 3b	Fig. 4	Fig. 5
LL	–36 degrees	–30 degrees	–30 degrees	–16 degrees	0 degrees	–49 degrees
L1–L4	–6 degrees	+7 degrees	–2 degrees	+16	+35 degrees	–19 degrees
L4–S1	–30 degrees	–38 degrees	–28 degrees	–32 degrees	–35 degrees	–30 degrees
PT	n.m.	n.m.	n.m.	n.m.	28 degrees	5 degrees
SS	30 degrees	16 degrees	18 degrees	12 degrees	2 degrees	25 degrees

Abbreviations: LL, lumbar lordosis; n.m., not measured; PT, pelvic tilt; SS, sacral slope.

more stable construct. It has been considered unnecessary to extend up to the high thoracic area, because the thoracic spine is considered to be flexible, and the thoracic flattened kyphosis has been considered a compensatory mechanism, not a surgical target in itself. This consideration limits the fusion area, which helps reduce the risk of complications.

The best way to evaluate the surgical result is to review the clinical photograph (**Fig. 15.5**); in this case, the compensatory mechanisms are no longer evident. Thoracic kyphosis is present, the pelvis and neck are in a neutral physiological position, and the knees are extended. If we measure the PT on the X-rays (**Fig. 15.5**), the value is 5 degrees, whereas in **Fig. 15.4** it is 28 degrees. It is possible to calculate a "theoretical" PT for a specific PI, using the formula of Vialle:

$$\text{PT expected} = 0.37(\text{PI}) - 7$$

The expected PT for our patient, using this formula, should have been ~ 4 degrees, whereas the actual one, after our revision, was 5 degrees. Restoration of a low PT is a known predictor of a good surgical outcome, and in this case the reduction is important and the final value is optimal. The achievement of an optimal correction is more important with younger patients than with the elderly,[20] and rigorous presurgical planning enables the surgeon to calculate the optimal correction as well as a range in which the correction should be.

A retrospective review of the presented case would be as follows: in the first presentation (**Fig. 15.1**) the surgical procedure of translaminar screwing created a fixed loss of lordosis in the L3-4 space. This was the driving force of a compensatory hyperlordosis in L4–S1. The L4-L5 disk is abnormal with a retrolisthesis (**Fig. 15.2**). If we carefully review the initial imaging (**Fig. 15.1**), L4-L5 is already abnormal and slightly slipped, so that a possible lesson here is to avoid leaving pathological adjacent levels uninstrumented. Moreover, after the second surgery (**Fig. 15.3**), the L3-L4 segmental lordosis is restored for only a short time, whereas the L4–S1 compensating hyperlordosis is fixed. At the 1-year follow-up, the upper lordosis angle was flat, and this is the possible reason for the worsening of the proximal junctional disease: the incorrect, fixed distribution of LL, resulting from the second surgery, caused the proximal junctional problem in the thoracolumbar area.

Chapter Summary

Repeated surgeries sometimes lead to deformity, as in the presented case. The incorrect use of instrumented fusion along the lumbar spine is responsible for the loss of the compensation ability at the adjacent levels. This ability is fundamental both in normal aging and in the degenerative spine. In this scenario, the loss of intrinsic compensation mechanisms leads to recruitment of compensation inside and outside the spine, and at the same time speeds up the clinical development of symptoms connected to these mechanisms.

Thus, the first important step is to correctly evaluate the patient's clinical condition. The differential diagnosis of low back pain is crucially important. The surgeon's experience and knowledge, and the careful observation and detailed interview of the patient are the tools to avoid misdiagnosis. A wrong diagnosis is usually the first step of a vicious circle of unsuccessful treatment.

After clinical evaluation, a consistent, systematic diagnostic workup should be done. The use of standing, full-spine plain films is often mandatory. This imaging provides the highest quality of information for evaluating spinal alignment in static conditions.

Surgery requires preoperative planning. The surgical targets and strategy form the basis for an effective procedure. Patients who have had multiple surgeries are often the victims of improper management and a confused interpretation of the presenting signs and symptoms. Thus, a methodical approach to surgical planning is mandatory.

Pearls

- Always check the surgical indications. Surgery should treat the patient, not the X-ray.
- Try to reconstruct the patient's history. The more detail you have about previous surgeries, the easier it is to understand what is needed in the revision.
- Discuss the risks, benefits, and possible complications with the patient and family.
- Be prepared to manage postoperative problems, and this kind of surgery is high-risk.
- Prepare a thorough, rigorous surgical plan. Identify the targets, measure all the required angles, and prepare a table with the expected values to be attained. This table presents the optimal correction. The final results should be as close as possible to this target.
- Carefully check the material to implant and to explant, ask for the manufacturer's technical support, especially if the previous surgery was done long ago by someone else. Different implants require different tools!
- Discuss the plan with the team. Revision surgery is demanding in terms of the surgeon's physical effort, surgical time, instrumentation needs, and anesthesiological management. Teamwork is fundamental.
- The younger the patient, the more rigorous the surgeon must be. Revision of young multi-operated patients requires an optimal final result. If the optimal alignment cannot be achieved, the clinical outcome will be problematic.

Pitfalls

- Surgery is not the answer for all problems.
- Do not trust the previous diagnosis. Usually it is wrong, and it is the cause of repeated, unsuccessful surgeries.
- Do not reduce surgical goals because they are technically too difficult.
- Do not underestimate the benefit of surgery in the elderly. They are the patients who most benefit from surgical correction of problems related to misalignment.

References

Five Must-Read References

1. Elfering A, Mannion AF. Epidemiology and risk factors of spinal disorders. In: Boos N, Aebi M, eds. Spinal Disorders: Fundamentals of Diagnosis and Treatment: Berlin: Springer; 2008:153–173
2. Diebo BG, Henry J, Lafage V, Berjano P. Sagittal deformities of the spine: factors influencing the outcomes and complications. Eur Spine J 2015;24(Suppl 1):S3–S15
3. Lamartina C, Berjano P. Spine alignment in adult trauma, degeneration and deformity. Eur Spine J 2014;23(6, Suppl 6):585–586
4. Mehta VA, Amin A, Omeis I, Gokaslan ZL, Gottfried ON. Implications of spinopelvic alignment for the spine surgeon. Neurosurgery 2015;76(Suppl 1):S42–S56, discussion S56 discussion S.
5. Maggio D, Ailon TT, Smith JS, et al; AOSpine North America; International Spine Study Group. Assessment of impact of standing long-cassette radiographs on surgical planning for lumbar pathology: an international survey of spine surgeons. J Neurosurg Spine 2015 Jul 31:1–8. [Epub ahead of print]
6. Vialle R, Levassor N, Rillardon L, Templier A, Skalli W, Guigui P. Radiographic analysis of the sagittal alignment and balance of the spine in asymptomatic subjects. J Bone Joint Surg Am 2005;87:260–267
7. Barrey C, Roussouly P, Le Huec J-C, D'Acunzi G, Perrin G. Compensatory mechanisms contributing to keep the sagittal balance of the spine. Eur Spine J 2013; 22(Suppl 6):S834–S841
8. Lamartina C, Berjano P. Classification of sagittal imbalance based on spinal alignment and compensatory mechanisms. Eur Spine J 2014;23:1177–1189
9. Lee S-H, Son E-S, Seo E-M, Suk K-S, Kim K-T. Factors determining cervical spine sagittal balance in asymptomatic adults: correlation with spinopelvic balance and thoracic inlet alignment. Spine J 2015;15:705–712
10. Roussouly P, Pinheiro-Franco JL. Biomechanical analysis of the spino-pelvic organization and adaptation in pathology. Eur Spine J 2011;20(Suppl 5):609–618
11. Nicholls F, Eksi MS, Ames CP, et al. Radiographic parameters associated with revision surgery for proximal junctional kyphosis. Spine J 2014;14:S38–S39
12. Katz JN, Stucki G, Lipson SJ, Fossel AH, Grobler LJ, Weinstein JN. Predictors of surgical outcome in degenerative lumbar spinal stenosis. Spine 1999;24: 2229–2233
13. Paul JC, Lonner BS, Goz V, et al. Complication rates are reduced for revision adult spine deformity surgery among high-volume hospitals and surgeons. Spine J 2015;15:1963–1972
14. Berjano P, Langella F, Ismael M-F, Damilano M, Scopetta S, Lamartina C. Successful correction of sagittal imbalance can be calculated on the basis of pelvic

incidence and age. Eur Spine J 2014;23(Suppl 6):587–596
15. Roussouly P, Gollogly S, Berthonnaud E, Dimnet J. Classification of the normal variation in the sagittal alignment of the human lumbar spine and pelvis in the standing position. Spine 2005;30:346–353
16. Boulay C, Tardieu C, Hecquet J, et al. Sagittal alignment of spine and pelvis regulated by pelvic incidence: standard values and prediction of lordosis. Eur Spine J 2006;15:415–422
17. Neal CJ, McClendon J, Halpin R, Acosta FL, Koski T, Ondra SL. Predicting ideal spinopelvic balance in adult spinal deformity. J Neurosurg Spine 2011;15:82–91
18. Schwab F, Patel A, Ungar B, Farcy J-P, Lafage V. Adult spinal deformity-postoperative standing imbalance: how much can you tolerate? An overview of key parameters in assessing alignment and planning corrective surgery. Spine 2010;35:2224–2231
19. Berjano P, Damilano M, Ismael M, Longo A, Bruno A, Lamartina C. Anterior column realignment (ACR) technique for correction of sagittal imbalance. Eur Spine J 2015;24(Suppl 3):451–453
20. Lafage R, Schwab F, Challier V, et al; International Spine Study Group. Defining spino-pelvic alignment thresholds: should operative goals in adult spinal deformity surgery account for age? Spine 2016;41:62–68

16

Chronic Back Pain, Failed Surgery, and What to Do When All Options Are Exhausted

Lawrence G. Lenke

Introduction

Despite the recognition of spine surgery as a unique discipline combining the best of orthopedic surgery and neurosurgery, spine surgery does not portend a perfect result for many patients. The rate of revision spine surgery is difficult to quantify, but it is not unusual for a busy spine surgery center to have many more patients undergoing surgery as a revision than as a primary. In all fairness to the spine surgery profession, even with successful spine surgery, at certain levels adjacent-segment pathology from progressive degeneration unrelated to the prior surgical procedure(s) can ensue at some point postoperatively, which may require further operative intervention. The term *failed back surgery syndrome* (FBSS) has been coined to depict a patient who has either not benefited from a spinal surgical procedure or who has had complications that led to a less than favorable outcome.[1–3] This chapter discusses the difficulty of managing patients who have chronic back pain or have failed spine surgery. How should these patients be evaluated, and what are the remaining treatment options? When would a potential surgical solution be advisable? FBSS patients are an important group to analyze to provide future guidance on not only the management but also the avoidance of this situation for future spine surgery patients. Also, the economic impact of caring for these patients long-term is not inconsequential and has negative impact on the spine surgery profession.[4]

Patient Management

For the chronic back pain patient, the key is to identify the pain generator. For most patients who have seen appropriate spine care physicians, the pain generator is an enigma. For patients who have a demonstrable pain generator, such as a large bulging disk, an inflamed sacroiliac joint, or a severely arthritic facet joint, various nonoperative treatments will provide at least partial relief. When a pain generator cannot be identified, then surgery should definitely not be offered, which should be a logical conclusion. A more difficult scenario is when there is a defined pain generator, such as a degenerated bulging disk, but confirming the physiological connection between the pathology and the pain is difficult. Because of the known common occurrence of spinal degenerative pathology and aging, and the inconsistent correlation with degenerative pathology seen on imaging and correlative symptoms, surgeons need to be very careful when offering surgery to patients with these common degenerative pathologies and chronic back pain.[5,6]

The workup of patients with chronic back pain to determine if surgery is indicated includes standard imaging such as plain upright radiographs, lumbar magnetic resonance imaging (MRI), and computed tomography (CT) scans. A technetium bone scan can highlight areas of increased metabolic uptake, with a potential correlation with pain generators that can be ameliorated by surgery. Diskography has fallen out of common practice due to the potentially deleterious effects of the annular puncture and nucleus disruption. Ultimately, the onus is on the spinal surgeon to sort out the merits of whether further surgery would be indicated and provide a good outcome. If the answer is no, which is usually the case, then the surgeon needs to provide the patient with other nonoperative options for managing the symptoms. Most spine centers are working with nonoperative specialists coming from disciplines such as pain management, physiatry, physical therapy, chiropractic medicine, and acupuncture, among others, and these practitioners should be consulted to provide additional diagnostic and potential therapeutic options to the patient.[7]

For patients with prior surgery, the list of potential pain generators expands dramatically. The workup of these patients begins by taking a thorough history beginning with the reason for the initial operation. For those who have had multiple spinal surgeries, the details regarding the indications for each procedure need to be delineated, if possible, along with the specific procedure(s) performed. Next, the chief complaint at the current time along with the time sequence of this problem needs to be determined. Unfortunately, with multiple spinal surgical procedures that have not helped the patient's symptoms, there are always psychological and emotional undertones that complicate the ability to determine if there is a structural or mechanical issue that can be resolved by additional surgery. Also, many of these patients are being co-managed by a pain management team, with resultant narcotic dependence that further complicates the ability of a spinal surgeon to sort out whether further surgery will be beneficial, even if there are obvious radiographic abnormalities that could be managed surgically. Thus, the evaluating spinal surgeon needs to be aware of all of these physical, psychological, and emotional overlays that contribute to the overall patient presentation.

Despite the multitude of negative implications of a multiply operated patient when contemplating additional surgery, there are distinct diagnoses that can benefit from additional surgery. These include obvious pseudarthrosis, especially when loose or misplaced instrumentation is confirmed, or when there is an obvious progression of altered spinal alignment from a segmental, regional, or global perspective. The optimal way to determine these conditions is with the evaluation of upright anteroposterior (AP) and lateral radiographs of the involved region of the spine. Occasionally comparing the upright radiographs to supine or prone radiographs will highlight an obvious area of pseudarthrosis by demonstrating a change in spinal alignment when gravity is removed from the upright posture. Obviously, when there is broken instrumentation, with a change in alignment from previous radiographs, spinal instability is then confirmed, and restoring stability and alignment can lead to a good result. This type of analysis is always important to do for patients presenting with long spinal instrumented constructs extending to the sacrum or pelvis, as these constructs are notorious for developing problems, especially at the bottom of the construct, where the stress and strain on the bony elements are tremendous. That region of the spine is also often best evaluated with a corresponding CT scan assessing the sacrum and pelvis. A sagittal CT reconstruction can highlight loose screws, L5-S1 pseudarthrosis, intradiskal pathology, and even sacral stress fractures (**Fig. 16.1**).

Regarding residual radicular problems, probably the most commonly missed diagnosis is lumbar foraminal stenosis in a revision setting.

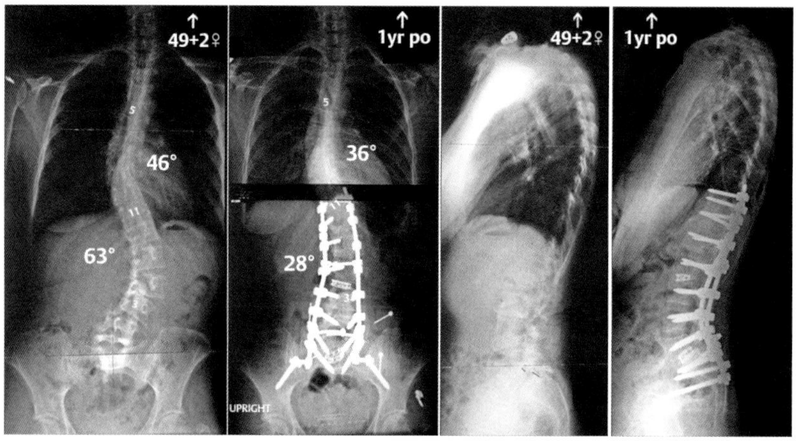

a

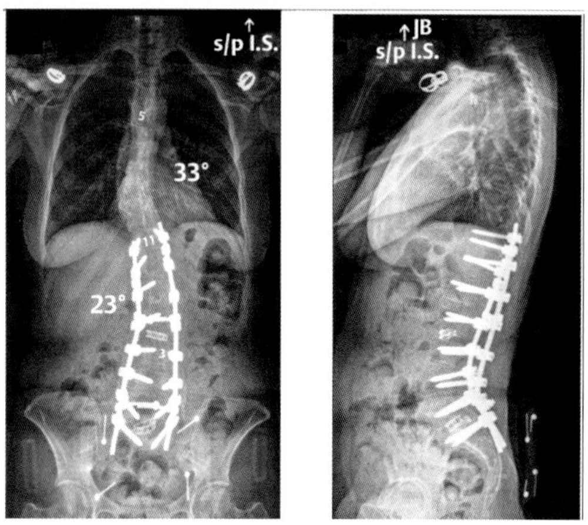

b

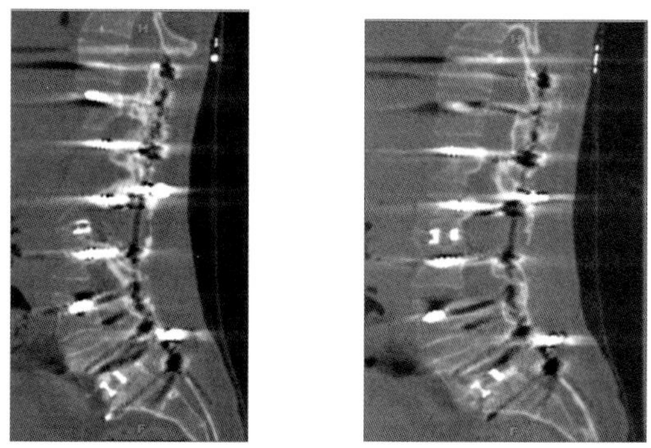

c

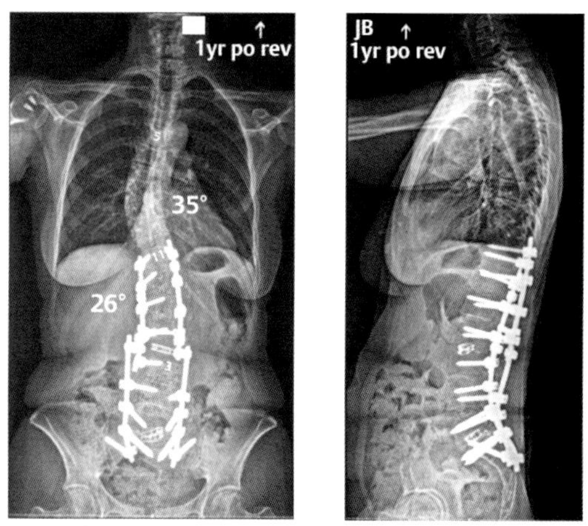

d

Fig. 16.1 **(a)** A 49-year-old woman presented with a history of back and bilateral leg pain. She had a lumbar scoliosis with rotatory subluxation and a low-grade isthmic spondylolisthesis at L5-S1. She underwent a posterior spinal fusion with instrumentation from T11 to the sacrum with iliac screws and transforaminal lumbar interbody fusions (TLIFs) at L2–L3 and L5-S1. At 3 years postoperative, she continued to complain of lumbosacral back pain. **(b)** She had her bilateral iliac screws removed at 3 years postoperative, without any change in her lumbosacral back pain. She then had a spine and pelvis bone scan, which showed increased uptake in the lumbosacral region. **(c)** A lumbar/sacral computed tomography (CT) scan was then performed, showing what appeared to be a solid anterior L5-S1 fusion. However, her symptoms persisted, and with the increased uptake at the lumbosacral junction, a lumbosacral pseudarthrosis was still high on the differential diagnosis list of the cause of her continued pain. **(d)** She then underwent a revision posterior spinal fusion (PSF) for a suspected pseudarthrosis confirmed at L5-S1. She had new implants placed, including bilateral sacral alar screws placed to support new bilateral S1 screws. At 2 months postoperative, she reported that her preoperative pain had completely subsided, and has remained absent at 2 years after the revision.

The neuroradiographic diagnosis can be challenging in the revision setting, as metal interposition can obscure visualization of the foraminal regions. Confirmation of temporary radicular pain relief by selective nerve root infiltration to both diagnose and potentially treat foraminal radicular pain can provide essential information to confirm this diagnosis in a primary or revision setting. CT myelography can also be helpful to confirm recurrent or continued stenosis in the lumbosacral spine. Once again, this can be followed by selective nerve root or transforaminal epidural steroid injections for confirmation of suspected radicular pain. Revision decompression of an area of recurrent/residual stenosis can produce an excellent outcome and should be considered in the right context.

For axial back pain complaints and implants that appear intact and without obvious problems, we often order a spine and pelvis technetium bone scan to identify any areas of increased uptake that may be indicative of a subtle problem such as micro-loosening of implants, sacroiliac joint abnormalities, and sacral stress fractures, among other pathologies. Often a focused CT scan follows the bone scan to further delineate areas of increased uptake. The surgeon then needs to determine if any of these abnormalities can be corrected with additional surgery leading to a satisfied patient and a favorable overall outcome.

In the situation when no treatable pathology is found from the above evaluations, then it is almost always best to avoid further surgery. The discussion of this topic is often very difficult, as these patients are miserable and often clinging to the hope of a quick fix provided by additional surgery. However, it is best to be open and forthright with the patient in explaining that additional surgery is not indicated and nonoperative care is the best option. At this point, I usually try and enlist a spinal physiatrist in the future evaluation and management of these patients. Additional assistance from pain management and physical therapists can be quite beneficial as well. Occasionally, patients will require psychological or psychiatric counseling as well to help with underlying depression or mood disorders that are quite common in this patient population.

Chapter Summary

The evaluation and treatment of a spine surgery patient who has had an unfavorable outcome is difficult and complex. Additional surgery may be indicated if a structural pathology can be identified that correlates with the patient's complaints and overall condition. In the absence of any definitive pathology that is amenable to further surgical intervention, then nonoperative care should be recommended. Spinal surgeons should collaborate with colleagues specializing in the nonoperative care of these patients for optimal treatment going forward for these very challenging patients.

Pearls

- A thorough workup of patients who have had prior spine surgery with continuing symptoms of axial or appendicular pain should be performed to identify potential correctable pain generators.
- Patients with structural abnormalities causing neural compression or segmental, regional, or global malalignment, or patients with failed fusion may benefit from revision surgery.
- The vast majority of patients with FBSS are best treated with nonoperative means if no structural or malalignment abnormalities can be determined from a thorough workup.
- A spine and pelvis bone scan can be useful as a screening test to highlight areas of physiological uptake/stress that would then be followed up with further tests, such as a CT or MRI scan for further delineation.

Pitfalls

- The term *failed back surgery syndrome* (FBSS) is comprehensive, as it describes any patient with a suboptimal outcome following spine surgery.
- Reoperating on a spine surgery patient without any demonstrable objective pathology that can be corrected is doomed to fail.

References

Five Must-Read References

1. Arts MP, Kols NI, Onderwater SM, Peul WC. Clinical outcome of instrumented fusion for the treatment of failed back surgery syndrome: a case series of 100 patients. Acta Neurochir (Wien) 2012;154:1213–1217
2. Schofferman J, Reynolds J, Herzog R, Covington E, Dreyfuss P, O'Neill C. Failed back surgery: etiology and diagnostic evaluation. Spine J 2003;3:400–403
3. Lucas AJ. Failed back surgery syndrome: whose failure? Time to discard a redundant term. Br J Pain 2012;6:162–165
4. Taylor RS, Taylor RJ. The economic impact of failed back surgery syndrome. Br J Pain 2012;6:174–181
5. Skaf G, Bouclaous C, Alaraj A, Chamoun R. Clinical outcome of surgical treatment of failed back surgery syndrome. Surg Neurol 2005;64:483–488, discussion 488–489
6. El-Sissy MH, Abdin MM, Abdel-Meguid A. Failed back surgery syndrome: evaluation of 100 cases. Med J Cairo Univ 2010;78:137–144
7. Anderson SR. A rationale for the treatment algorithm of failed back surgery syndrome. Curr Rev Pain 2000; 4:395–406

Index

Note: Page references followed by *f* or *t* indicate figures or tables, respectively